THE OFFICIAL
PATIENT'S SOURCEBOOK
on

CATARACT
SURGERY

JAMES N. PARKER, M.D.
AND PHILIP M. PARKER, PH.D., EDITORS

ICON Health Publications
ICON Group International, Inc.
4370 La Jolla Village Drive, 4th Floor
San Diego, CA 92122 USA

Printed in the United States of America.

Last digit indicates print number: 10 9 8 7 6 4 5 3 2 1

Publisher, Health Care: Philip Parker, Ph.D.
Editor(s): James Parker, M.D., Philip Parker, Ph.D.

Publisher's note: The ideas, procedures, and suggestions contained in this book are not intended as a substitute for consultation with your physician. All matters regarding your health require medical supervision. As new medical or scientific information becomes available from academic and clinical research, recommended treatments and drug therapies may undergo changes. The authors, editors, and publisher have attempted to make the information in this book up to date and accurate in accord with accepted standards at the time of publication. The authors, editors, and publisher are not responsible for errors or omissions or for consequences from application of the book, and make no warranty, expressed or implied, in regard to the contents of this book. Any practice described in this book should be applied by the reader in accordance with professional standards of care used in regard to the unique circumstances that may apply in each situation, in close consultation with a qualified physician. The reader is advised to always check product information (package inserts) for changes and new information regarding dose and contraindications before taking any drug or pharmacological product. Caution is especially urged when using new or infrequently ordered drugs, herbal remedies, vitamins and supplements, alternative therapies, complementary therapies and medicines, and integrative medical treatments.

Cataloging-in-Publication Data

Parker, James N., 1961-
Parker, Philip M., 1960-

The Official Patient's Sourcebook on Cataract Surgery: A Revised and Updated Directory for the Internet Age / James N. Parker and Philip M. Parker, editors
        p.   cm.
Includes bibliographical references, glossary and index.
ISBN: 0-497-00948-X
1. Cataract Surgery-Popular works.   I. Title.

Disclaimer

This publication is not intended to be used for the diagnosis or treatment of a health problem or as a substitute for consultation with licensed medical professionals. It is sold with the understanding that the publisher, editors, and authors are not engaging in the rendering of medical, psychological, financial, legal, or other professional services.

References to any entity, product, service, or source of information that may be contained in this publication should not be considered an endorsement, either direct or implied, by the publisher, editors or authors. ICON Group International, Inc., the editors, or the authors are not responsible for the content of any Web pages nor publications referenced in this publication.

Copyright Notice

Acknowledgements

The collective knowledge generated from academic and applied research summarized in various references has been critical in the creation of this sourcebook which is best viewed as a comprehensive compilation and collection of information prepared by various official agencies which directly or indirectly are dedicated to cataract surgery. All of the *Official Patient's Sourcebooks* draw from various agencies and institutions associated with the United States Department of Health and Human Services, and in particular, the Office of the Secretary of Health and Human Services (OS), the Administration for Children and Families (ACF), the Administration on Aging (AOA), the Agency for Healthcare Research and Quality (AHRQ), the Agency for Toxic Substances and Disease Registry (ATSDR), the Centers for Disease Control and Prevention (CDC), the Food and Drug Administration (FDA), the Healthcare Financing Administration (HCFA), the Health Resources and Services Administration (HRSA), the Indian Health Service (IHS), the institutions of the National Institutes of Health (NIH), the Program Support Center (PSC), and the Substance Abuse and Mental Health Services Administration (SAMHSA). In addition to these sources, information gathered from the National Library of Medicine, the United States Patent Office, the European Union, and their related organizations has been invaluable in the creation of this sourcebook. Some of the work represented was financially supported by the Research and Development Committee at INSEAD. This support is gratefully acknowledged. Finally, special thanks are owed to Tiffany Freeman for her excellent editorial support.

About the Editors

James N. Parker, M.D.

Dr. James N. Parker received his Bachelor of Science degree in Psychobiology from the University of California, Riverside and his M.D. from the University of California, San Diego. In addition to authoring numerous research publications, he has lectured at various academic institutions. Dr. Parker is the medical editor for the *Official Patient's Sourcebook* series published by ICON Health Publications.

Philip M. Parker, Ph.D.

Philip M. Parker is the Eli Lilly Chair Professor of Innovation, Business and Society at INSEAD (Fontainebleau, France and Singapore). Dr. Parker has also been Professor at the University of California, San Diego and has taught courses at Harvard University, the Hong Kong University of Science and Technology, the Massachusetts Institute of Technology, Stanford University, and UCLA. Dr. Parker is the associate editor for the *Official Patient's Sourcebook* series published by ICON Health Publications.

About ICON Health Publications

In addition to cataract surgery, *Official Patient's Sourcebooks* are available for the following related topics:

- The Official Patient's Sourcebook on Age-related Macular Degeneration
- The Official Patient's Sourcebook on Astigmatism
- The Official Patient's Sourcebook on Blepharitis
- The Official Patient's Sourcebook on Cataracts
- The Official Patient's Sourcebook on Conjunctivitis
- The Official Patient's Sourcebook on Corneal Transplant Surgery
- The Official Patient's Sourcebook on Diabetic Retinopathy
- The Official Patient's Sourcebook on Dry Eye
- The Official Patient's Sourcebook on Fuchs' Dystrophy
- The Official Patient's Sourcebook on Glaucoma
- The Official Patient's Sourcebook on Hyperopia
- The Official Patient's Sourcebook on Iridocorneal Endothelial Syndrome
- The Official Patient's Sourcebook on Keratitis
- The Official Patient's Sourcebook on Keratoconus
- The Official Patient's Sourcebook on Lasik Surgery
- The Official Patient's Sourcebook on Lattice Dystrophy
- The Official Patient's Sourcebook on Macular Holes
- The Official Patient's Sourcebook on Map-dot-fingerprint Dystrophy
- The Official Patient's Sourcebook on Myopia
- The Official Patient's Sourcebook on Ocular Herpes
- The Official Patient's Sourcebook on Ocular Histoplasmosis Syndrome
- The Official Patient's Sourcebook on Presbyopia
- The Official Patient's Sourcebook on Pterygium
- The Official Patient's Sourcebook on Retinal Detachment

To discover more about ICON Health Publications, simply check with your preferred online booksellers, including Barnes&Noble.com and Amazon.com which currently carry all of our titles. Or, feel free to contact us directly for bulk purchases or institutional discounts:

ICON Group International, Inc.
4370 La Jolla Village Drive, Fourth Floor
San Diego, CA 92122 USA
Fax: 858-546-4341
Web site: **www.icongrouponline.com/health**

Table of Contents

INTRODUCTION 1
  Overview *1*
  Organization *3*
  Scope *3*
  Moving Forward *4*

PART I: THE ESSENTIALS 7

CHAPTER 1. THE ESSENTIALS ON CATARACT SURGERY: GUIDELINES 9
  Overview *9*
  What Are Cataracts? *11*
  What Is the Lens? *11*
  How Do Cataracts Develop? *12*
  Who Is at Risk for Cataract? *13*
  What Are the Symptoms? *13*
  Are There Other Types of Cataract? *14*
  How Is a Cataract Detected? *14*
  How Is It Treated? *15*
  Is Cataract Surgery Effective? *15*
  Are There Different Types of Cataract Surgery? *16*
  What Are the Risks of Cataract Surgery? *16*
  What If I Have Other Eye Conditions and Need Cataract Surgery? ... *17*
  What Happens before Surgery? *17*
  What Happens during Surgery? *17*
  What Happens after Surgery? *18*
  Can Problems Develop after Surgery? *18*
  When Will My Vision Be Normal Again? *19*
  What Can I Do If I Already Have Lost Some Vision from Cataract? ... *19*
  What Research Is Being Done? *19*
  What Can I Do to Protect My Vision? *20*
  What Should I Ask My Eye Care Professional? *20*
  Where Can I Get More Information? *21*
  More Guideline Sources *22*
  Vocabulary Builder *25*

CHAPTER 2. SEEKING GUIDANCE 27
  Overview *27*
  Finding Associations *27*
  Finding an Eye Care Professional *29*
  Selecting Your Doctor *31*
  Working with Your Doctor *32*
  Broader Health-Related Resources *33*
  Vocabulary Builder *33*

PART II: ADDITIONAL RESOURCES AND ADVANCED MATERIAL 35

CHAPTER 3. STUDIES ON CATARACT SURGERY 37
Overview 37
The Combined Health Information Database 37
Federally Funded Research on Cataract Surgery 41
E-Journals: PubMed Central 55
The National Library of Medicine: PubMed 57
Vocabulary Builder 114

CHAPTER 4. PATENTS ON CATARACT SURGERY 119
Overview 119
Patents on Cataract Surgery 120
Patent Applications on Cataract Surgery 158
Keeping Current 172
Vocabulary Builder 172

CHAPTER 5. BOOKS ON CATARACT SURGERY 175
Overview 175
Book Summaries: Online Booksellers 175
Chapters on Cataract Surgery 180
General Home References 180

CHAPTER 6. PERIODICALS AND NEWS ON CATARACT SURGERY 183
Overview 183
News Services and Press Releases 183

CHAPTER 7. PHYSICIAN GUIDELINES AND DATABASES 189
Overview 189
NIH Guidelines 189
NIH Databases 190
Other Commercial Databases 193
Specialized References 194

PART III. APPENDICES 197

APPENDIX A. RESEARCHING YOUR MEDICATIONS 199
Overview 199
Your Medications: The Basics 199
Learning More about Your Medications 201
Commercial Databases 202
Contraindications and Interactions (Hidden Dangers) 203
A Final Warning 204
General References 205
Vocabulary Builder 206

APPENDIX B. RESEARCHING NUTRITION 207
Overview 207

Food and Nutrition: General Principles..207
Finding Studies on Cataract Surgery 212
Federal Resources on Nutrition...217
Additional Web Resources..218
Vocabulary Builder...219

APPENDIX C. FINDING MEDICAL LIBRARIES 221
Overview 221
Preparation 221
Finding a Local Medical Library...222
Medical Libraries in the U.S. and Canada 222

APPENDIX D. YOUR RIGHTS AND INSURANCE 229
Overview 229
Your Rights as a Patient 229
Patient Responsibilities 233
Choosing an Insurance Plan 234
Medicare and Medicaid 236
NORD's Medication Assistance Programs 239
Additional Resources...240

ONLINE GLOSSARIES...241
Online Dictionary Directories 242

CATARACT SURGERY GLOSSARY 243
General Dictionaries and Glossaries 248

INDEX 251

INTRODUCTION

Overview

Dr. C. Everett Koop, former U.S. Surgeon General, once said, "The best prescription is knowledge."[1] The Agency for Healthcare Research and Quality (AHRQ) of the National Institutes of Health (NIH) echoes this view and recommends that every patient incorporate education into the treatment process. According to the AHRQ:

> Finding out more about your condition is a good place to start. By contacting groups that support your condition, visiting your local library, and searching on the Internet, you can find good information to help guide your treatment decisions. Some information may be hard to find—especially if you don't know where to look.[2]

As the AHRQ mentions, finding the right information is not an obvious task. Though many physicians and public officials had thought that the emergence of the Internet would do much to assist patients in obtaining reliable information, in March 2001 the National Institutes of Health issued the following warning:

> The number of Web sites offering health-related resources grows every day. Many sites provide valuable information, while others may have information that is unreliable or misleading.[3]

---

[1] Quotation from **http://www.drkoop.com**.
[2] The Agency for Healthcare Research and Quality (AHRQ):
http://www.ahcpr.gov/consumer/diaginfo.htm.
[3] From the NIH, National Cancer Institute (NCI):
http://cancertrials.nci.nih.gov/beyond/evaluating.html.

Since the late 1990s, physicians have seen a general increase in patient Internet usage rates. Patients frequently enter their doctor's offices with printed Web pages of home remedies in the guise of latest medical research. This scenario is so common that doctors often spend more time dispelling misleading information than guiding patients through sound therapies. *The Official Patient's Sourcebook on Cataract Surgery* has been created for patients who have decided to make education and research an integral part of the treatment process. The pages that follow will tell you where and how to look for information covering virtually all topics related to cataract surgery, from the essentials to the most advanced areas of research.

The title of this book includes the word "official." This reflects the fact that the sourcebook draws from public, academic, government, and peer-reviewed research. Selected readings from various agencies are reproduced to give you some of the latest official information available to date on cataract surgery.

Given patients' increasing sophistication in using the Internet, abundant references to reliable Internet-based resources are provided throughout this sourcebook. Where possible, guidance is provided on how to obtain free-of-charge, primary research results as well as more detailed information via the Internet. E-book and electronic versions of this sourcebook are fully interactive with each of the Internet sites mentioned (clicking on a hyperlink automatically opens your browser to the site indicated). Hard copy users of this sourcebook can type cited Web addresses directly into their browsers to obtain access to the corresponding sites. Since we are working with ICON Health Publications, hard copy *Sourcebooks* are frequently updated and printed on demand to ensure that the information provided is current.

In addition to extensive references accessible via the Internet, every chapter presents a "Vocabulary Builder." Many health guides offer glossaries of technical or uncommon terms in an appendix. In editing this sourcebook, we have decided to place a smaller glossary within each chapter that covers terms used in that chapter. Given the technical nature of some chapters, you may need to revisit many sections. Building one's vocabulary of medical terms in such a gradual manner has been shown to improve the learning process.

We must emphasize that no sourcebook on cataract surgery should affirm that a specific diagnostic procedure or treatment discussed in a research study, patent, or doctoral dissertation is "correct" or your best option. This sourcebook is no exception. Each patient is unique. Deciding on appropriate options is always up to the patient in consultation with their physician and healthcare providers.

Organization

This sourcebook is organized into three parts. Part I explores basic techniques to researching cataract surgery (e.g. finding guidelines on cataract surgery), followed by a number of topics, including information on how to get in touch with organizations and associations that dedicate their work to cataract surgery. It also gives you sources of information that can help you find a doctor in your local area specializing in cataract surgery. Collectively, the material presented in Part I is a complete primer on basic research topics for patients having cataract surgery.

Part II moves on to advanced research dedicated to cataract surgery. Part II is intended for those willing to invest many hours of hard work and study. It is here that we direct you to the latest scientific and applied research on cataract surgery. When possible, contact names, links via the Internet, and summaries are provided. It is in Part II where the vocabulary process becomes important as authors publishing advanced research frequently use highly specialized language. In general, every attempt is made to recommend "free-to-use" options.

Part III provides appendices of useful background reading for all patients undergoing cataract surgery. The appendices are dedicated to more pragmatic issues faced by many patients having cataract surgery. Accessing materials via medical libraries may be the only option for some readers, so a guide is provided for finding local medical libraries which are open to the public. Part III, therefore, focuses on advice that goes beyond the biological and scientific issues facing patients having cataract surgery.

Scope

While this sourcebook covers cataract surgery, your doctor, research publications, and specialists may refer to your treatment plan using a variety of terms. Therefore, you should understand that cataract surgery is often considered a synonym closely related to the following:

- Cataract Extraction
- Cataract Removal

For the purposes of this sourcebook, we have attempted to be as inclusive as possible, looking for official information for all of the synonyms relevant to cataract surgery. You may find it useful to refer to synonyms when accessing databases or interacting with healthcare professionals and medical librarians.

Moving Forward

Since the 1980s, the world has seen a proliferation of healthcare guides. Some are written by patients or their family members. These generally take a layperson's approach to understanding and coping with a medical procedure or treatment. They can be uplifting, encouraging, and highly supportive. Other guides are authored by physicians or other healthcare providers who have a more clinical outlook. Each of these two styles of guide has its purpose and can be quite useful.

As editors, we have chosen a third route. We have chosen to expose you to as many sources of official and peer-reviewed information as practical, for the purpose of educating you about basic and advanced knowledge as recognized by medical science today. You can think of this sourcebook as your personal Internet age reference librarian.

Why "Internet age"? All too often, patients having cataract surgery will log on to the Internet, type words into a search engine, and receive several Web site listings which are mostly irrelevant or redundant. These patients are left to wonder where the relevant information is, and how to obtain it. Since only the smallest fraction of information dealing with cataract surgery is even indexed in search engines, a non-systematic approach often leads to frustration and disappointment. With this sourcebook, we hope to direct you to the information you need that you would not likely find using popular Web directories. Beyond Web listings, in many cases we will reproduce brief summaries or abstracts of available reference materials. These abstracts often contain distilled information on topics of discussion.

While we focus on the more scientific aspects of cataract surgery, there is, of course, the emotional side to consider. Later in the sourcebook, we provide a chapter dedicated to helping you find peer groups and associations that can provide additional support beyond research produced by medical science. We hope that the choices we have made give you the most options available in moving forward with your decision process. In this way, we wish you the best in your efforts to incorporate this educational approach into your treatment plan.

The Editors

PART I: THE ESSENTIALS

ABOUT PART I

Part I has been edited to give you access to what we feel are "the essentials" on cataract surgery. The essentials of a procedure typically include the definition or description of the procedure and a discussion of who requires it. Your doctor or healthcare provider may have already explained the essentials of cataract surgery to you or even given you a pamphlet or brochure describing cataract surgery. Now you are searching for more in-depth information. As editors, we have decided, nevertheless, to include a discussion on where to find essential information that can complement what your doctor has already told you. In this section we recommend a process, not a particular Web site or reference book. The process ensures that, as you search the Web, you gain background information in such a way as to maximize your understanding.

CHAPTER 1. THE ESSENTIALS ON CATARACT SURGERY: GUIDELINES

Overview

Official agencies, as well as federally funded institutions supported by national grants, frequently publish a variety of guidelines on cataract surgery. These are typically called "Fact Sheets" or "Guidelines." They can take the form of a brochure, information kit, pamphlet, or flyer. Often they are only a few pages in length. The great advantage of guidelines over other sources is that they are often written with the patient in mind. Since new guidelines on cataract surgery can appear at any moment and be published by a number of sources, the best approach to finding guidelines is to systematically scan the Internet-based services that post them.

The National Institutes of Health (NIH)[4]

The National Institutes of Health (NIH) is the first place to search for relatively current patient guidelines and fact sheets on cataract surgery. Originally founded in 1887, the NIH is one of the world's foremost medical research centers and the federal focal point for medical research in the United States. At any given time, the NIH supports some 35,000 research grants at universities, medical schools, and other research and training institutions, both nationally and internationally. The rosters of those who have conducted research or who have received NIH support over the years include the world's most illustrious scientists and physicians. Among them are 97 scientists who have won the Nobel Prize for achievement in medicine.

---

[4] Adapted from the NIH: **http://www.nih.gov/about/NIHoverview.html**.

There is no guarantee that any one Institute will have a guideline on a specific diagnostic or therapeutic procedure, though the National Institutes of Health collectively publish many guidelines for both common and lesser-known procedures. The best way to access NIH guidelines is via the Internet. Although the NIH is organized into many different Institutes and Offices, the following is a list of key Web sites where you are most likely to find NIH clinical guidelines and publications dealing with cataract surgery and associated procedures:

- Office of the Director (OD); guidelines consolidated across agencies available at **http://www.nih.gov/health/consumer/conkey.htm**

- National Eye Institute (NEI); guidelines available at **http://www.nei.nih.gov/publications/publications.htm**

- National Library of Medicine (NLM); extensive encyclopedia (A.D.A.M., Inc.) with guidelines available at **http://www.nlm.nih.gov/medlineplus/healthtopics.html**

Among those listed above, the National Eye Institute is especially noteworthy. Established by Congress in 1968 to protect and prolong the vision of the American people, the National Eye Institute (NEI), one of the Federal government's National Institutes of Health (NIH), conducts and supports research that helps prevent and treat eye diseases and other disorders of vision.[5] Vision research is supported by the NEI through approximately 1600 research grants and training awards made to scientists at more than 250 medical centers, hospitals, universities, and other institutions across the country and around the world. The NEI also conducts laboratory and patient-oriented research at its own facilities located on the NIH campus in Bethesda, Maryland. This research leads to sight-saving treatments, reduces visual impairment and blindness, and improves the quality of life for people of all ages. NEI-supported research has advanced our knowledge of how the eye functions in health and disease. Another part of the NEI mission is to conduct public and professional education programs that help

---

[5] Throughout the sourcebook, some of the text has been "adapted" from various official or governmental sources. Adapted signifies "reproduced" or "reproduced with minor editorial adjustments." This paragraph has been adapted from the NEI: **http://www.nei.nih.gov/about/mission.htm**; the NEI has also established the National Eye Health Education Program (NEHEP), a partnership of about 60 professional, civic, and voluntary organizations and government agencies concerned with eye health. The program represents a natural extension of the NEI's support of vision research -- a final step in the research continuum, where results are disseminated to health professionals, patients, and the public. Other NEI public education activities include a traveling exhibit, which have been viewed by more than 3.8 million people nationwide; and a school curriculum on vision for grades 4-8.

prevent blindness, reduce visual impairment, and increase awareness of services and devices that are available for people with low vision.

The National Institutes of Health has recently published the following guideline for cataract surgery:

What Are Cataracts?[6]

A cataract is a clouding of the lens in the eye that affects vision. Most cataracts are related to aging. Cataracts are very common in older people. By age 80, more than half of all Americans either have a cataract or have had cataract surgery.

A cataract can occur in either or both eyes. It cannot spread from one eye to the other.

What Is the Lens?

The lens is a clear part of the eye that helps to focus light, or an image, on the retina. The retina is the light-sensitive tissue at the back of the eye.

In a normal eye, light passes through the transparent lens to the retina. Once it reaches the retina, light is changed into nerve signals that are sent to the brain.

The lens must be clear for the retina to receive a sharp image. If the lens is cloudy from a cataract, the image you see will be blurred.

---

[6] Adapted from the National Eye Institute:
http://www.nei.nih.gov/health/cataract/cataract_facts.htm.

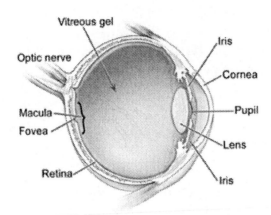

How Do Cataracts Develop?

Age-related cataracts develop in two ways:

- Clumps of protein reduce the sharpness of the image reaching the retina.
- The clear lens slowly changes to a yellowish/brownish color, adding a brownish tint to vision.

Clumps of Protein Reduce the Sharpness of the Image Reaching the Retina

The lens consists mostly of water and protein. When the protein clumps up, it clouds the lens and reduces the light that reaches the retina. The clouding may become severe enough to cause blurred vision. Most age-related cataracts develop from protein clumpings.

When a cataract is small, the cloudiness affects only a small part of the lens. You may not notice any changes in your vision. Cataracts tend to "grow" slowly, so vision gets worse gradually. Over time, the cloudy area in the lens may get larger, and the cataract may increase in size. Seeing may become more difficult. Your vision may get duller or blurrier.

The Clear Lens Slowly Changes to a Yellowish/Brownish Color, Adding a Brownish Tint to Vision

As the clear lens slowly colors with age, your vision gradually may acquire a brownish shade. At first, the amount of tinting may be small and may not cause a vision problem. Over time, increased tinting may make it more difficult to read and perform other routine activities. This gradual change in the amount of tinting does not affect the sharpness of the image transmitted to the retina.

If you have advanced lens discoloration, you may not be able to identify blues and purples. You may be wearing what you believe to be a pair of black socks, only to find out from friends that you are wearing purple socks.

Who Is at Risk for Cataract?

The risk of cataract increases as you get older. Other risk factors for cataract include:

- Certain diseases (for example, diabetes)
- Personal behavior (smoking, alcohol use)
- The environment (prolonged exposure to ultraviolet sunlight)

What Are the Symptoms?

The most common symptoms of a cataract are:

- Cloudy or blurry vision.
- Colors seem faded.
- Glare. Headlights, lamps, or sunlight may appear too bright. A halo may appear around lights.
- Poor night vision.
- Double vision or multiple images in one eye. (This symptom may clear as the cataract gets larger.)
- Frequent prescription changes in your eyeglasses or contact lenses.

These symptoms can also be a sign of other eye problems. If you have any of these symptoms, check with your eye care professional.

Are There Other Types of Cataract?

Yes. Although most cataracts are related to aging, there are other types of cataract:

- Secondary cataract. Cataracts can form after surgery for other eye problems, such as glaucoma. Cataracts also can develop in people who have other health problems, such as diabetes. Cataracts are sometimes linked to steroid use.

- Traumatic cataract. Cataracts can develop after an eye injury, sometimes years later.

- Congenital cataract. Some babies are born with cataracts or develop them in childhood, often in both eyes. These cataracts may be so small that they do not affect vision. If they do, the lenses may need to be removed.

- Radiation cataract. Cataracts can develop after exposure to some types of radiation.

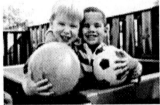   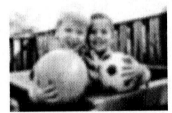

Normal vision   *The same scene as viewed by a person with cataract*

How Is a Cataract Detected?

To detect a cataract, an eye care professional examines the lens. A comprehensive eye examination usually includes:

- **Visual acuity test:** This eye chart test measures how well you see at various distances.

- **Pupil dilation:** The pupil is widened with eyedrops to allow your eye care professional to see more of the lens and retina and look for other eye problems.

- **Tonometry:** This is a standard test to measure fluid pressure inside the eye. Increased pressure may be a sign of glaucoma.

Your eye care professional may also do other tests to learn more about the structure and health of your eye.

How Is It Treated?

The symptoms of early cataract may be improved with new eyeglasses, brighter lighting, anti-glare sunglasses, or magnifying lenses. If these measures do not help, surgery is the only effective treatment. Surgery involves removing the cloudy lens and replacing it with an artificial lens.

A cataract needs to be removed only when vision loss interferes with your everyday activities, such as driving, reading, or watching TV. You and your eye care professional can make this decision together. Once you understand the benefits and risks of surgery, you can make an informed decision about whether cataract surgery is right for you. In most cases, delaying cataract surgery will not cause long-term damage to your eye or make the surgery more difficult. You do not have to rush into surgery.

Sometimes a cataract should be removed even if it does not cause problems with your vision. For example, a cataract should be removed if it prevents examination or treatment of another eye problem, such as age-related macular degeneration or diabetic retinopathy.

If you choose surgery, your eye care professional may refer you to a specialist to remove the cataract.

If you have cataracts in both eyes that require surgery, the surgery will be performed on each eye at separate times, usually four to eight weeks apart.

Is Cataract Surgery Effective?

Cataract removal is one of the most common operations performed in the United States. It also is one of the safest and most effective types of surgery. In about 90 percent of cases, people who have cataract surgery have better vision afterward.

Are There Different Types of Cataract Surgery?

There are two types of cataract surgery. Your doctor can explain the differences and help determine which is better for you:

- **Phacoemulsification, or phaco.** A small incision is made on the side of the cornea, the clear, dome-shaped surface that covers the front of the eye. Your doctor inserts a tiny probe into the eye. This device emits ultrasound waves that soften and break up the lens so that it can be removed by suction. Most cataract surgery today is done by phacoemulsification, also called "small incision cataract surgery."

- **Extracapsular surgery.** Your doctor makes a longer incision on the side of the cornea and removes the cloudy core of the lens in one piece. The rest of the lens is removed by suction.

After the natural lens has been removed, it often is replaced by an artificial lens, called an intraocular lens (IOL). An IOL is a clear, plastic lens that requires no care and becomes a permanent part of your eye. Light is focused clearly by the IOL onto the retina, improving your vision. You will not feel or see the new lens.

Some people cannot have an IOL. They may have another eye disease or have problems during surgery. For these patients, a soft contact lens, or glasses that provide high magnification, may be suggested.

What Are the Risks of Cataract Surgery?

As with any surgery, cataract surgery poses risks, such as infection and bleeding. Before cataract surgery, your doctor may ask you to temporarily stop taking certain medications that increase the risk of bleeding during surgery. After surgery, you must keep your eye clean, wash your hands before touching your eye, and use the prescribed medications to help minimize the risk of infection. Serious infection can result in loss of vision.

Cataract surgery slightly increases your risk of retinal detachment. Other eye disorders, such as high myopia (nearsightedness), can further increase your risk of retinal detachment after cataract surgery. One sign of a retinal detachment is a sudden increase in flashes or floaters. Floaters are little "cobwebs" or specks that seem to float about in your field of vision. If you notice a sudden increase in floaters or flashes, see an eye care professional immediately. A retinal detachment is a medical emergency. If necessary, go to an emergency service or hospital. Your eye must be examined by an eye surgeon as soon as possible. A retinal detachment causes no pain. Early treatment for retinal detachment often can prevent permanent loss of vision. The longer the retina stays detached, the less likely you will regain good vision once you are treated. Even if you are treated promptly, some vision may be lost.

Talk to your eye care professional about these risks. Make sure cataract surgery is right for you.

What If I Have Other Eye Conditions and Need Cataract Surgery?

Many people who need cataract surgery also have other eye conditions, such as age-related macular degeneration or glaucoma. If you have other eye conditions in addition to cataract, talk with your doctor. Learn about the risks, benefits, alternatives, and expected results of cataract surgery.

What Happens before Surgery?

A week or two before surgery, your doctor will do some tests. These tests may include measuring the curve of the cornea and the size and shape of your eye. This information helps your doctor choose the right type of IOL.

You may be asked not to eat or drink anything 12 hours before your surgery.

What Happens during Surgery?

At the hospital or eye clinic, drops will be put into your eye to dilate the pupil. The area around your eye will be washed and cleansed.

The operation usually lasts less than one hour and is almost painless. Many people choose to stay awake during surgery. Others may need to be put to sleep for a short time. If you are awake, you will have an anesthetic to numb the nerves in and around your eye.

After the operation, a patch may be placed over your eye. You will rest for a while. Your medical team will watch for any problems, such as bleeding. Most people who have cataract surgery can go home the same day. You will need someone to drive you home.

What Happens after Surgery?

Itching and mild discomfort are normal after cataract surgery. Some fluid discharge is also common. Your eye may be sensitive to light and touch. If you have discomfort, your doctor can suggest treatment. After one or two days, moderate discomfort should disappear.

For a few days after surgery, your doctor may ask you to use eyedrops to help healing and decrease the risk of infection. Ask your doctor about how to use your eyedrops, how often to use them, and what effects they can have. You will need to wear an eye shield or eyeglasses to help protect your eye. Avoid rubbing or pressing on your eye.

When you are home, try not to bend from the waist to pick up objects on the floor. Do not lift any heavy objects. You can walk, climb stairs, and do light household chores.

In most cases, healing will be complete within eight weeks. Your doctor will schedule exams to check on your progress.

Can Problems Develop after Surgery?

Problems after surgery are rare, but they can occur. These problems can include infection, bleeding, inflammation (pain, redness, swelling), loss of vision, double vision, and high or low eye pressure. With prompt medical attention, these problems usually can be treated successfully.

Sometimes the eye tissue that encloses the IOL becomes cloudy and may blur your vision. This condition is called an after-cataract. An after-cataract can develop months or years after cataract surgery.

An after-cataract is treated with a laser. Your doctor uses a laser to make a tiny hole in the eye tissue behind the lens to let light pass through. This outpatient procedure is called a YAG laser capsulotomy. It is painless and rarely results in increased eye pressure or other eye problems. As a precaution, your doctor may give you eyedrops to lower your eye pressure before or after the procedure.

When Will My Vision Be Normal Again?

You can return quickly to many everyday activities, but your vision may be blurry. The healing eye needs time to adjust so that it can focus properly with the other eye, especially if the other eye has a cataract. Ask your doctor when you can resume driving.

If you received an IOL, you may notice that colors are very bright. The IOL is clear, unlike your natural lens that may have had a yellowish/brownish tint. Within a few months after receiving an IOL, you will become used to improved color vision. Also, when your eye heals, you may need new glasses or contact lenses.

What Can I Do If I Already Have Lost Some Vision from Cataract?

If you have lost some sight from cataract or cataract surgery, ask your eye care professional about low vision services and devices that may help you make the most of your remaining vision. Ask for a referral to a specialist in low vision. Many community organizations and agencies offer information about low vision counseling, training, and other special services for people with visual impairments. A nearby school of medicine or optometry may provide low vision services.

What Research Is Being Done?

The National Eye Institute is conducting and supporting a number of studies focusing on factors associated with the development of age-related cataract. These studies include:

- The effect of sunlight exposure, which may be associated with an increased risk of cataract.
- Vitamin supplements, which have shown varying results in delaying the progression of cataract.
- Genetic studies, which show promise for better understanding cataract development.

What Can I Do to Protect My Vision?

Wearing sunglasses and a hat with a brim to block ultraviolet sunlight may help to delay cataract. If you smoke, stop. Researchers also believe good nutrition can help reduce the risk of age-related cataract. They recommend eating green leafy vegetables, fruit, and other foods with antioxidants.

If you are age 60 or older, you should have a comprehensive dilated eye exam at least once every two years. In addition to cataract, your eye care professional can check for signs of age-related macular degeneration, glaucoma, and other vision disorders. Early treatment for many eye diseases may save your sight.

What Should I Ask My Eye Care Professional?

You can protect yourself against vision loss by working in partnership with your eye care professional. Ask questions and get the information you need to take care of yourself and your family.

What Are Some Questions to Ask?

About my eye disease or disorder...
- What is my diagnosis?
- What caused my condition?
- Can my condition be treated?
- How will this condition affect my vision now and in the future?
- Should I watch for any particular symptoms and notify you if they occur?
- Should I make any lifestyle changes?

About my treatment...
- What is the treatment for my condition?
- When will the treatment start and how long will it last?
- What are the benefits of this treatment and how successful is it?
- What are the risks and side effects associated with this treatment?
- Are there foods, drugs, or activities I should avoid while I'm on this treatment?

- If my treatment includes taking medicine, what should I do if I miss a dose?

- Are other treatments available?

About my tests...

- What kinds of tests will I have?

- What can I expect to find out from these tests?

- When will I know the results?

- Do I have to do anything special to prepare for any of the tests?

- Do these tests have any side effects or risks?

- Will I need more tests later?

Other Suggestions

- If you don't understand your eye care professional's responses, ask questions until you do understand.

- Take notes or get a friend or family member to take notes for you. Or, bring a tape recorder to help you remember the discussion.

- Ask your eye care professional to write down his or her instructions to you.

- Ask your eye care professional for printed material about your condition.

- If you still have trouble understanding your eye care professional's answers, ask where you can go for more information.

- Other members of your health care team, such as nurses and pharmacists, can be good sources of information. Talk to them, too.

Today, patients take an active role in their health care. Be an active patient about your eye care.

Where Can I Get More Information?

For more information about cataracts, you may wish to contact:

American Academy of Ophthalmology
655 Beach Street
San Francisco, CA 94109-7424

(415) 561-8500
http://www.eyenet.org

American Optometric Association
243 Lindbergh Boulevard
St. Louis, MO 63141
(314) 991-4100
http://www.aoanet.org

National Eye Institute
2020 Vision Place
Bethesda, MD 20892-3655
(301) 496-5248
http://www.nei.nih.gov

Prevent Blindness America
500 East Remington Road
Schaumburg, IL 60173
1-800-331-2020
(847) 843-2020
http://www.preventblindness.org

For more information about IOLs, contact:

U.S. Food and Drug Administration
Office of Consumer Affairs
Parklawn Building (HFE-88)
5600 Fishers Lane
Rockville, MD 20857
1-800-532-4440
(301) 827-4420
http://www.fda.gov

More Guideline Sources

The guideline above on cataract surgery is only one example of the kind of material that you can find online and free of charge. The remainder of this chapter will direct you to other sources which either publish or can help you find additional guidelines on topics related to cataract surgery. Many of the guidelines listed below address topics that may be of particular relevance to your specific situation or of special interest to only some patients having cataract surgery. Due to space limitations these sources are listed in a concise manner. Do not hesitate to consult the following sources by either using the Internet hyperlink provided, or, in cases where the contact information is provided, contacting the publisher or author directly.

Topic Pages: MEDLINEplus

For patients wishing to go beyond guidelines published by specific Institutes of the NIH, the National Library of Medicine has created a vast and patient-oriented healthcare information portal called MEDLINEplus. Within this Internet-based system are "health topic pages." You can think of a health topic page as a guide to patient guides. To access this system, log on to **http://www.nlm.nih.gov/medlineplus/healthtopics.html**. From there you can either search using the alphabetical index or browse by broad topic areas. Recently, MEDLINEplus listed the following as being relevant to cataract surgery:

Cataract
http://www.nlm.nih.gov/medlineplus/cataract.html

Eye Diseases
http://www.nlm.nih.gov/medlineplus/eyediseases.html

Eye Wear
http://www.nlm.nih.gov/medlineplus/eyewear.html

Glaucoma
http://www.nlm.nih.gov/medlineplus/glaucoma.html

Laser Eye Surgery
http://www.nlm.nih.gov/medlineplus/lasereyesurgery.html

Macular Degeneration
http://www.nlm.nih.gov/medlineplus/maculardegeneration.html

Refractive Errors
http://www.nlm.nih.gov/medlineplus/refractiveerrors.html

You may also choose to use the search utility provided by MEDLINEplus at the following Web address: **http://www.nlm.nih.gov/medlineplus/**. Simply type a keyword into the search box and click "Search." This utility is similar to the NIH search utility, with the exception that it only includes materials that are linked within the MEDLINEplus system (mostly patient-oriented information). It also has the disadvantage of generating unstructured results. We recommend, therefore, that you use this method only if you have a very targeted search.

The Combined Health Information Database (CHID)

CHID Online is a reference tool that maintains a database directory of thousands of journal articles and patient education guidelines on cataract surgery. One of the advantages of CHID over other sources is that it offers summaries that describe the guidelines available, including contact information and pricing. CHID's general Web site is **http://chid.nih.gov/**. To search this database, go to **http://chid.nih.gov/detail/detail.html**. In particular, you can use the advanced search options to look up pamphlets, reports, brochures, and information kits. The following was recently posted in this archive:

- **When You Need an Operation: About Cataract Surgery in Adults**

  Source: Chicago, IL: American College of Surgeons. 1995. 14 p.

  Contact: Available from American College of Surgeons. 55 East Erie Street, Chicago, IL 60611. (312) 664-4050. PRICE: Single copy free; bulk copies available. Item number PI-11.

  Summary: This booklet provides information for people who are about to undergo **cataract surgery.** The booklet explains why cataract operations are performed; how the surgical procedure is performed; and what to expect before and after the operation. Topics include: the causes of cataracts, typical symptoms, non-surgical treatments for cataracts, timing **cataract surgery,** recovery concerns, complications, and post-surgery ongoing care. Although the booklet is designed for all patients undergoing **cataract surgery,** the authors also refer to the special needs of patients with diabetes. The booklet encourages patients to bring any questions to their health care providers. 1 figure.

The NIH Search Utility

After browsing the references listed at the beginning of this chapter, you may want to explore the NIH search utility. This allows you to search for documents on over 100 selected Web sites that comprise the NIH-WEB-SPACE. Each of these servers is "crawled" and indexed on an ongoing basis. Your search will produce a list of various documents, all of which will relate in some way to cataract surgery. The drawbacks of this approach are that the information is not organized by theme and that the references are often a mix of information for professionals and patients. Nevertheless, a large number of the listed Web sites provide useful background information. To use the

NIH   search   utility,   visit   the   following   Web   page: http://search.nih.gov/index.html.

Additional Web Sources

A number of Web sites that often link to government sites are available to the public. These can also point you in the direction of essential information. The following is a representative sample:

- AOL: **http://search.aol.com/cat.adp?id=168&layer=&from=subcats**
- Family Village: **http://www.familyvillage.wisc.edu/specific.htm**
- Google: **http://directory.google.com/Top/Health/Conditions_and_Diseases/**
- Med Help International: **http://www.medhelp.org/HealthTopics/A.html**
- Open Directory Project: **http://dmoz.org/Health/Conditions_and_Diseases/**
- Yahoo.com: **http://health.yahoo.com/health**
- WebMD®Health: **http://my.webmd.com/health_topics**

Vocabulary Builder

The material in this chapter may have contained a number of unfamiliar words. The following Vocabulary Builder introduces you to terms used in this chapter that have not been covered in the previous chapter:

Cataracts: In medicine, an opacity of the crystalline lens of the eye obstructing partially or totally its transmission of light. [NIH]

Cornea: The transparent anterior portion of the fibrous coat of the eye consisting of five layers. [NIH]

Impairment: In the context of health experience, an impairment is any loss or abnormality of psychological, physiological, or anatomical structure or function. [NIH]

Myopia: Astigmatism in which one principal meridian is myopic and the other enmetropic, or in which both meridians are myopic. [NIH]

Need: A state of tension or dissatisfaction felt by an individual that impels him to action toward a goal he believes will satisfy the impulse. [NIH]

Nerve: A cordlike structure of nervous tissue that connects parts of the nervous system with other tissues of the body and conveys nervous impulses to, or away from, these tissues. [NIH]

Outpatient: A patient who is not an inmate of a hospital but receives diagnosis or treatment in a clinic or dispensary connected with the hospital. [NIH]

Patch: A piece of material used to cover or protect a wound, an injured part, etc.: a patch over the eye. [NIH]

Probe: An instrument used in exploring cavities, or in the detection and dilatation of strictures, or in demonstrating the potency of channels; an elongated instrument for exploring or sounding body cavities. [NIH]

Refer: To send or direct for treatment, aid, information, de decision. [NIH]

Sharpness: The apparent blurring of the border between two adjacent areas of a radiograph having different optical densities. [NIH]

Specialist: In medicine, one who concentrates on 1 special branch of medical science. [NIH]

CHAPTER 2. SEEKING GUIDANCE

Overview

Some patients are comforted by the knowledge that a number of organizations dedicate their resources to helping people. These associations can become invaluable sources of information and advice. Many associations offer aftercare support, financial assistance, and other important services.[7] In addition to support groups, your physician can be a valuable source of guidance and support. Therefore, finding a physician that can work with your unique situation is a very important aspect of your care.

In this chapter, we direct you to resources that can help you find patient organizations and medical specialists. We begin by describing how to find associations and peer groups that can help you better understand cataract surgery. The chapter ends with a discussion on how to find a doctor that is right for you.

Finding Associations

There are a several Internet directories that provide lists of medical associations with information on or resources relating to cataract surgery. By consulting all of associations listed in this chapter, you will have nearly exhausted all sources for patient associations concerned with cataract surgery.

---

[7] Churches, synagogues, and other houses of worship might also have groups that can offer you the social support you need.

The National Health Information Center (NHIC)

The National Health Information Center (NHIC) offers a free referral service to help people find organizations that provide information about cataract surgery. For more information, see the NHIC's Web site at **http://www.health.gov/NHIC/** or contact an information specialist by calling 1-800-336-4797.

DIRLINE

A comprehensive source of information on associations is the DIRLINE database maintained by the National Library of Medicine. The database comprises some 10,000 records of organizations, research centers, and government institutes and associations which primarily focus on health and biomedicine. DIRLINE is available via the Internet at the following Web site: **http://dirline.nlm.nih.gov/**. Simply type in "cataract surgery" (or a synonym) or the name of a topic, and the site will list information contained in the database on all relevant organizations.

The Combined Health Information Database

Another comprehensive source of information on healthcare associations is the Combined Health Information Database. Using the "Detailed Search" option, you will need to limit your search to "Organizations" and "cataract surgery". Type the following hyperlink into your Web browser: **http://chid.nih.gov/detail/detail.html**. To find associations, use the drop boxes at the bottom of the search page where "You may refine your search by." For publication date, select "All Years." Then, select your preferred language and the format option "Organization Resource Sheet." By making these selections and typing in "cataract surgery" (or synonyms) into the "For these words:" box, you will only receive results on organizations dealing with cataract surgery. You should check back periodically with this database since it is updated every 3 months.

Online Support Groups

In addition to support groups, commercial Internet service providers offer forums and chat rooms for people having different illnesses and conditions. WebMD®, for example, offers such a service at its Web site: **http://boards.webmd.com/roundtable**. These online self-help communities can help you connect with a network of people whose concerns are similar to yours. Online support groups are places where people can talk informally. If you read about a novel approach, consult with your doctor or other healthcare providers, as the treatments or discoveries you hear about may not be scientifically proven to be safe and effective.

Finding an Eye Care Professional[8]

The National Eye Institute does not provide referrals nor recommend specific eye care professionals. However, you may wish to consider the following ways of finding a professional to provide your eye care. You can:

- Ask family members and friends about eye care professionals they use.

- Ask your family doctor for the name of a local eye care specialist.

- Call the department of ophthalmology or optometry at a nearby hospital or university medical center.

- Contact a state or county association of ophthalmologists or optometrists. These groups, usually called academies or societies, may have lists of eye care professionals with specific information on specialty and experience.

- Contact your insurance company or health plan to learn whether it has a list of eye care professionals that are covered under your plan.

- At a bookstore or library, check on available journals and books about choosing physicians and medical treatments. Here are some examples:

  - Most large libraries have the reference set *The ABMS Compendium of Certified Medical Professionals*, which lists board-certified ophthalmologists, each with a small amount of biographical information. A library reference specialist can also help you identify other books on finding healthcare professionals or help you seek additional information about local eye physicians using the Internet.

  - Each year, usually in August, the magazine *U.S. News and World Report* features an article that rates hospitals in the United States.

For more specific information, the following sources may prove useful:

- The American Academy of Ophthalmology coordinates an online listing called **Find an Ophthalmologist** that contains information on member ophthalmologists practicing in the United States and abroad. This service is designed to help the general public locate ophthalmologists within a specific region. Web site: **http://www.eyenet.org/**.

---

[8] This section has been adapted from **http://www.nei.nih.gov/health/findprofessional.htm**.

- The **International Society of Refractive Surgery** maintains a comprehensive directory of surgeons around the world who are currently performing refractive surgery. Telephone: (407) 786-7446. E-mail: isrshq@isrs.org. Web site: **http://www.isrs.org.**

- The **Blue Book of Optometrists** and the **Red Book of Ophthalmologists,** now available online, can be used to find doctors in the U.S., Puerto Rico, and Canada. This resource is helpful when you know the doctor's name, but need contact information.
  Web site: **http://www.eyefind.com/.**

- Administrators in Medicine and the Association of State Medical Board Executive Directors have launched **DocFinder,** an online database that helps consumers learn whether any malpractice actions have been taken against a particular doctor. The site provides links to the licensing boards in the participating states.
  Web site: **http://www.docboard.org/.**

- The **American Association of Eye and Ear Hospitals (AAEEH)** is comprised of the premier centers for specialized eye and ear procedures in the world. Association members are major referral centers that offer some of the most innovative teaching programs, and routinely treat the most severely ill eye and ear patients. Telephone: (202) 347-1993. Web site: **http://www.aaeeh.org/locations.html.**

Additional steps you can take to locate doctors include the following:

- Information on doctors in some states is available on the Internet at **http://www.docboard.org.** This Web site is run by "Administrators in Medicine," a group of state medical board directors.

- The American Board of Medical Specialties can tell you if your doctor is board certified. "Certified" means that the doctor has completed a training program in a specialty and has passed an exam, or "board," to assess his or her knowledge, skills, and experience to provide quality patient care in that specialty. Primary care doctors may also be certified as specialists. The AMBS Web site is located at **http://www.abms.org/newsearch.asp.**[9] You can also contact the ABMS by phone at 1-866-ASK-ABMS.

- You can call the American Medical Association (AMA) at 800-665-2882 for information on training, specialties, and board certification for many licensed doctors in the United States. This information also can be found in "Physician Select" at the AMA's Web site: **http://www.ama-assn.org/aps/amahg.htm.**

---

[9] While board certification is a good measure of a doctor's knowledge, it is possible to receive quality care from doctors who are not board certified.

If the previous sources did not meet your needs, you may want to log on to the Web site of the National Organization for Rare Disorders (NORD) at **http://www.rarediseases.org/**. NORD maintains a database of doctors with expertise in various rare diseases. The Metabolic Information Network (MIN), 800-945-2188, also maintains a database of physicians with expertise in various metabolic diseases.

Selecting Your Doctor[10]

When you have compiled a list of prospective doctors, call each of their offices. First, ask if the doctor accepts your health insurance plan and if he or she is taking new patients. If the doctor is not covered by your plan, ask yourself if you are prepared to pay the extra costs. The next step is to schedule a visit with your chosen physician. During the first visit you will have the opportunity to evaluate your doctor and to find out if you feel comfortable with him or her. Ask yourself, did the doctor:

- Give me a chance to ask questions about cataract surgery?

- Really listen to my questions?

- Answer in terms I understood?

- Show respect for me?

- Ask me questions?

- Make me feel comfortable?

- Address the health problem(s) I came with?

- Ask me my preferences about different alternatives to cataract surgery?

- Spend enough time with me?

Trust your instincts when deciding if the doctor is right for you. But remember, it might take time for the relationship to develop. It takes more than one visit for you and your doctor to get to know each other.

---

[10] This section has been adapted from the AHRQ:
www.ahrq.gov/consumer/qntascii/qntdr.htm.

Working with Your Doctor[11]

Research has shown that patients who have good relationships with their doctors tend to be more satisfied with their care and have better results. Here are some tips to help you and your doctor become partners:

- You know important things about your symptoms and your health history. Tell your doctor what you think he or she needs to know.

- It is important to tell your doctor personal information, even if it makes you feel embarrassed or uncomfortable.

- Bring a "health history" list with you (and keep it up to date).

- Always bring any medications you are currently taking with you to the appointment, or you can bring a list of your medications including dosage and frequency information. Talk about any allergies or reactions you have had to your medications.

- Tell your doctor about any natural or alternative medicines you are taking.

- Bring other medical information, such as x-ray films, test results, and medical records.

- Ask questions. If you don't, your doctor will assume that you understood everything that was said.

- Write down your questions before your visit. List the most important ones first to make sure that they are addressed.

- Consider bringing a friend with you to the appointment to help you ask questions. This person can also help you understand and/or remember the answers.

- Ask your doctor to draw pictures if you think that this would help you understand.

- Take notes. Some doctors do not mind if you bring a tape recorder to help you remember things, but always ask first.

- Let your doctor know if you need more time. If there is not time that day, perhaps you can speak to a nurse or physician assistant on staff or schedule a telephone appointment.

- Take information home. Ask for written instructions. Your doctor may also have brochures and audio and videotapes that can help you.

---

[11] This section has been adapted from the AHRQ: **www.ahrq.gov/consumer/qntascii/qntdr.htm**.

- After leaving the doctor's office, take responsibility for your care. If you have questions, call. If your symptoms get worse or if you have problems with your medication, call. If you had tests and do not hear from your doctor, call for your test results. If your doctor recommended that you have certain tests, schedule an appointment to get them done. If your doctor said you should see an additional specialist, make an appointment.

By following these steps, you will enhance the relationship you will have with your physician.

Broader Health-Related Resources

In addition to the references above, the NIH has set up guidance Web sites that can help patients find healthcare professionals. These include:[12]

- Caregivers:
  http://www.nlm.nih.gov/medlineplus/caregivers.html
- Choosing a Doctor or Healthcare Service:
  http://www.nlm.nih.gov/medlineplus/choosingadoctororhealthcareserv ice.html
- Hospitals and Health Facilities:
  http://www.nlm.nih.gov/medlineplus/healthfacilities.html

Vocabulary Builder

The following vocabulary builder provides definitions of words used in this chapter that have not been defined in previous chapters:

Consultation: A deliberation between two or more physicians concerning the diagnosis and the proper method of treatment in a case. [NIH]

---

[12] You can access this information at
http://www.nlm.nih.gov/medlineplus/healthsystem.html.

PART II: ADDITIONAL RESOURCES AND ADVANCED MATERIAL

ABOUT PART II

In Part II, we introduce you to additional resources and advanced research on cataract surgery. All too often, patients who conduct their own research are overwhelmed by the difficulty in finding and organizing information. The purpose of the following chapters is to provide you an organized and structured format to help you find additional information resources on cataract surgery. In Part II, as in Part I, our objective is not to interpret the latest advances on cataract surgery or render an opinion. Rather, our goal is to give you access to original research and to increase your awareness of sources you may not have already considered. In this way, you will come across the advanced materials often referred to in pamphlets, books, or other general works. Once again, some of this material is technical in nature, so consultation with a professional familiar with cataract surgery is suggested.

CHAPTER 3. STUDIES ON CATARACT SURGERY

Overview

Every year, academic studies are published on cataract surgery or related procedures. Broadly speaking, there are two types of studies. The first are peer reviewed. Generally, the content of these studies has been reviewed by scientists or physicians. Peer-reviewed studies are typically published in scientific journals and are usually available at medical libraries. The second type of studies is non-peer reviewed. These works include summary articles that do not use or report scientific results. These often appear in the popular press, newsletters, or similar periodicals.

In this chapter, we will show you how to locate peer-reviewed references and studies on cataract surgery. We will begin by discussing research that has been summarized and is free to view by the public via the Internet. We then show you how to generate a bibliography on cataract surgery and teach you how to keep current on new studies as they are published or undertaken by the scientific community.

The Combined Health Information Database

The Combined Health Information Database summarizes studies across numerous federal agencies. To limit your investigation to research studies and cataract surgery, you will need to use the advanced search options. First, go to **http://chid.nih.gov/index.html**. From there, select the "Detailed Search" option (or go directly to that page with the following hyperlink: **http://chid.nih.gov/detail/detail.html**). The trick in extracting studies is found in the drop boxes at the bottom of the search page where "You may refine your search by." Select the dates and language you prefer, and the format option "Journal Article." At the top of the search form, select the number of records you would like to see (we recommend 100) and check the box to display "whole records." We recommend that you type in "cataract surgery" (or synonyms) into the "For these words:" box. Consider using the option "anywhere in record" to make your search as broad as possible. If you want to limit the search to only a particular field, such as the title of the journal, then select this option in the "Search in these fields" drop box. The following is a sample of what you can expect from this type of search:

- **Health of Family Members Caring for Elderly Persons With Dementia: A Longitudinal Study**

  Source: Annals of Internal Medicine. 120(2): 126-132. January 15, 1994.

  Summary: Researchers estimated changes in depression and physical symptoms for 1 year in caregivers for older people with dementia and in a comparison group. They examined the relationship between changes in caregiver health and certain characteristics of patients with dementia. Two hundred eighteen close family members of patients with dementia and patients consecutively undergoing **cataract surgery** were interviewed soon after referral of patients to the study (time 1). Of these, 86 caregivers (family members of patients with dementia) and 95 comparison participants (family members of patients with cataracts) were interviewed about 1 year later (time 2). Measurements included those for depression, consumption of prescription medications by caregivers and comparison participants, coping efficacy of both subject populations, and the severity of cognitive impairment in patients with dementia. A higher level of behavioral disturbance in patients with dementia at time 1 and institutionalization of patients between time 1 and time 2 predicted worsening caregiver depression and physical symptoms during the study period. Overall mean changes in depression and physical symptoms during 1 year were small for caregivers and comparison participants. However, peoples' responses to the caregiving situation differ substantially. 6 tables, 49 references.

- **Association of Ocular Disease and Mortality in a Diabetic Population**

  Source: Archives of Ophthalmology. 117(11): 1487-1494. November 1999.

  Contact: Available from American Medical Association. Subscriber Services Center, P.O. Box 10945, Chicago, IL 60610. (800) AMA-2350 or (312) 670-7827. Fax (312) 464-5831. E-mail: ama-subs@ama-assn.org.

  Summary: This article describes a study that investigated the association of retinopathy and other eye conditions with all-cause and cause specific mortality in a population of people who have diabetes from 11 counties in southern Wisconsin. Participants in the younger-onset group were diagnosed as having diabetes at less than 30 years of age and were taking insulin, and participants in the older-onset group were diagnosed as having diabetes at 30 years of age or older. Diabetic retinopathy, macular edema, visual acuity, and cataract were measured using standardized protocols at baseline examinations from 1980 to 1982, in which 996 younger-onset and 1,370 older-onset persons participated. Participants were followed up for 16 years. In the younger-onset group, after controlling for age and gender, retinopathy severity, macular edema, cataract, history of **cataract surgery,** and history of glaucoma at baseline were associated with all-cause and ischemic heart disease mortality. In the older-onset group, after controlling for age and gender, retinopathy and visual impairment were related to all-cause, ischemic heart disease, and stroke mortality. No ocular variable under study was related to cancer mortality in the older-onset group. After controlling for systemic risk factors, visual impairment was associated with all-cause and ischemic heart disease mortality in the younger onset group. In the older-onset group, retinopathy severity was related to all-cause and stroke mortality, and visual impairment was related to all-cause, ischemic heart disease, and stroke mortality. The article concludes that the presence of more severe retinopathy or visual impairment in patients who have diabetes is a risk indicator for increased risk of ischemic heart disease death. The presence of these ocular conditions may identify individuals who should be under care for cardiovascular disease. 4 figures. 6 tables. 57 references. (AA-M).

- **Opportunistic Fungal Infections: Superficial and Systemic Candidiasis**

Source: Geriatrics. 52(10): 50-54, 59. October 1997.

Summary: This article is the second in a series on opportunistic fungal infections in the older adult. The authors focus on those aspects of infection due to Candida that are of special relevance to physicians caring for the older population, with emphasis on clinical presentation and treatment. They note that age alone is not usually sufficient for the development of disease due to Candida, but it appears to be associated with increased morbidity and mortality. Mucocutaneous Candida infections such as thrush and denture stomatitis are associated with local and mechanical factors, including xerostomia (dry mouth), the use of broad-spectrum antibiotics, inhaled corticosteroids, and diminished cell-mediated immunity. In an older adult, oral thrush (in the absence of an obvious cause or extension to involve the esophagus) may herald underlying immunosuppression in the form of cancer or AIDS. A rare and sight-threatening complication of **cataract surgery** is Candida endophthalmitis. Systemic Candida infections are becoming more common due to the increasing use of immunosuppressive drugs and the increasing risk of nosocomial candidiasis in the intensive care unit. In addition, candiduria is increasingly common in older patients with diabetes mellitus, indwelling urinary catheters, and a history of antibiotic therapy. 3 figures. 22 references. (AA-M).

• **Eye Care**

Source: Diabetes in the News. 10(3): 52. June 1991.

Contact: Available from Ames Center for Diabetes Education. Ames Division, Miles Laboratories, P.O. Box 3115, Elkhart, IN 46515. (312) 664-9782 or (800) 348-8100.

Summary: This brief article details the ins and outs of protecting the eyes from the sun's ultraviolet (UV) light. The advice in this article is especially important for people with diabetic retinopathy, those who have had **cataract surgery,** or those with other risk factors, such as taking certain medications. Topics include the dangers of overexposure to UV light, the development of cataracts, UV-caused damage to the retina, and some simple precautions to protect the eyes from overexposure to UV light. The author briefly considers the role of sunglasses and how to purchase a pair that will provide adequate protection.

• **Association Among Visual Hallucinations, Visual Acuity, and Specific Eye Pathologies in Alzheimer's Disease: Treatment Implications**

Source: American Journal of Psychiatry. 156(12): 1983-1985. December 1999.

Summary: This journal article examines the associations of visual acuity and specific eye pathologies with visual hallucinations in people with Alzheimer's disease (AD). Fifty patients with probable AD (20 with and 30 without visual hallucinations) were evaluated for psychotic symptoms with Columbia University Scale for Psychopathology in Alzheimer's Disease. Cognitive function was assessed with the cognitive section of the Cambridge Examination for Mental Disorders of the Elderly. Visual acuity was measured before and after refraction, and patients received standardized assessments for cataracts and macular degeneration. Impaired visual acuity and the severity of cognitive impairment were significantly associated with visual hallucinations. No patient with normal acuity (6/5 or 6/6 on the Snellen chart) had these symptoms. Impaired acuity improved with refraction in 60 percent of the patients with visual hallucinations. Of the specific eye pathologies, only cataracts were significantly associated with visual hallucinations. The authors conclude that glasses and **cataract surgery** should be investigated as prophylactic or adjunctive treatments for visual hallucinations in patients with probable AD. 1 table, 11 references.

Federally Funded Research on Cataract Surgery

The U.S. Government supports a variety of research studies relating to cataract surgery and associated procedures. These studies are tracked by the Office of Extramural Research at the National Institutes of Health.[13] CRISP (Computerized Retrieval of Information on Scientific Projects) is a searchable database of federally funded biomedical research projects conducted at universities, hospitals, and other institutions. Visit CRISP at **http://crisp.cit.nih.gov/crisp/crisp_query.generate_screen**. You can perform targeted searches by various criteria including geography, date, as well as topics related to cataract surgery and related treatments.

For most of the studies, the agencies reporting into CRISP provide summaries or abstracts. As opposed to clinical trial research using patients, many federally funded studies use animals or simulated models to explore cataract surgery and related treatments. In some cases, therefore, it may be difficult to understand how some basic or fundamental research could eventually translate into medical practice. The following sample is typical of the type of information found when searching the CRISP database for cataract surgery:

- **Project Title: A CELL-BASED THERAPY FOR CATARACTS**

  Principal Investigator & Institution: Lang, Richard A.; Associate Professor; Children's Hospital Med Ctr (Cincinnati) 3333 Burnet Ave Cincinnati, Oh 452293039

  Timing: Fiscal Year 2003; Project Start 01-AUG-2003; Project End 31-JUL-2006

  Summary: (provided by applicant): Our long term objective is to develop a cell-based therapy for cataracts. In the case of the cataractous lens in adults, this approach offers the advantage, when compared with plastic prosthetic lenses, that the regenerated lens would be entirely natural in function and would accommodate normally. The regenerated organ

---

[13] Healthcare projects are funded by the National Institutes of Health (NIH), Substance Abuse and Mental Health Services (SAMHSA), Health Resources and Services Administration (HRSA), Food and Drug Administration (FDA), Centers for Disease Control and Prevention (CDCP), Agency for Healthcare Research and Quality (AHRQ), and Office of Assistant Secretary of Health (OASH).

would also be young in cellular terms and would therefore have extended function even in an environment, such as the diabetic patient, that favored the formation of cataracts. A cell-based therapy would also offer a unique advantage for the treatment of cataracts in newborns where conventional intraocular lens implantation is complicated by the rapid growth of the immature eye (a newborn's eye is 17 mm in length but grows to 22 mm by the end of the second year). The experimental strategy is to develop the techniques for production, identification and isolation of lens progenitor cells from mouse embryonic stem cells, and then to determine whether lens progenitors will form a lens in situ after implantation in the empty lens capsule of an experimental animal. Three Aims are designed to lead us towards this long-term goal. Aim 1 - to derive ES cell lines that give lens progenitor-GFP expression in chimeric mice. To prepare for the derivation on lens progenitor cells in culture, we will generate ES celt lines that give the normal Pax6 ectoderm enhancer expression pattern in chimeric mice. Aim 2 - To determine whether lens progenitor cells can be identified and isolated from embryonic stem cells. We will ask whether mouse embryonic stem cells are a source of lens progenitor cells using a variety of differentiation conditions in culture. Aim 3 - To determine whether lens progenitors will form a lens in situ. We will determine if lens progenitors isolated according to Aim 2 can generate a lens when placed in the empty lens capsule in nude (immune deficient) rats. If we are able to observe lens development from implanted progenitors, we will have established the basis of a cell-based therapy. Once established in animal models, the techniques described would be used with human ES cells and additional steps taken toward a practical therapy.

Website: http://crisp.cit.nih.gov/crisp/Crisp_Query.Generate_Screen

- **Project Title: A NEW THERAPY FOR DIABETIC MACULAR EDEMA**

    Principal Investigator & Institution: Ma, Jian-Xing; Laureate Professor; Medicine; University of Oklahoma Hlth Sciences Ctr Health Sciences Center Oklahoma City, Ok 73126

    Timing: Fiscal Year 2003; Project Start 30-SEP-2003; Project End 31-AUG-2005

    Summary: (provided by applicant): This is a R21/R33 phase-combined proposal aiming to develop a new treatment for diabetic macular edema using peptide angiogenic inhibitors. Vascular leakage is an early feature of diabetic retinopathy and can result in diabetic macular edema. Over-expression of VEGF is a major causative factor leading to vascular leakage in diabetic retinopathy. Currently, there is no satisfactory treatment for macular edema which remains a major cause of vision loss in diabetic patients. Plasminogen kringle 5 (K5) is a potent angiogenic inhibitor. Our recent studies have shown that K5 significantly decreases vascular leakage in the retina in the experimental diabetes, laser-induced choroid neovascularization and oxygen-induced retinopathy rat models. The K5- induced reduction of vascular leakage requires only less than one-tenth of the dose needed for the inhibition of neovascularization. Furthermore, our preliminary data suggest that the K5-induced reduction of vascular leakage may be through blocking hypoxia-induced VEGF over-expression in the retina, primarily in Muller cells. We hypothesize that a sustained ocular delivery of K5 may induce a long-term reduction of vascular leakage in diabetic retina and thus, may have therapeutic effect on cyctoid macular edema (CME) secondary to **cataract surgery** and diabetic macular edema. In the R21 phase, we propose to first reveal the mechanisms for the K5-induced down-regulation of VEGF expression and identify the receptor or binding protein on the cell surface which mediates the K.5-induced reduction of permeability. As diabetic macular edema is a chronic complication of diabetes and requires a long-term treatment, we propose to develop a KS-polymer pellet to achieve a sustained release of K5. The ocular delivery routes of the K5 pellet will be optimized and the pharmacokinetics will be studied in rats. The long-term effect of the K5 pellet on vascular leakage will be determined in a diabetic rat model. The R21 phase will achieve the following goals: 1),to reveal the mechanism and identify the receptor mediating the K5 action, 2) to develop a sustained delivery system for K5 and 3) to prove the concept that a sustained delivery of K5 can induce a prolonged reduction of vascular leakage, The R21 phase will provide essential tools and information for starting the R33 phase. In the R33 phase, we will study the pharmacokinetics of K5 in ocular tissues and optimize the delivery route in normal dogs, With the optimized delivery route, the efficacy of K5 on reduction of vascular leakage will be confirmed in a dog model of vascular leakage induced by intravitreal injection of IGF-1. The possible toxicity of K5 to the retinal vasculature and retinal structure will be examined in both rats and dogs by histochemistry. The retinal function will be examined by ERG recoding. Although this project does not reach clinical trials, the proposed studies will obtain pre-clinical data such as pharmacokinetics, delivery route, efficacy and toxicity from more than one species, which are essential and useful for starting clinical trials. These studies will contribute to the development of a new treatment for CME and for diabetic macular edema. This new treatment will use natural human peptides and will be less invasive. This new therapy, if successful, can prevent vision loss from macular edema in diabetic patients.

Website: http://crisp.cit.nih.gov/crisp/Crisp_Query.Generate_Screen

- **Project Title: ABERRATIONS OF EYES IN NORMAL AND CLINICAL POPULATIONS**

Principal Investigator & Institution: Applegate, Raymond A.; Professor; None; University of Houston 4800 Calhoun Rd Houston, Tx 77004

Timing: Fiscal Year 2002; Project Start 01-APR-1991; Project End 29-FEB-2004

Summary: (Adapted From The Applicant's Abstract): In the United States, **cataract surgery** is the most frequently performed surgical procedure among 30 million Medicare beneficiaries at an estimated cost of $3.5 billion per year. In the Baltimore Eye Survey, cataract is reported as the leading cause of blindness in those over the age of 40, and to be four times more common in African-Americans than in Caucasian-Americans. In the world, cataract is the leading cause of blindness. The proposed research is designed to take a significant step toward reducing blindness resulting from cataract. To evaluate the effectiveness of preventative therapy designed to delay or prevent cataract formation, new sensitive markers of early cataract development and progression need to be identified. This need is specifically recognized and reflected in Objective 1 of the Report of the Lens and Cataract Panel in: Vision Research, A National Plan: 1999-2003. Objective 1 of the NEI report is to: "Determine if there are novel markers that differentiate the normal aging process from the diseased (cataractous) state." To meet objective 1, the Report identifies the need for the development of "morphological and optical markers that can be visualized by noninvasive techniques." The specific aims of the resubmission are to demonstrate that: wavefront sensing can quantify the optical aberrations and local scattering properties of early cataract formation; wavefront sensing can differentiate the normal aging process from the cataractous state; wavefront sensing has the accuracy and precision to be an effective monitoring tool in longitudinal studies of new therapy designed to delay, prevent, or slow cataract formation and progression. These specific aims will be accomplished by modifying Hartmann/Shack wavefront sensor technology to quantify the optical aberrations and local scattering properties of eyes with early cataract and eyes of normals in the 4th, 5th and 6th decades of life.

Website: http://crisp.cit.nih.gov/crisp/Crisp_Query.Generate_Screen

- **Project Title: CHARACTERISTICS OF T CELL RECEPTORS**

Principal Investigator & Institution: Marrack, Philippa C.; Investigator; National Jewish Medical & Res Ctr and Research Center Denver, Co 80206

Timing: Fiscal Year 2003; Project Start 01-MAY-1982; Project End 30-APR-2006

Summary: T cells bearing alphabeta T cell receptors react with antigen in the form of peptides bound to major histocompatibility complex proteins (MHC). This reaction is crucial to the ability of T cells to orchestrate destruction of invading organisms. It is also involved in graft rejection and in T cell attacks on the tissues of their own host in autoimmune disease. Several aspects of T cell reaction with MHC are not understood. The projects in this application will study two of these aspects. The first set of experiments will study the ways in which T cells are selected to react with peptides bond to MHC in the thymus. A major focus of these experiments will be the role of the peptides bound to MHC. Mice will be created in which a single peptide is firmly bound to an MHC protein, and the ability of this MHC/single peptide combination to select T cells studied. The second set of experiments will investigate the relationship between T cell receptors and MHC. It is thought that the two sets of proteins may have an intrinsic affinity for each other. Experiments proposed here will try to find out if this is so. T cells from the MHV/single peptide mice, which are very reactive with MHC proteins, will be used to study the phenomenon.

Website: http://crisp.cit.nih.gov/crisp/Crisp_Query.Generate_Screen

- **Project Title: ELECTRICAL ALTERNATIVE LASERS INTRAOCULAR MICROSURGERY**

Principal Investigator & Institution: Palanker, Daniel V.; Ophthalmology; Stanford University Stanford, Ca 94305

Timing: Fiscal Year 2002; Project Start 01-JAN-2001; Project End 31-DEC-2003

Summary: We propose to develop and evaluate a precise yet low cost electric operative cutting instrument for ophthalmic surgery based on pulsed plasma-mediated dissection of soft tissue in liquid medium. One of the first applications of this device will be in vitreoretinal surgery, namely, for tractionless removal of vitreoretinal membranes. The common techniques for treatment of vitreoretinal membranes are mechanical segmentation, peeling or delamination where a significant degree of traction is often applied to the underlying retinal tissue, and this can induce damage to the internal layers, iatrogenic tears and bleeding. Several attempts to develop laser- based instrumentation for vitreoretinal surgery have been undertaken, but all these systems have failed so far to achieve widespread acceptance due to either extensive collateral tissue damage, or high cost and low efficiency of these systems. One of the most powerful mechanisms of laser-tissue interaction in liquid medium is dielectric breakdown-based plasma generation. This approach, based on application of tightly focused short pulse lasers, has not been accepted clinically in vitreoretinal surgery due to difficulties with tight focusing of the laser beam near the retina in real operational conditions. We propose to use a similar interaction mechanism but without lasers. A sub-microsecond high voltage discharge applied via an intraocular microelectrode will generate plasma in liquid medium and can allow for precise cutting of soft tissue. The energy deposition is confined to the area determined by the size of the electrode - on the order of a few micrometers - thus allowing for very low threshold energy and very fine control of the penetration depth. This system combining high precision, reliability and versatility with low cost will allow for widespread acceptance in operating practice. Applicability of this approach to vitreoretinal surgery and other intraocular procedures, such as capsulotomy and **cataract surgery** will be tested in-vitro and on animal models including histological analysis, scanning electron microscopy and physiological tests.

Website: http://crisp.cit.nih.gov/crisp/Crisp_Query.Generate_Screen

- **Project Title: FUNCTION OF ADHESION MOLECULES IN LENS DEVELOPMENT**

Principal Investigator & Institution: Menko, Allyn Sue.; Pathology, Anat/Cell Biology; Thomas Jefferson University Office of Research Administration Philadelphia, Pa 191075587

Timing: Fiscal Year 2002; Project Start 01-AUG-1993; Project End 31-MAR-2006

Summary: (provided by applicant): The long-term goals of this application are to examine how a6 integrin signaling pathways regulate lens cell differentiation and to determine how changes in this integrin signaling pathway may mediate cell migration that leads to posterior capsule opacification (PCO) following **cataract surgery.** During the last funding period we demonstrated that a6 integrin is required for lens cell differentiation. We then began our investigation of potential a6 integrin signaling pathways in the developing lens, focusing on the relationship between a6 integrin and growth factor signaling. We have discovered that the insulin-like growth factor-1 receptor (IGF-1R) becomes associated with a6 integrin during lens cell differentiation and that the IGF-1R in this a6 integrin signaling complex is tyrosine phosphorylated. We determined that other molecules known to be downstream of the IGF-1R signaling pathway, Shc and extracellular signal-regulated kinase (ERK), were also associated with a6 integrin in the embryonic lens. These investigations led us to examine potential regulators of a6 integrin/IGF-IR signaling in the lens. A role was identified for the Src family kinases (SFKs) in regulation of both lens cell proliferation and differentiation. We have made significant advances in determining the requisite role for a6 integrin in lens cell differentiation and defining the components of the a6 integrin signaling complex. This continuation application is focused on mapping a6 integrin signaling pathways and determining how they are regulated in order to understand a6 integrin function in mediating lens cell differentiation. We propose an integrated approach to map the signaling pathways including genetic, biochemical and cell biological studies. a6 integrin, through its association with different signaling pathways, also could play role a role in mediating the migration of lens epithelial cells along the posterior capsule as occurs in PCO following **cataract surgery.** We will use a model for PCO to investigate whether changes in a6 integrin signaling mediate cell migration in PCO. We will also investigate possible therapies to block integrin-mediated cell migration in PCO. The specific aims are: 1) Investigate the hypothesis that the activation of a6 integrin induces a signaling pathway involving activation of IGF-1R and its downstream signaling effectors; 2) Examine the hypothesis that Src family kinases play a central role in lens cell differentiation through their regulation of a6 integrin/IGF-1R coordinated signaling; and 3) Examine the hypothesis that PCO is triggered by changes in a6 integrin/IGF-1R signaling which lead to the acquisition of a migratory phenotype by lens epithelial cells. These studies also will examine whether inhibition of SFKS could prevent PCO.

Website: http://crisp.cit.nih.gov/crisp/Crisp_Query.Generate_Screen

- **Project Title: GENETIC BASIS OF NANOPHTHALMOS**

Principal Investigator & Institution: Sundin, Olof H.; Assistant Professor; Ophthalmology; Johns Hopkins University 3400 N Charles St Baltimore, Md 21218

Timing: Fiscal Year 2002; Project Start 15-AUG-2001; Project End 30-JUN-2004

Summary: (provided by applicant): Nanophthalmos is a rare developmental disorder in which the eye is much smaller than normal, and the retina is placed unusually close to the lens. The result of this is profound hyperopia (farsightedness) in the range of +8 to +24 diopters, a condition apparent at birth and maintained throughout life. The eye is formed intact and functional, typically without disorders elsewhere in the body. This is in contrast to microphthalmia, in which small eyes are associated with more serious structural malformations. The nanophthalmic eye exhibits a thick iris and a lens displaced towards the anterior chamber, features thought to contribute to the high incidence of angle closure glaucoma among these patients. Another characteristic of the disease is massive thickening of the choroid and sclera, which may be associated with a tendency of the eye to develop exudative retinal detachment, especially as a complication of glaucoma or **cataract surgery.** The disease is usually inherited as an autosomal recessive. There is also an autosomal dominant form of the disease, which has recently been mapped by genetic linkage to an interval on chromosome 11p. The identity of this gene remains unknown, and no locus has yet been reported for the recessive form of the disease. This application focuses on detailed linkage mapping and isolation of the gene for recessive nanophthalmos. Once this is accomplished, we will investigate its pattern of expression and the subcellular localization of the gene product. Identification of a gene for nanophthalmos would provide a starting point for the genetic diagnosis and rational development of treatments for this rare ocular disease. It also promises insights into the developmental mechanisms by which the eye normally regulates its size and shape in order to adjust its optical properties.

Website: http://crisp.cit.nih.gov/crisp/Crisp_Query.Generate_Screen

- **Project Title: INTERVENTIONS FOR VISUAL LOSS IN NURSING HOME RESIDENTS**

Principal Investigator & Institution: West, Sheila K.; Professor; Ophthalmology; Johns Hopkins University 3400 N Charles St Baltimore, Md 21218

Timing: Fiscal Year 2002; Project Start 01-MAY-1999; Project End 30-APR-2004

Summary: (adapted from investigator's abstract): The burden of visual impairment among older persons is considerable, with especially high rates reported among nursing home residents. Causes of visual impairment are largely remediable with refraction and **cataract surgery,** or the functional impact lessened with appropriate low vision aids. Yet, no intervention trial to determine methods to improve visual status in nursing home residents has ever been carried out. Moreover, the impact of improving visual status on socialization and functional status in nursing homes is unknown. In this project the investigators propose to measure the impact on socialization, and a variety of other measures of function, of a visual impairment intervention program. Nursing homes will be randomized into a group receiving standard care and a group receiving a visual impairment intervention program, and outcomes compared at 6 and 12 months after the intervention. The intervention program consists of 3 tracks depending on the cause of vision loss: free refraction and subsidized spectacles; transportation in connection with

cataract surgery; and free training and subsidized low vision aids. From 28 nursing homes on the Lower Eastern Shore of Maryland, the investigators will assess visual impairment and the causes of visual loss in the residents. They expect to identify 578 persons with presenting acuity worse than 20/40 in the better eye, and an equal sample of 578 persons with no visual loss. Baseline comparisons of difference between those with visual impairment and those with no visual loss will determine the impact of visual loss on functional status. Those with visual loss will be randomized, by nursing home, into treatment arms for prospective determination of the impact of impairment in visual status on function. The primary outcome measure is improved socialization scores, using a scale of observed resident behavior with nursing home staff respondents. Secondary outcomes include utilization of appropriate eye care services in both treatment arms, change in physical function and mobility, changes in depressive symptomatology, and changes in psychoactive drug use. Prospective change will be measured among intervention and control groups, including both visually impaired and non-impaired. The cost-effectiveness of the intervention strategy will be determined. Optimizing eye care services for nursing home residents will become increasingly important as the size of this population increases. This trial will answer timely questions of the impact on the functional status of the most frail elderly of modest, potentially sustainable inputs into improving the appropriate utilization of eye care services.

Website: http://crisp.cit.nih.gov/crisp/Crisp_Query.Generate_Screen

- **Project Title: MULTIDIMENSIONAL INTERVENTION FOR VISION-IMPAIRED ELDERS**

Principal Investigator & Institution: Coleman, Anne L.; Assistant Professor; University of California Los Angeles 10920 Wilshire Blvd., Suite 1200 Los Angeles, Ca 90024

Timing: Fiscal Year 2002

Summary: (provided by the applicant) Visual impairment is very common in older persons and is associated with decreased vision-specific and overall functioning. Two of the most common causes of visual impairment, uncorrected refractive error and cataracts, are reversible, while the others, such as glaucoma and age-related macular degeneration, are not. No matter whether visual impairment is irreversible or reversible, visual functioning may improve with increased lighting and the use of low vision aids. The proposed Intervention Development Study (IDS) is designed to provide enough information to support an application for a Randomized Clinical Trial (RCT) to determine whether visual and overall functioning of older persons can be enhanced through a multi-dimensional intervention that corrects reversible causes of visual impairment, improves lighting in the home environment, and provides access to low vision aids. The IDS is designed so that it will provide critical information about the feasibility, recruitment rates, expected effect sizes, and costs that would be associated with a RCT. During phase I, participants will have their visual functioning optimized through **cataract surgery** or new eye glasses. Subjects with visually significant cataracts will be referred for **cataract surgery.** Subjects in whom their vision can be improved with new eyeglasses (uncorrected refractive error) will be randomized to either receive an updated prescription and voucher for new eyeglasses immediately or receive the updated prescription and voucher for new eyeglasses 3 months later. The impact of correction of uncorrected refractive error (e.g., new eyeglasses) on vision-related quality of life measures will be investigated in phase I. Subjects with visual functioning that cannot be improved with **cataract surgery** or new eye glasses because of age-related macular degeneration or glaucoma will be followed during phase I. In phase II, all participants will be randomized to either an intervention aiming to improve lighting conditions in the home environment or a control condition of changing existing light bulbs in the home. Following a factorial design, a subset of individuals with near vision worse than 20/40 will be randomized to the provision of low vision aids and training on their use. Primary outcomes of the study will be measures of vision-related quality of life and measures of functioning.

Website: http://crisp.cit.nih.gov/crisp/Crisp_Query.Generate_Screen

- **Project Title: NEW BIOMATERIALS FOR SUTURELESS OPHTHALMIC SURGERIES**

Principal Investigator & Institution: Grinstaff, Mark W.; Associate Professor; Chemistry; Duke University Durham, Nc 27706

Timing: Fiscal Year 2002; Project Start 01-FEB-2002; Project End 31-JAN-2006

Summary: We propose a systematic study to test the hypothesis that light-activated polymers can replace or supplement conventional sutures in ophthalmic surgeries. Specifically we have synthesized novel dendrimers, termed biodendrimers, composed of biocompatible monomers such as glycerol and lactic acid. We will take advantage of the favorable chemical and physical properties of these photocrosslinkable biodendrimers to seal corneal perforations and to secure corneal autografts in human enucleated eyes and chicken eyes in vivo. Accordingly, answers will be sought to the following questions: 1. Can the chemical structure of a biodendrimer be optimized to afford specific properties required for sutureless ophthalmic surgeries? 2. Will a biodendrimer seal a 3 mm full thickness linear or stellate corneal perforation? 3. Will a biodendrimer secure a corneal autograft? Corneal perforation and corneal transplantation are two models of corneal tissue injury that are ideal for testing new tissue sealants. The traditional approach to repair both these injuries involves sutures, yet the use of sutures affords a number of limitations and complications. Tissue adhesives such as cyanoacrylate are becoming more widely accepted in various corneal procedures, however these materials have only met with marginal success. Improvements made to the composition and/or to the method of application can potentially enhance the effectiveness of tissue sealants for treating wounds and even broaden the scope of clinical use. Potential indications in other ophthalmic areas include ruptured globe repair, wound closure in **cataract surgery,** and wound modulation in glaucoma filtering surgery. The novel photocrosslinkable biodendrimers described in this proposal represent a new class of ophthalmic tissue adhesives that may accomplish the objectives cited above sealing corneal perforations, and securing corneal autografts. Successful completion of these studies may lead to new ophthalmic surgical techniques, procedures, and treatments using unique, custom-designed biomaterials.

Website: http://crisp.cit.nih.gov/crisp/Crisp_Query.Generate_Screen

- **Project Title: PATHOGENESIS OF CORNEAL EDEMA AFTER INTRAOCULAR SURGERY**

Principal Investigator & Institution: Edelhauser, Henry F.; Professor; Ophthalmology; Emory University 1784 North Decatur Road Atlanta, Ga 30322

Timing: Fiscal Year 2002; Project Start 01-JUL-1989; Project End 30-APR-2007

Summary: (provided by applicant): The objective of this study is to understand the pathogenesis of corneal edema which occurs, in some patients, following intraocular surgery. At greatest risk are diabetic patients, patients with guttata, maltino implant patients and possibly long-term contact lens wearers, all of whom have severe endothelial polymegathism, particularly as they approach the age for **cataract surgery.** Our basic premise is that the cornea of these patients have a compromised endothelium and additional stress such as intraocular surgery, postoperative inflammation and increases in intraocular pressure will affect the metabolic pump and barrier functions of the compromised endothelium resulting in postoperative corneal edema. The proposed studies should further our understanding of the pathogenesis of corneal edema and the prevention of postsurgical corneal edema. We propose to test the following hypothesis about the specific effects of each of three factors on the compromised corneal endothelium. (1) that the corneal endothelium has a regeneration zone (stem cells) that maintains a constant supply of new cells to enable endothelial cell migration from the peripheral limbal region to the central region of the cornea: these studies will evaluate endothelial cells that are transit amphifying cells, terminally differential cells, the effect of mitomycin C, glaucoma drainage implants and polymegathism on the endothelial cell population in the three zones of endothelial cells: regenerative, storage and migration. (2) that glutathoine will protect corneal endothelial cells against apoptosis and that the cellular levels of reduced glutathione (GSH) will modulate Fas-mediated apoptosis. And (3) that endotoxin (LPS) produced during inflammation in the presence of the binding protein (LPB) and the anchoring glycoprotein CD-14 causes the release of cytokines from the corneal endothelial cells which can result in corneal edema. The results of these studies should provide a better understanding of the corneal endothelial response following intraocular surgery and in the prevention of postoperative corneal edema that can occur in stressed corneas with low cell numbers and following gram negative intraocular inflammation.

Website: http://crisp.cit.nih.gov/crisp/Crisp_Query.Generate_Screen

- **Project Title: PATIENT ORIENTED OPHTHALMIC RESEARCH AND MENTORSHIP**

Principal Investigator & Institution: Schein, Oliver D.; Professor; Ophthalmology; Johns Hopkins University 3400 N Charles St Baltimore, Md 21218

Timing: Fiscal Year 2002; Project Start 30-SEP-1999; Project End 29-SEP-2004

Summary: Since completing my clinical training in 1989, my research career has been devoted to clinical ophthalmic research that has used a variety of epidemiologic methodologies to study therapeutic interventions, assess new technologies, and better understand mechanisms of disease. To a large extent, by productivity can be attributed to mentorship I received early in my career and the accessibility of skilled colleagues with multidisciplinary skills at the Johns Hopkins Schools of Medicine and Hygiene and Public Health. My clinical and administrative responsibilities have increased annually. The K24 can provide an ideal mechanism to allow me to continue to prioritize patient-oriented clinical research and mentorship. My 5-year plans include 1) the completion and dissemination of results of a large clinical trial on the value of medical testing for **cataract surgery;** 2) the conduct of a large prospective study on the progression and risk factors for posterior capsular opacification, using a digital system we have designed; 3) studying patient function and preferences related to refractive error and its correction using a questionnaire we have developed and validated; 4) initiating clinical trials comparing alternative treatments for dry eye; and 5) developing new methodologies to facilitate the postmarket surveillance of new ophthalmic technologies to assess safety. Effective mentorship of junior physicians will be achieved by incorporating them into the above research plans; acting as a liaison for them to related programs in the Schools of Medicine and Hygiene and Public Health; conducting the Public Health Ophthalmology fellowship; securing departmental and other pilot funds to initiate junior faculty clinical research and providing assistance with grant application. Both a firm commitment and additional linked support have been pledged by the Chairman of my department and the Deans' offices of the Johns Hopkins Schools of Medicine and Hygiene and Public Health.

Website: http://crisp.cit.nih.gov/crisp/Crisp_Query.Generate_Screen

- **Project Title: POSTOPERATIVE ADJUSTMENT OF INTRAOCULAR LENS POWER**

Principal Investigator & Institution: Chang, Shiao H.;; Calhoun Vision, Inc. 2555 E Colorado Blvd, Ste 400 Pasadena, Ca 911076620

Timing: Fiscal Year 2002; Project Start 01-FEB-2000; Project End 29-SEP-2003

Summary: (From the Applicant's Abstract): For patients over 60-years old, **cataract surgery** with Intraocular lens (IOL) implantation is the most commonly-performed surgical procedure. Unfortunately, the calculation of IOL power is often imprecise due to pre-operative measurement error, post-operative astigmatism from irregular wound healing, or variability in the placement of an IOL. As a result, most cataract patients need to wear spectacles in order to achieve optimal vision. The objective of this project is to develop a light-adjustable Intraocular lens (LAL). The LAL is an IOL whose power can be precisely adjusted with light 2-4 weeks after **cataract surgery** to correct refractive errors such as tilt, power, and astigmatism which may have been induced by the procedure or through subsequent wound healing. By post-operatively modifying IOL power and precisely correcting refractive error, the LAL will enable cataract patients to predictably achieve best-possible vision without the need for spectacles. The project has three aims: (1)Develop and optimize a silicone LAL composition, including matrix, macromer, photoinitiator, and UV absorber; (2)Optically test and differentiate and LAL via characterization, irradiation protocol, and a treatment nomogram; and (3)Conduct pre-

Clinical animal studies regarding the LAL's biocompatibility and safety. PROPOSED COMMERCIAL APPLICATION: NOT AVAILABLE

Website: http://crisp.cit.nih.gov/crisp/Crisp_Query.Generate_Screen

- **Project Title: PROTEOLYTIC ENZYMES AND CATARACTOGENESIS**

Principal Investigator & Institution: Wagner, B J.; Professor; Biochem and Molecular Biology; Univ of Med/Dent Nj Newark Newark, Nj 07107

Timing: Fiscal Year 2003; Project Start 01-JAN-1978; Project End 30-JUN-2006

Summary: (provided by applicant): The long-term goal of this project is to test proteasome inhibitors as potential therapeutic agents for ocular lens disorders. Posterior capsular opacification (PCO) and anterior polar and subcapsular cataract manifest abnormal proliferation or apoptosis. The proteasome is a key factor in proliferation and apoptosis in many cell types. Several classes of powerful anti-proteasome drugs are under development or in clinical trial for treatment of disparate diseases. Proteasome inhibition may stop abnormal proliferation or apoptosis in PCO and cataractogenesis, and prevent or delay opacification. The specific aims are to answer the following questions about PCO and anterior polar and subcapsular cataracts: Is there altered Ubiquitin-Proteasome pathway activity? Proteolytic activity will be quantitated using chromogenic and/or fluorescent substrates. Are levels of pro- or anti-apoptotic proteasome substrates altered? Expression and function of regulatory proteins will be determined and correlated with apoptosis and markers of cataract. Do proteasome inhibitors prevent changes associated with opacification? Well-defined classes of proteasome inhibitors will be tested for the ability to prevent or delay changes associated with cataract formation. TGF-beta will be used to induce PCO and cataract like changes in an eye bank donor lens capsular bag model, a rat lens explant model, and in cultured HLE B-3 cells. Anterior capsules obtained during **cataract surgery** will be analyzed for markers of cataract and apoptosis. These experiments will for the first time address the role of the proteasome in lens pathology. If an abnormal balance between proliferation and apoptosis is part of opacification, the proteasome is an important therapeutic target, and these studies may provide the basis for a novel, effective pharmacological treatment of PCO and cataract.

Website: http://crisp.cit.nih.gov/crisp/Crisp_Query.Generate_Screen

- **Project Title: ULTRASONIC SYSTEM FOR OCULAR VISUALIZATION AND BIOMETRY**

Principal Investigator & Institution: Wiseman, George D.;; Ultralink, Llc 2083 Hawaii Ave Ne Saint Petersburg, Fl 33703

Timing: Fiscal Year 2002; Project Start 01-FEB-2002; Project End 31-JUL-2002

Summary: (Provided by Applicant): The long-term objective of this program is a commercially viable system that will play a key role in restoring and preserving vision for millions of patients in this country and abroad. The system will couple high-frequency ultrasound (40 MHz) with novel signal processing to provide accurate, precise biometry of the cornea and anterior chamber. Measurements will be used by ophthalmologists to: 1) plan refractive laser surgery of the cornea (for vision correction and restoration); 2) select the appropriate type and size of recently developed intra-ocular lenses (IOL) to correct refractive errors or restore vision following **cataract surgery;** and, 3) document causes of undesired side-effects following laser and IOL procedures, so that corrective actions can be initiated promptly. The system will incorporate advanced, patented methodology developed by the Weill Medical College of Cornell University (WMC) and Riverside Research Institute (RRI). Ultralink, Inc. has already implemented an initial "proof-of-concept" system that successfully demonstrated the practicality of these objectives. This innovative system functioned extremely well, but it also identified several practical issues that will be addressed in this program so that these techniques can realize their full clinical and commercial potentials. The program will integrate system design (Phase I), and development and testing (Phase II) at Ultralink, WMC, and RRI. PROPOSED COMMERCIAL APPLICATION: The research will provide advanced ultrasonic systems to provide precise biometric data that is essential for optimal laser?refractive surgery and intraocular lens implants.

Website: http://crisp.cit.nih.gov/crisp/Crisp_Query.Generate_Screen

E-Journals: PubMed Central[14]

PubMed Central (PMC) is a digital archive of life sciences journal literature developed and managed by the National Center for Biotechnology

---

[14] Adapted from the National Library of Medicine:
http://www.pubmedcentral.nih.gov/about/intro.html.

Information (NCBI) at the U.S. National Library of Medicine (NLM).[15] Access to this growing archive of e-journals is free and unrestricted.[16] To search, go to **http://www.ncbi.nlm.nih.gov/entrez/query.fcgi?db=Pmc**, and type "cataract surgery" (or synonyms) into the search box. This search gives you access to full-text articles. The following is a sample of items found for cataract surgery in the PubMed Central database:

- **Abiotrophia Species as a Cause of Endophthalmitis Following Cataract Extraction.** by Namdari H, Kintner K, Jackson BA, Namdari S, Hughes JL, Peairs RR, Savage DJ.; 1999 May;
  http://www.pubmedcentral.gov/articlerender.fcgi?tool=pmcentrez&artid=84829

- **Iris recognition as a biometric method after cataract surgery.** by Roizenblatt R, Schor P, Dante F, Roizenblatt J, Belfort R Jr.; 2004;
  http://www.pubmedcentral.gov/articlerender.fcgi?tool=pmcentrez&artid=333428

- **Longitudinal study on visual outcome and spectacle use after intracapsular cataract extraction in Northern India.** by Gupta SK, Murthy GV, Sharma N.; 2003;
  http://www.pubmedcentral.gov/articlerender.fcgi?tool=pmcentrez&artid=183851

- **Outbreak of Candida parapsilosis endophthalmitis after cataract extraction and intraocular lens implantation..** by McCray E, Rampell N, Solomon SL, Bond WW, Martone WJ, O'Day D.; 1986 Oct;
  http://www.pubmedcentral.gov/picrender.fcgi?tool=pmcentrez&action=stream&blobtype=pdf&artid=268984

- **Prioritization for cataract surgery.** by Sanmugasunderam S, Romanchuk K.; 2001 Oct 2;
  http://www.pubmedcentral.gov/articlerender.fcgi?tool=pmcentrez&artid=81486

- **Prioritization for cataract surgery.** by Bellan L, Mathen M.; 2001 Oct 2;
  http://www.pubmedcentral.gov/articlerender.fcgi?tool=pmcentrez&artid=81487

---

[15] With PubMed Central, NCBI is taking the lead in preservation and maintenance of open access to electronic literature, just as NLM has done for decades with printed biomedical literature. PubMed Central aims to become a world-class library of the digital age.

[16] The value of PubMed Central, in addition to its role as an archive, lies the availability of data from diverse sources stored in a common format in a single repository. Many journals already have online publishing operations, and there is a growing tendency to publish material online only, to the exclusion of print.

- **Rhizobium (Agrobacterium) radiobacter Identified as a Cause of Chronic Endophthalmitis Subsequent to Cataract Extraction.** by Namdari H, Hamzavi S, Peairs RR.; 2003 Aug;
  http://www.pubmedcentral.gov/articlerender.fcgi?tool=pmcentrez&arti d=179851

- **Visual outcome of cataract surgery with pupillary sphincterotomy in eyes with coexisting corneal opacity.** by Sinha R, Sharma N, Vajpayee RB.; 2004;
  http://www.pubmedcentral.gov/articlerender.fcgi?tool=pmcentrez&arti d=400508

The National Library of Medicine: PubMed

One of the quickest and most comprehensive ways to find academic studies in both English and other languages is to use PubMed, maintained by the National Library of Medicine. The advantage of PubMed over previously mentioned sources is that it covers a greater number of domestic and foreign references. It is also free to the public.[17] If the publisher has a Web site that offers full text of its journals, PubMed will provide links to that site, as well as to sites offering other related data. User registration, a subscription fee, or some other type of fee may be required to access the full text of articles in some journals.

To generate your own bibliography of studies relating to cataract surgery, simply go to the PubMed Web site at **www.ncbi.nlm.nih.gov/pubmed**. Type "cataract surgery" (or synonyms) into the search box, and click "Go." The following is the type of output you can expect from PubMed for "cataract surgery" (hyperlinks lead to article summaries):

- **A 10 year retrospective survey of cataract surgery and endophthalmitis in a single eye unit: injectable lenses lower the incidence of endophthalmitis.**
  Author(s): Mayer E, Cadman D, Ewings P, Twomey JM, Gray RH, Claridge KG, Hakin KN, Bates AK.
  Source: The British Journal of Ophthalmology. 2003 July; 87(7): 867-9.
  http://www.ncbi.nlm.nih.gov/entrez/query.fcgi?cmd=Retrieve&db=pu bmed&dopt=Abstract&list_uids=12812888

---

[17] PubMed was developed by the National Center for Biotechnology Information (NCBI) at the National Library of Medicine (NLM) at the National Institutes of Health (NIH). The PubMed database was developed in conjunction with publishers of biomedical literature as a search tool for accessing literature citations and linking to full-text journal articles at Web sites of participating publishers. Publishers that participate in PubMed supply NLM with their citations electronically prior to or at the time of publication.

- **A comparison of anterior chamber and posterior chamber intraocular lenses after vitreous presentation during cataract surgery: the Department of Veterans Affairs Cooperative Cataract Study.**
  Author(s): Collins JF, Gaster RN, Krol WF, Colling CL, Kirk GF, Smith TJ; Department of Veterans Affairs Cooperative Cataract Study.
  Source: American Journal of Ophthalmology. 2003 July; 136(1): 1-9.
  http://www.ncbi.nlm.nih.gov/entrez/query.fcgi?cmd=Retrieve&db=pubmed&dopt=Abstract&list_uids=12834663

- **A comparison of cataract surgery under topical anaesthesia with and without intracameral lignocaine.**
  Author(s): Roberts T, Boytell K.
  Source: Clinical & Experimental Ophthalmology. 2002 February; 30(1): 19-22.
  http://www.ncbi.nlm.nih.gov/entrez/query.fcgi?cmd=Retrieve&db=pubmed&dopt=Abstract&list_uids=11885789

- **A hand to hold: communication during cataract surgery.**
  Author(s): Astbury N.
  Source: Eye (London, England). 2004 February; 18(2): 115-6.
  http://www.ncbi.nlm.nih.gov/entrez/query.fcgi?cmd=Retrieve&db=pubmed&dopt=Abstract&list_uids=14762399

- **A histological analysis of lens capsules stained with trypan blue for capsulorrhexis in phacoemulsification cataract surgery.**
  Author(s): Singh AJ, Sarodia UA, Brown L, Jagjivan R, Sampath R.
  Source: Eye (London, England). 2003 July; 17(5): 567-70.
  http://www.ncbi.nlm.nih.gov/entrez/query.fcgi?cmd=Retrieve&db=pubmed&dopt=Abstract&list_uids=12855960

- **A nationwide survey of post-operative instructions following uncomplicated phacoemulsification cataract surgery.**
  Author(s): Wu G, Morrell A.
  Source: Eye (London, England). 2001 December; 15(Pt 6): 723-7.
  http://www.ncbi.nlm.nih.gov/entrez/query.fcgi?cmd=Retrieve&db=pubmed&dopt=Abstract&list_uids=11826990

- **A population based eye survey of older adults in Tirunelveli district of south India: blindness, cataract surgery, and visual outcomes.**
  Author(s): Nirmalan PK, Thulasiraj RD, Maneksha V, Rahmathullah R, Ramakrishnan R, Padmavathi A, Munoz SR, Ellwein LB.
  Source: The British Journal of Ophthalmology. 2002 May; 86(5): 505-12.
  http://www.ncbi.nlm.nih.gov/entrez/query.fcgi?cmd=Retrieve&db=pubmed&dopt=Abstract&list_uids=11973242

- **A prospective study of the rate of falls before and after cataract surgery.**
  Author(s): Brannan S, Dewar C, Sen J, Clarke D, Marshall T, Murray PI.
  Source: The British Journal of Ophthalmology. 2003 May; 87(5): 560-2.
  http://www.ncbi.nlm.nih.gov/entrez/query.fcgi?cmd=Retrieve&db=pubmed&dopt=Abstract&list_uids=12714392

- **A prospective, case controlled study of the natural history of diabetic retinopathy and maculopathy after uncomplicated phacoemulsification cataract surgery in patients with type 2 diabetes.**
  Author(s): Squirrell D, Bhola R, Bush J, Winder S, Talbot JF.
  Source: The British Journal of Ophthalmology. 2002 May; 86(5): 565-71.
  http://www.ncbi.nlm.nih.gov/entrez/query.fcgi?cmd=Retrieve&db=pubmed&dopt=Abstract&list_uids=11973256

- **A self-administered health questionnaire for the preoperative risk stratification of patients undergoing cataract surgery.**
  Author(s): Reeves SW, Tielsch JM, Katz J, Bass EB, Schein OD.
  Source: American Journal of Ophthalmology. 2003 May; 135(5): 599-606.
  http://www.ncbi.nlm.nih.gov/entrez/query.fcgi?cmd=Retrieve&db=pubmed&dopt=Abstract&list_uids=12719065

- **Actual and intended refraction after cataract surgery.**
  Author(s): Kaye SB.
  Source: Journal of Cataract and Refractive Surgery. 2003 November; 29(11): 2189-94.
  http://www.ncbi.nlm.nih.gov/entrez/query.fcgi?cmd=Retrieve&db=pubmed&dopt=Abstract&list_uids=14670430

- **Acute comitant esotropia after cataract surgery.**
  Author(s): Zafirakis P, Voudouri A, Livir-Rallatos G, Livir-Rallatos C, Theodossiadis P, Vergados I, Baltatzis S.
  Source: Journal of Cataract and Refractive Surgery. 2002 February; 28(2): 373-5.
  http://www.ncbi.nlm.nih.gov/entrez/query.fcgi?cmd=Retrieve&db=pubmed&dopt=Abstract&list_uids=11821225

- **Anaesthesia-related diplopia after cataract surgery.**
  Author(s): Mather C, McSwiney M.
  Source: British Journal of Anaesthesia. 2003 July; 91(1): 152; Author Reply 152-3.
  http://www.ncbi.nlm.nih.gov/entrez/query.fcgi?cmd=Retrieve&db=pubmed&dopt=Abstract&list_uids=12862027

- **Anaesthesia-related diplopia after cataract surgery.**
  Author(s): Lanigan LP, Hammond CJ.
  Source: British Journal of Anaesthesia. 2003 July; 91(1): 152; Author Reply 152-3.
  http://www.ncbi.nlm.nih.gov/entrez/query.fcgi?cmd=Retrieve&db=pubmed&dopt=Abstract&list_uids=12821574

- **Anesthetic management of cardiac patient for cataract surgery.**
  Author(s): Farooq FB, Sultan ST.
  Source: J Coll Physicians Surg Pak. 2003 September; 13(9): 522-3.
  http://www.ncbi.nlm.nih.gov/entrez/query.fcgi?cmd=Retrieve&db=pubmed&dopt=Abstract&list_uids=12971874

- **Anterior and posterior capsulorhexis in pediatric cataract surgery with or without trypan blue dye: randomized prospective clinical study.**
  Author(s): Saini JS, Jain AK, Sukhija J, Gupta P, Saroha V.
  Source: Journal of Cataract and Refractive Surgery. 2003 September; 29(9): 1733-7.
  http://www.ncbi.nlm.nih.gov/entrez/query.fcgi?cmd=Retrieve&db=pubmed&dopt=Abstract&list_uids=14522292

- **Anterior vitreous face behavior with AcrySof in pediatric cataract surgery.**
  Author(s): Vasavada AR, Nath VC, Trivedi RH.
  Source: J Aapos. 2003 December; 7(6): 384-8.
  http://www.ncbi.nlm.nih.gov/entrez/query.fcgi?cmd=Retrieve&db=pubmed&dopt=Abstract&list_uids=14730289

- **Aqueous humor levels of topically applied bupivacaine 0.75% in cataract surgery.**
  Author(s): Lagnado R, Tan J, Cole R, Sampath R.
  Source: Journal of Cataract and Refractive Surgery. 2003 September; 29(9): 1767-70.
  http://www.ncbi.nlm.nih.gov/entrez/query.fcgi?cmd=Retrieve&db=pubmed&dopt=Abstract&list_uids=14522298

- **Articaine versus lidocaine plus bupivacaine for peribulbar anaesthesia in cataract surgery.**
  Author(s): Ozdemir M, Ozdemir G, Zencirci B, Oksuz H.
  Source: British Journal of Anaesthesia. 2004 February; 92(2): 231-4.
  http://www.ncbi.nlm.nih.gov/entrez/query.fcgi?cmd=Retrieve&db=pubmed&dopt=Abstract&list_uids=14722174

- **Astigmatism outcomes of horizontal temporal versus nasal clear corneal incision cataract surgery.**
  Author(s): Barequet IS, Yu E, Vitale S, Cassard S, Azar DT, Stark WJ.
  Source: Journal of Cataract and Refractive Surgery. 2004 February; 30(2): 418-23.
  http://www.ncbi.nlm.nih.gov/entrez/query.fcgi?cmd=Retrieve&db=pubmed&dopt=Abstract&list_uids=15030834

- **Bacterial contamination of the anterior chamber during phacoemulsification cataract surgery.**
  Author(s): Leong JK, Shah R, McCluskey PJ, Benn RA, Taylor RF.
  Source: Journal of Cataract and Refractive Surgery. 2002 May; 28(5): 826-33.
  http://www.ncbi.nlm.nih.gov/entrez/query.fcgi?cmd=Retrieve&db=pubmed&dopt=Abstract&list_uids=11978463

- **Bacterial endophthalmitis following cataract surgery in an eye with a preexisting Molteno implant.**
  Author(s): Ellis BD, Varley GA, Kalenak JW, Meisler DM, Huang SS.
  Source: Ophthalmic Surg. 1993 February; 24(2): 117-8.
  http://www.ncbi.nlm.nih.gov/entrez/query.fcgi?cmd=Retrieve&db=pubmed&dopt=Abstract&list_uids=8446345

- **Bacterial endophthalmitis following sutureless cataract surgery.**
  Author(s): Perlstein SH, Edelstein MS, Chubak GS.
  Source: Archives of Ophthalmology. 1994 March; 112(3): 301-2.
  http://www.ncbi.nlm.nih.gov/entrez/query.fcgi?cmd=Retrieve&db=pu
  bmed&dopt=Abstract&list_uids=8129649

- **Bacterial endophthalmitis following sutureless cataract surgery.**
  Author(s): Miller KM, Glasgow BJ.
  Source: Archives of Ophthalmology. 1993 March; 111(3): 377-9.
  http://www.ncbi.nlm.nih.gov/entrez/query.fcgi?cmd=Retrieve&db=pu
  bmed&dopt=Abstract&list_uids=8447751

- **Bacterial endophthalmitis prophylaxis for cataract surgery: an evidence-based update.**
  Author(s): Ciulla TA, Starr MB, Masket S.
  Source: Ophthalmology. 2002 January; 109(1): 13-24. Review.
  http://www.ncbi.nlm.nih.gov/entrez/query.fcgi?cmd=Retrieve&db=pu
  bmed&dopt=Abstract&list_uids=11772573

- **Barriers to acceptance of cataract surgery among patients presenting to district hospitals in rural Malawi.**
  Author(s): Courtright P, Kanjaloti S, Lewallen S.
  Source: Trop Geogr Med. 1995; 47(1): 15-8.
  http://www.ncbi.nlm.nih.gov/entrez/query.fcgi?cmd=Retrieve&db=pu
  bmed&dopt=Abstract&list_uids=7747324

- **Barriers to the uptake of cataract surgery.**
  Author(s): Johnson JG, Goode Sen V, Faal H.
  Source: Trop Doct. 1998 October; 28(4): 218-20.
  http://www.ncbi.nlm.nih.gov/entrez/query.fcgi?cmd=Retrieve&db=pu
  bmed&dopt=Abstract&list_uids=9803842

- **Bilateral cataract surgery combined with implantation of a brown diaphragm intraocular lens after trabeculectomy for congenital aniridia.**
  Author(s): Esquenazi S, Amador S.
  Source: Ophthalmic Surgery and Lasers. 2002 November-December; 33(6): 514-7.
  http://www.ncbi.nlm.nih.gov/entrez/query.fcgi?cmd=Retrieve&db=pu
  bmed&dopt=Abstract&list_uids=12449232

- **Bilateral cataract surgery in adult and pediatric patients in a single session.**
  Author(s): Totan Y, Bayramlar H, Cekic O, Aydin E, Erten A, Daglioglu MC.
  Source: Journal of Cataract and Refractive Surgery. 2000 July; 26(7): 1008-11.
  http://www.ncbi.nlm.nih.gov/entrez/query.fcgi?cmd=Retrieve&db=pubmed&dopt=Abstract&list_uids=10946191

- **Bilateral cataract surgery.**
  Author(s): Misson GP, Pearce JL, Fielder AR.
  Source: Lancet. 1992 March 7; 339(8793): 623.
  http://www.ncbi.nlm.nih.gov/entrez/query.fcgi?cmd=Retrieve&db=pubmed&dopt=Abstract&list_uids=1347129

- **Bilateral corneal decompensation after bilateral simultaneous cataract surgery.**
  Author(s): McDonnell PJ.
  Source: Journal of Cataract and Refractive Surgery. 1999 August; 25(8): 1038.
  http://www.ncbi.nlm.nih.gov/entrez/query.fcgi?cmd=Retrieve&db=pubmed&dopt=Abstract&list_uids=10445184

- **Brimonidine and postoperative pressure spikes in cataract surgery.**
  Author(s): Whitehouse G.
  Source: Clinical & Experimental Ophthalmology. 2000 October; 28(5): 364-6.
  http://www.ncbi.nlm.nih.gov/entrez/query.fcgi?cmd=Retrieve&db=pubmed&dopt=Abstract&list_uids=11097284

- **Broken intraocular lens during cataract surgery.**
  Author(s): Kirkpatrick JN, Cook SD.
  Source: The British Journal of Ophthalmology. 1992 August; 76(8): 509.
  http://www.ncbi.nlm.nih.gov/entrez/query.fcgi?cmd=Retrieve&db=pubmed&dopt=Abstract&list_uids=1390540

- **By the way, doctor. I'm about to have cataract surgery. I wasn't too concerned until someone told me that 30%-50% of people who have it need a laser operation that can cause blindness! Now I'm not so sure about going through with it.**
  Author(s): Hutchinson BT.
  Source: Harvard Health Letter / from Harvard Medical School. 2002 July; 27(9): 8.
  http://www.ncbi.nlm.nih.gov/entrez/query.fcgi?cmd=Retrieve&db=pubmed&dopt=Abstract&list_uids=12138039

- **Capsular apposition after cataract surgery.**
  Author(s): Werblin TP.
  Source: Ophthalmology. 2004 February; 111(2): 409; Author Reply 409-10.
  http://www.ncbi.nlm.nih.gov/entrez/query.fcgi?cmd=Retrieve&db=pubmed&dopt=Abstract&list_uids=15019404

- **Carticaine versus lidocaine for peribulbar anesthesia in cataract surgery.**
  Author(s): Fathi AA, Soliman MM.
  Source: Journal of Cataract and Refractive Surgery. 2002 March; 28(3): 513-6.
  http://www.ncbi.nlm.nih.gov/entrez/query.fcgi?cmd=Retrieve&db=pubmed&dopt=Abstract&list_uids=11973100

- **Case-control study of endophthalmitis after cataract surgery comparing scleral tunnel and clear corneal wounds.**
  Author(s): Chung CF, Lam DS.
  Source: American Journal of Ophthalmology. 2004 March; 137(3): 598-9; Author Reply 599.
  http://www.ncbi.nlm.nih.gov/entrez/query.fcgi?cmd=Retrieve&db=pubmed&dopt=Abstract&list_uids=15013914

- **Cataract surgery in allogeneic bone marrow transplant recipients with graft-versus-host disease(1).**
  Author(s): Penn EA, Soong HK.
  Source: Journal of Cataract and Refractive Surgery. 2002 March; 28(3): 417-20.
  http://www.ncbi.nlm.nih.gov/entrez/query.fcgi?cmd=Retrieve&db=pubmed&dopt=Abstract&list_uids=11973086

- **Cataract surgery in cataracta membranacea.**
  Author(s): Heuring AH, Menkhaus S, Walter S, Behrens-Baumann W.
  Source: Journal of Cataract and Refractive Surgery. 2002 June; 28(6): 1065-8.
  http://www.ncbi.nlm.nih.gov/entrez/query.fcgi?cmd=Retrieve&db=pubmed&dopt=Abstract&list_uids=12036656

- **Cataract surgery in patients with Behcet's disease.**
  Author(s): Kadayifcilar S, Gedik S, Eldem B, Irkec M.
  Source: Journal of Cataract and Refractive Surgery. 2002 February; 28(2): 316-20.
  http://www.ncbi.nlm.nih.gov/entrez/query.fcgi?cmd=Retrieve&db=pubmed&dopt=Abstract&list_uids=11821216

- **Cataract surgery on diabetic patients. A prospective evaluation of risk factors and complications.**
  Author(s): Flesner P, Sander B, Henning V, Parving HH, Dornonville de la Cour M, Lund-Andersen H.
  Source: Acta Ophthalmologica Scandinavica. 2002 February; 80(1): 19-24.
  http://www.ncbi.nlm.nih.gov/entrez/query.fcgi?cmd=Retrieve&db=pubmed&dopt=Abstract&list_uids=11906299

- **Cataract surgery: expectations of patients assisted during a community project in Sao Paulo, state of Sao Paulo, Brazil.**
  Author(s): Kara-Junior N, Temporini ER, Kara-Jose N.
  Source: Revista Do Hospital Das Clinicas. 2001 November-December; 56(6): 163-8.
  http://www.ncbi.nlm.nih.gov/entrez/query.fcgi?cmd=Retrieve&db=pubmed&dopt=Abstract&list_uids=11836538

- **Cataract surgical coverage and outcome of cataract surgery in a rural district in Malawi.**
  Author(s): Courtright P, Metcalfe N, Hoechsmann A, Chirambo M, Lewallen S, Barrows J, Witte C; Chikwawa Survey Team.
  Source: Can J Ophthalmol. 2004 February; 39(1): 25-30.
  http://www.ncbi.nlm.nih.gov/entrez/query.fcgi?cmd=Retrieve&db=pubmed&dopt=Abstract&list_uids=15040611

- **Changes in astigmatism after congenital cataract surgery and foldable intraocular lens implantation.**
  Author(s): Spierer A, Bar-Sela S.
  Source: Journal of Pediatric Ophthalmology and Strabismus. 2004 January-February; 41(1): 35-8.
  http://www.ncbi.nlm.nih.gov/entrez/query.fcgi?cmd=Retrieve&db=pubmed&dopt=Abstract&list_uids=14974833

- **Clinical and theoretical results of intraocular lens power calculation for cataract surgery after photorefractive keratectomy for myopia.**
  Author(s): Odenthal MT, Eggink CA, Melles G, Pameyer JH, Geerards AJ, Beekhuis WH.
  Source: Archives of Ophthalmology. 2002 April; 120(4): 431-8.
  http://www.ncbi.nlm.nih.gov/entrez/query.fcgi?cmd=Retrieve&db=pubmed&dopt=Abstract&list_uids=11934316

- **Clinical applications of capsular tension rings in cataract surgery.**
  Author(s): Gimbel HV, Sun R.
  Source: Ophthalmic Surgery and Lasers. 2002 January-February; 33(1): 44-53. Review.
  http://www.ncbi.nlm.nih.gov/entrez/query.fcgi?cmd=Retrieve&db=pubmed&dopt=Abstract&list_uids=11820662

- **Combined cataract surgery and vitrectomy for breakthrough vitreous hemorrhage from age-related macular degeneration.**
  Author(s): Chaudhry NA, Flynn HW, Murray TG, Belfort A.
  Source: Ophthalmic Surgery and Lasers. 2002 January-February; 33(1): 16-8.
  http://www.ncbi.nlm.nih.gov/entrez/query.fcgi?cmd=Retrieve&db=pubmed&dopt=Abstract&list_uids=11820658

- **Combined strabismus and phacoemulsification cataract surgery: a useful option in selected patients.**
  Author(s): Squirrell D, Edwards M, Burke J.
  Source: Eye (London, England). 2001 December; 15(Pt 6): 736-8.
  http://www.ncbi.nlm.nih.gov/entrez/query.fcgi?cmd=Retrieve&db=pubmed&dopt=Abstract&list_uids=11826993

- **Comments on anesthesia for cataract surgery.**
  Author(s): Livingston M.
  Source: Journal of Cataract and Refractive Surgery. 2002 May; 28(5): 736-7.
  http://www.ncbi.nlm.nih.gov/entrez/query.fcgi?cmd=Retrieve&db=pubmed&dopt=Abstract&list_uids=11978447

- **Complications in the first year following cataract surgery with and without IOL in infants and older children.**
  Author(s): Plager DA, Yang S, Neely D, Sprunger D, Sondhi N.
  Source: J Aapos. 2002 February; 6(1): 9-14.
  http://www.ncbi.nlm.nih.gov/entrez/query.fcgi?cmd=Retrieve&db=pubmed&dopt=Abstract&list_uids=11907473

- **Corneal endothelial cell density after trypan blue capsule staining in cataract surgery.**
  Author(s): van Dooren BT, de Waard PW, Poort-van Nouhuys H, Beekhuis WH, Melles GR.
  Source: Journal of Cataract and Refractive Surgery. 2002 April; 28(4): 574-5.
  http://www.ncbi.nlm.nih.gov/entrez/query.fcgi?cmd=Retrieve&db=pubmed&dopt=Abstract&list_uids=11955881

- **Corneal endothelial cell morphology in patients undergoing cataract surgery.**
  Author(s): Inoue K, Tokuda Y, Inoue Y, Amano S, Oshika T, Inoue J.
  Source: Cornea. 2002 May; 21(4): 360-3.
  http://www.ncbi.nlm.nih.gov/entrez/query.fcgi?cmd=Retrieve&db=pubmed&dopt=Abstract&list_uids=11973383

- **Corneal toxicity secondary to inadvertent use of benzalkonium chloride preserved viscoelastic material in cataract surgery.**
  Author(s): Eleftheriadis H, Cheong M, Sandeman S, Syam PP, Brittain P, Klintworth GK, Lloyd A, Liu C.
  Source: The British Journal of Ophthalmology. 2002 March; 86(3): 299-305.
  http://www.ncbi.nlm.nih.gov/entrez/query.fcgi?cmd=Retrieve&db=pubmed&dopt=Abstract&list_uids=11864888

- **Cost-effectiveness of the AMOArray multifocal intraocular lens in cataract surgery.**
  Author(s): Orme ME, Paine AC, Teale CW, Kennedy LM.
  Source: Journal of Refractive Surgery (Thorofare, N.J. : 1995). 2002 March-April; 18(2): 162-8.
  http://www.ncbi.nlm.nih.gov/entrez/query.fcgi?cmd=Retrieve&db=pubmed&dopt=Abstract&list_uids=11934206

- **Day 1 review following cataract surgery: are we seeing the precise details?**
  Author(s): Goh D, Lim N.
  Source: The British Journal of Ophthalmology. 2002 April; 86(4): 481-2.
  http://www.ncbi.nlm.nih.gov/entrez/query.fcgi?cmd=Retrieve&db=pubmed&dopt=Abstract&list_uids=11914232

- **Deep lamellar keratoplasty combined with cataract surgery.**
  Author(s): Muraine MC, Collet A, Brasseur G.
  Source: Archives of Ophthalmology. 2002 June; 120(6): 812-5.
  http://www.ncbi.nlm.nih.gov/entrez/query.fcgi?cmd=Retrieve&db=pubmed&dopt=Abstract&list_uids=12049588

- **Delayed allergic reaction to hyaluronidase: a rare sequel to cataract surgery.**
  Author(s): Ahluwalia HS, Lukaris A, Lane CM.
  Source: Eye (London, England). 2003 March; 17(2): 263-6. Review.
  http://www.ncbi.nlm.nih.gov/entrez/query.fcgi?cmd=Retrieve&db=pubmed&dopt=Abstract&list_uids=12640426

- **Delayed orbital hemorrhage after cataract surgery in a patient with an acquired factor VIII inhibitor.**
  Author(s): White WL, Mundis RJ.
  Source: American Journal of Ophthalmology. 2001 November; 132(5): 785-6.
  http://www.ncbi.nlm.nih.gov/entrez/query.fcgi?cmd=Retrieve&db=pubmed&dopt=Abstract&list_uids=11704045

- **Descemet membrane tear after cataract surgery.**
  Author(s): Nouri M, Pineda R Jr, Azar D.
  Source: Seminars in Ophthalmology. 2002 September-December; 17(3-4): 115-9.
  http://www.ncbi.nlm.nih.gov/entrez/query.fcgi?cmd=Retrieve&db=pubmed&dopt=Abstract&list_uids=12759838

- **Descemet's membrane detachment after cataract surgery: management and outcome.**
  Author(s): Marcon AS, Rapuano CJ, Jones MR, Laibson PR, Cohen EJ.
  Source: Ophthalmology. 2002 December; 109(12): 2325-30.
  http://www.ncbi.nlm.nih.gov/entrez/query.fcgi?cmd=Retrieve&db=pu bmed&dopt=Abstract&list_uids=12466178

- **Developing cataract surgery priority criteria: results from the Western Canada Waiting List Project.**
  Author(s): Romanchuk KG, Sanmugasunderam S, Hadorn DC; Steering Committee of the Western Canada Waiting List Project.
  Source: Can J Ophthalmol. 2002 April; 37(3): 145-54.
  http://www.ncbi.nlm.nih.gov/entrez/query.fcgi?cmd=Retrieve&db=pu bmed&dopt=Abstract&list_uids=12083473

- **Development and assessment of a priority score for cataract surgery.**
  Author(s): Fantini MP, Negro A, Accorsi S, Cisbani L, Taroni F, Grilli R.
  Source: Can J Ophthalmol. 2004 February; 39(1): 48-55.
  http://www.ncbi.nlm.nih.gov/entrez/query.fcgi?cmd=Retrieve&db=pu bmed&dopt=Abstract&list_uids=15040614

- **Development of day case cataract surgery: a literature review.**
  Author(s): Cooper JM.
  Source: British Journal of Nursing (Mark Allen Publishing). 1996 November 28-December 11; 5(21): 1327-33. Review.
  http://www.ncbi.nlm.nih.gov/entrez/query.fcgi?cmd=Retrieve&db=pu bmed&dopt=Abstract&list_uids=9015989

- **Development of exudative age-related macular degeneration after cataract surgery.**
  Author(s): Pollack A, Marcovich A, Bukelman A, Zalish M, Oliver M.
  Source: Eye (London, England). 1997; 11 (Pt 4): 523-30.
  http://www.ncbi.nlm.nih.gov/entrez/query.fcgi?cmd=Retrieve&db=pu bmed&dopt=Abstract&list_uids=9425419

- **Diabetic maculopathy and cataract surgery.**
  Author(s): Gupta A, Gupta V.
  Source: Ophthalmology Clinics of North America. 2001 December; 14(4): 625-37. Review.
  http://www.ncbi.nlm.nih.gov/entrez/query.fcgi?cmd=Retrieve&db=pu bmed&dopt=Abstract&list_uids=11787742

- **Different opening techniques in cataract surgery.**
  Author(s): Vamosi P, Lampe Z, Berta A.
  Source: Acta Chir Hung. 1997; 36(1-4): 378-80.
  http://www.ncbi.nlm.nih.gov/entrez/query.fcgi?cmd=Retrieve&db=pubmed&dopt=Abstract&list_uids=9408409

- **Diplopia after cataract surgery.**
  Author(s): Rahman W, Gregson RM.
  Source: British Journal of Anaesthesia. 2004 January; 92(1): 153-4.
  http://www.ncbi.nlm.nih.gov/entrez/query.fcgi?cmd=Retrieve&db=pubmed&dopt=Abstract&list_uids=14665574

- **Diplopia after cataract surgery: comparative results after topical or regional injection anesthesia.**
  Author(s): Yanguela J, Gomez-Arnau JI, Martin-Rodrigo JC, Andueza A, Gili P, Paredes B, Porras MC, Gonzalez del Valle F, Arias A.
  Source: Ophthalmology. 2004 April; 111(4): 686-92.
  http://www.ncbi.nlm.nih.gov/entrez/query.fcgi?cmd=Retrieve&db=pubmed&dopt=Abstract&list_uids=15051199

- **Discontinuing aspirin or warfarin optional before cataract surgery.**
  Author(s): Mounsey A.
  Source: The Journal of Family Practice. 2003 December; 52(12): 933-5.
  http://www.ncbi.nlm.nih.gov/entrez/query.fcgi?cmd=Retrieve&db=pubmed&dopt=Abstract&list_uids=14653976

- **Dissatisfaction with cataract surgery in relation to visual results in a population-based study in Sweden.**
  Author(s): Monestam E, Wachtmeister L.
  Source: Journal of Cataract and Refractive Surgery. 1999 August; 25(8): 1127-34.
  http://www.ncbi.nlm.nih.gov/entrez/query.fcgi?cmd=Retrieve&db=pubmed&dopt=Abstract&list_uids=10445200

- **Do patients with age related maculopathy and cataract benefit from cataract surgery?**
  Author(s): Ambrecht AM, Findlay C, Aspinall P, Dhillon B.
  Source: The British Journal of Ophthalmology. 1999 February; 83(2): 253-4.
  http://www.ncbi.nlm.nih.gov/entrez/query.fcgi?cmd=Retrieve&db=pubmed&dopt=Abstract&list_uids=10396210

- **Documentation patterns before cataract surgery at ten academic centers.**
  Author(s): Lee PP, Hilborne L, McDonald L, Tobacman JK, Kolder H, Johnson T, Brook RH.
  Source: Ophthalmology. 1996 August; 103(8): 1179-83.
  http://www.ncbi.nlm.nih.gov/entrez/query.fcgi?cmd=Retrieve&db=pubmed&dopt=Abstract&list_uids=8764784

- **Does prospective monitoring improve cataract surgery outcomes in Africa?**
  Author(s): Yorston D, Gichuhi S, Wood M, Foster A.
  Source: The British Journal of Ophthalmology. 2002 May; 86(5): 543-7.
  http://www.ncbi.nlm.nih.gov/entrez/query.fcgi?cmd=Retrieve&db=pubmed&dopt=Abstract&list_uids=11973251

- **Double-ring and double-layer sign of the anterior lens capsule during cataract surgery.**
  Author(s): Abe T, Hirata H, Hayasaka S.
  Source: Japanese Journal of Ophthalmology. 2001 November-December; 45(6): 657-8.
  http://www.ncbi.nlm.nih.gov/entrez/query.fcgi?cmd=Retrieve&db=pubmed&dopt=Abstract&list_uids=11754912

- **Early objective assessment of intraocular inflammation after phacoemulsification cataract surgery.**
  Author(s): Findl O, Amon M, Petternel V, Kruger A.
  Source: Journal of Cataract and Refractive Surgery. 2003 November; 29(11): 2143-7.
  http://www.ncbi.nlm.nih.gov/entrez/query.fcgi?cmd=Retrieve&db=pubmed&dopt=Abstract&list_uids=14670423

- **Effect of a capsular tension ring on intraocular lens decentration and tilting after cataract surgery.**
  Author(s): Lee DH, Shin SC, Joo CK.
  Source: Journal of Cataract and Refractive Surgery. 2002 May; 28(5): 843-6.
  http://www.ncbi.nlm.nih.gov/entrez/query.fcgi?cmd=Retrieve&db=pubmed&dopt=Abstract&list_uids=11978466

- **Effect of a fixed dorzolamide-timolol combination on intraocular pressure after small-incision cataract surgery with Viscoat.**
  Author(s): Rainer G, Menapace R, Findl O, Sacu S, Schmid K, Petternel V, Kiss B, Georgopoulos M.
  Source: Journal of Cataract and Refractive Surgery. 2003 September; 29(9): 1748-52.
  http://www.ncbi.nlm.nih.gov/entrez/query.fcgi?cmd=Retrieve&db=pubmed&dopt=Abstract&list_uids=14522295

- **Effect of cataract surgery on IOP after trabeculectomy.**
  Author(s): Rebolleda G, Munoz-Negrete FJ.
  Source: Journal of Cataract and Refractive Surgery. 2003 November; 29(11): 2043; Author Reply 2043.
  http://www.ncbi.nlm.nih.gov/entrez/query.fcgi?cmd=Retrieve&db=pubmed&dopt=Abstract&list_uids=14670402

- **Effect of cataract surgery on the corneal endothelium: modern phacoemulsification compared with extracapsular cataract surgery.**
  Author(s): Bourne RR, Minassian DC, Dart JK, Rosen P, Kaushal S, Wingate N.
  Source: Ophthalmology. 2004 April; 111(4): 679-85.
  http://www.ncbi.nlm.nih.gov/entrez/query.fcgi?cmd=Retrieve&db=pubmed&dopt=Abstract&list_uids=15051198

- **Effect of cataract surgery on the progression of diabetic retinopathy.**
  Author(s): Chung J, Kim MY, Kim HS, Yoo JS, Lee YC.
  Source: Journal of Cataract and Refractive Surgery. 2002 April; 28(4): 626-30.
  http://www.ncbi.nlm.nih.gov/entrez/query.fcgi?cmd=Retrieve&db=pubmed&dopt=Abstract&list_uids=11955902

- **Effect of central corneal thickness on surgically induced astigmatism in cataract surgery.**
  Author(s): Woo SJ, Lee JH.
  Source: Journal of Cataract and Refractive Surgery. 2003 December; 29(12): 2401-6.
  http://www.ncbi.nlm.nih.gov/entrez/query.fcgi?cmd=Retrieve&db=pubmed&dopt=Abstract&list_uids=14709304

- **Effect of eye patching on postoperative inflammation after cataract surgery.**
  Author(s): Honda S, Matsuo A, Toda H, Saito I.
  Source: Journal of Cataract and Refractive Surgery. 2004 January; 30(1): 273-4.
  http://www.ncbi.nlm.nih.gov/entrez/query.fcgi?cmd=Retrieve&db=pubmed&dopt=Abstract&list_uids=14967304

- **Effect of haptic design on change in axial lens position after cataract surgery.**
  Author(s): Wirtitsch MG, Findl O, Menapace R, Kriechbaum K, Koeppl C, Buehl W, Drexler W.
  Source: Journal of Cataract and Refractive Surgery. 2004 January; 30(1): 45-51.
  http://www.ncbi.nlm.nih.gov/entrez/query.fcgi?cmd=Retrieve&db=pubmed&dopt=Abstract&list_uids=14967267

- **Effect of midazolam on anxiety level and pain perception in cataract surgery with topical anesthesia.**
  Author(s): Habib NE, Mandour NM, Balmer HG.
  Source: Journal of Cataract and Refractive Surgery. 2004 February; 30(2): 437-43.
  http://www.ncbi.nlm.nih.gov/entrez/query.fcgi?cmd=Retrieve&db=pubmed&dopt=Abstract&list_uids=15030838

- **Effect of prophylactic antibiotics on antimicrobial resistance of viridans streptococci in the normal flora of cataract surgery patients.**
  Author(s): Seppala H, Al-Juhaish M, Jarvinen H, Laitinen R, Huovinen P.
  Source: Journal of Cataract and Refractive Surgery. 2004 February; 30(2): 307-15.
  http://www.ncbi.nlm.nih.gov/entrez/query.fcgi?cmd=Retrieve&db=pubmed&dopt=Abstract&list_uids=15030817

- **Effectiveness and tolerance of piroxicam 0.5% and diclofenac sodium 0.1% in controlling inflammation after cataract surgery.**
  Author(s): Scuderi B, Driussi GB, Chizzolini M, Salvetat ML, Beltrame G.
  Source: Eur J Ophthalmol. 2003 July; 13(6): 536-40.
  http://www.ncbi.nlm.nih.gov/entrez/query.fcgi?cmd=Retrieve&db=pubmed&dopt=Abstract&list_uids=12948311

- **Efficacy and safety of rimexolone 1% versus prednisolone acetate 1% in the control of postoperative inflammation following phacoemulsification cataract surgery.**
  Author(s): Yaylali V, Ozbay D, Tatlipinar S, Yildirim C, Ozden S.
  Source: International Ophthalmology. 2004; 25(1): 65-8.
  http://www.ncbi.nlm.nih.gov/entrez/query.fcgi?cmd=Retrieve&db=pubmed&dopt=Abstract&list_uids=15085979

- **Elimination of routine testing in patients undergoing cataract surgery allows substantial savings in laboratory costs. A brief report.**
  Author(s): Imasogie N, Wong DT, Luk K, Chung F.
  Source: Canadian Journal of Anaesthesia = Journal Canadien D'anesthesie. 2003 March; 50(3): 246-8.
  http://www.ncbi.nlm.nih.gov/entrez/query.fcgi?cmd=Retrieve&db=pubmed&dopt=Abstract&list_uids=12620946

- **Endoillumination-assisted cataract surgery in a patient with corneal opacity.**
  Author(s): Nishimura A, Kobayashi A, PhD, Segawa Y, PhD, Sugiyama K, PhD.
  Source: Journal of Cataract and Refractive Surgery. 2003 December; 29(12): 2277-80.
  http://www.ncbi.nlm.nih.gov/entrez/query.fcgi?cmd=Retrieve&db=pubmed&dopt=Abstract&list_uids=14709285

- **Endophthalmitis after contemporary cataract surgery: defining incidence and risk factors.**
  Author(s): McGhee CN, Ormonde S.
  Source: Clinical & Experimental Ophthalmology. 2003 June; 31(3): 176-8. Review.
  http://www.ncbi.nlm.nih.gov/entrez/query.fcgi?cmd=Retrieve&db=pubmed&dopt=Abstract&list_uids=12786765

- **Evaluation of telemedicine for slit lamp examination of the eye following cataract surgery.**
  Author(s): Smith LF, Bainbridge J, Burns J, Stevens J, Taylor P, Murdoch I.
  Source: The British Journal of Ophthalmology. 2003 April; 87(4): 502-3.
  http://www.ncbi.nlm.nih.gov/entrez/query.fcgi?cmd=Retrieve&db=pubmed&dopt=Abstract&list_uids=12642321

- **Evaluation of the Greenbaum sub-tenon's block: a role in anticoagulated patients presenting for cataract surgery.**
  Author(s): Berrington JS.
  Source: British Journal of Anaesthesia. 2002 March; 88(3): 457; Author Reply 457.
  http://www.ncbi.nlm.nih.gov/entrez/query.fcgi?cmd=Retrieve&db=pubmed&dopt=Abstract&list_uids=11990292

- **Excessive fibrin after cataract surgery associated with aminocaproic acid use.**
  Author(s): Jabbur NS.
  Source: Journal of Cataract and Refractive Surgery. 2003 August; 29(8): 1636-7.
  http://www.ncbi.nlm.nih.gov/entrez/query.fcgi?cmd=Retrieve&db=pubmed&dopt=Abstract&list_uids=12954320

- **Extracapsular cataract surgery compared with manual small incision cataract surgery in community eye care setting in western India: a randomised controlled trial.**
  Author(s): Gogate PM, Deshpande M, Wormald RP, Deshpande R, Kulkarni SR.
  Source: The British Journal of Ophthalmology. 2003 June; 87(6): 667-72.
  http://www.ncbi.nlm.nih.gov/entrez/query.fcgi?cmd=Retrieve&db=pubmed&dopt=Abstract&list_uids=12770957

- **Factors associated with second eye cataract surgery.**
  Author(s): Castells X, Alonso J, Ribo C, Nara D, Teixido A, Castilla M.
  Source: The British Journal of Ophthalmology. 2000 January; 84(1): 9-12.
  http://www.ncbi.nlm.nih.gov/entrez/query.fcgi?cmd=Retrieve&db=pubmed&dopt=Abstract&list_uids=10611090

- **Factors leading to reduced intraocular pressure after combined trabeculotomy and cataract surgery.**
  Author(s): Tanito M, Ohira A, Chihara E.
  Source: Journal of Glaucoma. 2002 February; 11(1): 3-9.
  http://www.ncbi.nlm.nih.gov/entrez/query.fcgi?cmd=Retrieve&db=pubmed&dopt=Abstract&list_uids=11821682

- **Factors related to fear in patients undergoing cataract surgery: a qualitative study focusing on factors associated with fear and reassurance among patients who need to undergo cataract surgery.**
  Author(s): Nijkamp MD, Ruiter RA, Roeling M, van den Borne B, Hiddema F, Hendrikse F, Nuijts RM.
  Source: Patient Education and Counseling. 2002 July; 47(3): 265-72.
  http://www.ncbi.nlm.nih.gov/entrez/query.fcgi?cmd=Retrieve&db=pubmed&dopt=Abstract&list_uids=12088605

- **Factors that influence the surgical effects of astigmatic keratotomy after cataract surgery.**
  Author(s): Inoue T, Maeda N, Sasaki K, Watanabe H, Inoue Y, Nishida K, Inoue Y, Yamamoto S, Shimomura Y, Tano Y.
  Source: Ophthalmology. 2001 July; 108(7): 1269-74.
  http://www.ncbi.nlm.nih.gov/entrez/query.fcgi?cmd=Retrieve&db=pubmed&dopt=Abstract&list_uids=11425686

- **Features of a modern retrobulbar anesthetic injection for cataract surgery.**
  Author(s): Davison JA.
  Source: Journal of Cataract and Refractive Surgery. 1993 March; 19(2): 284-9.
  http://www.ncbi.nlm.nih.gov/entrez/query.fcgi?cmd=Retrieve&db=pubmed&dopt=Abstract&list_uids=8487175

- **First results of cataract surgery and implantation of negative power intraocular lenses in highly myopic eyes.**
  Author(s): Kohnen S, Brauweiler P.
  Source: Journal of Cataract and Refractive Surgery. 1996 May; 22(4): 416-20.
  http://www.ncbi.nlm.nih.gov/entrez/query.fcgi?cmd=Retrieve&db=pubmed&dopt=Abstract&list_uids=8733843

- **Five year incidence of cataract surgery: the Blue Mountains Eye Study.**
  Author(s): Panchapakesan J, Mitchell P, Tumuluri K, Rochtchina E, Foran S, Cumming RG.
  Source: The British Journal of Ophthalmology. 2003 February; 87(2): 168-72.
  http://www.ncbi.nlm.nih.gov/entrez/query.fcgi?cmd=Retrieve&db=pubmed&dopt=Abstract&list_uids=12543745

- **Five year study of astigmatic stability after cataract surgery with intraocular lens implantation: comparison of wound sizes.**
  Author(s): Drews RC.
  Source: Journal of Cataract and Refractive Surgery. 2000 February; 26(2): 250-3.
  http://www.ncbi.nlm.nih.gov/entrez/query.fcgi?cmd=Retrieve&db=pubmed&dopt=Abstract&list_uids=10683793

- **Fixed-dose combination of 0.1% diclofenac plus 0.3% tobramycin ophthalmic solution for inflammation after cataract surgery: a randomized, comparative, active treatment-controlled trial.**
  Author(s): Barraquer RI, Alvarez de Toledo JP, Montane D, Escoto RM, Garcia Torres C, Bennani-Tazzi M.
  Source: Eur J Ophthalmol. 1998 July-September; 8(3): 173-8.
  http://www.ncbi.nlm.nih.gov/entrez/query.fcgi?cmd=Retrieve&db=pubmed&dopt=Abstract&list_uids=9793772

- **Flare-cell meter measurement of inflammation after uneventful cataract surgery with intraocular lens implantation.**
  Author(s): Alio JL, Sayans JA, Chipont E.
  Source: Journal of Cataract and Refractive Surgery. 1997 July-August; 23(6): 935-9.
  http://www.ncbi.nlm.nih.gov/entrez/query.fcgi?cmd=Retrieve&db=pubmed&dopt=Abstract&list_uids=9292681

- **Flared phacoemulsification tips to decrease ultrasound time and energy in cataract surgery.**
  Author(s): McNeill JI.
  Source: Journal of Cataract and Refractive Surgery. 2001 September; 27(9): 1433-6.
  http://www.ncbi.nlm.nih.gov/entrez/query.fcgi?cmd=Retrieve&db=pubmed&dopt=Abstract&list_uids=11566528

- **Floaters after cataract surgery.**
  Author(s): Chignell A.
  Source: Journal of the Royal Society of Medicine. 1996 June; 89(6): 332.
  http://www.ncbi.nlm.nih.gov/entrez/query.fcgi?cmd=Retrieve&db=pubmed&dopt=Abstract&list_uids=8758192

- **Foreign objects in clear corneal cataract surgery wounds.**
  Author(s): Stewart JM, Hollander DA.
  Source: Journal of Cataract and Refractive Surgery. 2003 November; 29(11): 2045-6.
  http://www.ncbi.nlm.nih.gov/entrez/query.fcgi?cmd=Retrieve&db=pubmed&dopt=Abstract&list_uids=14670405

- **Frequency and predictors of glaucoma after pediatric cataract surgery.**
  Author(s): Rabiah PK.
  Source: American Journal of Ophthalmology. 2004 January; 137(1): 30-7.
  http://www.ncbi.nlm.nih.gov/entrez/query.fcgi?cmd=Retrieve&db=pubmed&dopt=Abstract&list_uids=14700641

- **Functional improvement after phacoemulsification cataract surgery.**
  Author(s): Chang-Godinich A, Ou RJ, Koch DD.
  Source: Journal of Cataract and Refractive Surgery. 1999 September; 25(9): 1226-31.
  http://www.ncbi.nlm.nih.gov/entrez/query.fcgi?cmd=Retrieve&db=pubmed&dopt=Abstract&list_uids=10476506

- **Functional vision, wavefront sensing, and cataract surgery.**
  Author(s): Packer M, Fine IH, Hoffman RS.
  Source: International Ophthalmology Clinics. 2003 Spring; 43(2): 79-91. Review.
  http://www.ncbi.nlm.nih.gov/entrez/query.fcgi?cmd=Retrieve&db=pubmed&dopt=Abstract&list_uids=12711904

- **Fungal and bacterial chronic endophthalmitis following cataract surgery.**
  Author(s): Bourcier T, Scheer S, Chaumeil C, Morel C, Borderie V, Laroche L.
  Source: The British Journal of Ophthalmology. 2003 March; 87(3): 372-3.
  http://www.ncbi.nlm.nih.gov/entrez/query.fcgi?cmd=Retrieve&db=pubmed&dopt=Abstract&list_uids=12598469

- **Fungal endophthalmitis following cataract surgery: clinical presentation, microbiological spectrum, and outcome.**
  Author(s): Narang S, Gupta A, Gupta V, Dogra MR, Ram J, Pandav SS, Chakrabarti A.
  Source: American Journal of Ophthalmology. 2001 November; 132(5): 609-17.
  http://www.ncbi.nlm.nih.gov/entrez/query.fcgi?cmd=Retrieve&db=pubmed&dopt=Abstract&list_uids=11704021

- **Fungal infection of sutureless self-sealing incision for cataract surgery.**
  Author(s): Garg P, Mahesh S, Bansal AK, Gopinathan U, Rao GN.
  Source: Ophthalmology. 2003 November; 110(11): 2173-7.
  http://www.ncbi.nlm.nih.gov/entrez/query.fcgi?cmd=Retrieve&db=pubmed&dopt=Abstract&list_uids=14597526

- **Fusidic acid prophylaxis before cataract surgery: patient self-administration.**
  Author(s): Gray TB, Keenan JI, Clemett RS, Allardyce RA.
  Source: Australian and New Zealand Journal of Ophthalmology. 1993 May; 21(2): 99-103.
  http://www.ncbi.nlm.nih.gov/entrez/query.fcgi?cmd=Retrieve&db=pubmed&dopt=Abstract&list_uids=8333941

- **Gains from cataract surgery: visual function and quality of life.**
  Author(s): Desai P, Reidy A, Minassian DC, Vafidis G, Bolger J.
  Source: The British Journal of Ophthalmology. 1996 October; 80(10): 868-73.
  http://www.ncbi.nlm.nih.gov/entrez/query.fcgi?cmd=Retrieve&db=pubmed&dopt=Abstract&list_uids=8976696

- **Gender and cataract surgery in Sweden 1992-1997. A retrospective observational study based on the Swedish National Cataract Register.**
  Author(s): Lundstrom M, Stenevi U, Thorburn W.
  Source: Acta Ophthalmologica Scandinavica. 1999 April; 77(2): 204-8.
  http://www.ncbi.nlm.nih.gov/entrez/query.fcgi?cmd=Retrieve&db=pubmed&dopt=Abstract&list_uids=10321540

- **Gender and referral to cataract surgery in Sweden.**
  Author(s): Olofsson P, Lundstrom M, Stenevi U.
  Source: Acta Ophthalmologica Scandinavica. 2001 August; 79(4): 350-3.
  http://www.ncbi.nlm.nih.gov/entrez/query.fcgi?cmd=Retrieve&db=pubmed&dopt=Abstract&list_uids=11453852

- **General anaesthesia for day-case cataract surgery.**
  Author(s): Whitehead PN.
  Source: British Journal of Anaesthesia. 1995 August; 75(2): 252-3.
  http://www.ncbi.nlm.nih.gov/entrez/query.fcgi?cmd=Retrieve&db=pu
  bmed&dopt=Abstract&list_uids=7577268

- **General practitioners' awareness of different techniques of cataract surgery: implications for quality of care.**
  Author(s): Potamitis T, Fouladi M, Aggarwal RK, Jones HS, Fielder AR.
  Source: Bmj (Clinical Research Ed.). 1994 May 21; 308(6940): 1334-5.
  http://www.ncbi.nlm.nih.gov/entrez/query.fcgi?cmd=Retrieve&db=pu
  bmed&dopt=Abstract&list_uids=8019220

- **General versus regional anaesthesia for cataract surgery: effects on neutrophil apoptosis and the postoperative pro-inflammatory state.**
  Author(s): Goto Y, Ho SL, McAdoo J, Fanning NF, Wang J, Redmond HP, Shorten GD.
  Source: European Journal of Anaesthesiology. 2000 August; 17(8): 474-80.
  http://www.ncbi.nlm.nih.gov/entrez/query.fcgi?cmd=Retrieve&db=pu
  bmed&dopt=Abstract&list_uids=10998029

- **Gentamicin retinal toxicity after cataract surgery in an eye that underwent vitrectomy.**
  Author(s): Rosenbaum JD, Krumholz DM, Metz DM.
  Source: Ophthalmic Surgery and Lasers. 1997 March; 28(3): 236-8.
  http://www.ncbi.nlm.nih.gov/entrez/query.fcgi?cmd=Retrieve&db=pu
  bmed&dopt=Abstract&list_uids=9076799

- **Geographic variation in utilization of cataract surgery.**
  Author(s): Javitt JC, Kendix M, Tielsch JM, Steinwachs DM, Schein OD, Kolb MM, Steinberg EP.
  Source: Medical Care. 1995 January; 33(1): 90-105.
  http://www.ncbi.nlm.nih.gov/entrez/query.fcgi?cmd=Retrieve&db=pu
  bmed&dopt=Abstract&list_uids=7823650

- **Giant retinal tear as a complication of attempted removal of intravitreal lens fragments during cataract surgery.**
  Author(s): Aaberg TM Jr, Rubsamen PE, Flynn HW Jr, Chang S, Mieler WF, Smiddy WE.
  Source: American Journal of Ophthalmology. 1997 August; 124(2): 222-6.
  http://www.ncbi.nlm.nih.gov/entrez/query.fcgi?cmd=Retrieve&db=pu
  bmed&dopt=Abstract&list_uids=9262547

- **Glare disability and contrast sensitivity before and after cataract surgery.**
  Author(s): Superstein R, Boyaner D, Overbury O, Collin C.
  Source: Journal of Cataract and Refractive Surgery. 1997 March; 23(2): 248-53.
  http://www.ncbi.nlm.nih.gov/entrez/query.fcgi?cmd=Retrieve&db=pubmed&dopt=Abstract&list_uids=9113577

- **Glare measurements before and after cataract surgery.**
  Author(s): Hard AL, Beckman C, Sjostrand J.
  Source: Acta Ophthalmol (Copenh). 1993 August; 71(4): 471-6.
  http://www.ncbi.nlm.nih.gov/entrez/query.fcgi?cmd=Retrieve&db=pubmed&dopt=Abstract&list_uids=8249576

- **Glaucoma after congenital cataract surgery.**
  Author(s): Asrani SG, Wilensky JT.
  Source: Ophthalmology. 1995 June; 102(6): 863-7.
  http://www.ncbi.nlm.nih.gov/entrez/query.fcgi?cmd=Retrieve&db=pubmed&dopt=Abstract&list_uids=7777291

- **Glaucoma following childhood cataract surgery.**
  Author(s): Mills MD, Robb RM.
  Source: Journal of Pediatric Ophthalmology and Strabismus. 1994 November-December; 31(6): 355-60; Discussion 361.
  http://www.ncbi.nlm.nih.gov/entrez/query.fcgi?cmd=Retrieve&db=pubmed&dopt=Abstract&list_uids=7714698

- **Glaucoma following congenital cataract surgery.**
  Author(s): Lee AF, Lee SM, Chou JC, Liu JH.
  Source: Zhonghua Yi Xue Za Zhi (Taipei). 1998 February; 61(2): 65-70.
  http://www.ncbi.nlm.nih.gov/entrez/query.fcgi?cmd=Retrieve&db=pubmed&dopt=Abstract&list_uids=9532867

- **Glaucoma following congenital cataract surgery: an 18-year longitudinal follow-up.**
  Author(s): Magnusson G, Abrahamsson M, Sjostrand J.
  Source: Acta Ophthalmologica Scandinavica. 2000 February; 78(1): 65-70.
  http://www.ncbi.nlm.nih.gov/entrez/query.fcgi?cmd=Retrieve&db=pubmed&dopt=Abstract&list_uids=10726793

- **Guidelines. Cataract surgery and beyond.**
  Author(s): Lee PP.
  Source: Archives of Ophthalmology. 1993 May; 111(5): 597-8.
  http://www.ncbi.nlm.nih.gov/entrez/query.fcgi?cmd=Retrieve&db=pu
  bmed&dopt=Abstract&list_uids=8489433

- **Healon GV versus Healon in demanding cataract surgery.**
  Author(s): Caporossi A, Baiocchi S, Sforzi C, Frezzotti R.
  Source: Journal of Cataract and Refractive Surgery. 1995 November; 21(6): 710-3.
  http://www.ncbi.nlm.nih.gov/entrez/query.fcgi?cmd=Retrieve&db=pu
  bmed&dopt=Abstract&list_uids=8551453

- **Healon5 versus Viscoat during cataract surgery: intraocular pressure, laser flare and corneal changes.**
  Author(s): Schwenn O, Dick HB, Krummenauer F, Christmann S, Vogel A, Pfeiffer N.
  Source: Graefe's Archive for Clinical and Experimental Ophthalmology = Albrecht Von Graefes Archiv Fur Klinische Und Experimentelle Ophthalmologie. 2000 October; 238(10): 861-7.
  http://www.ncbi.nlm.nih.gov/entrez/query.fcgi?cmd=Retrieve&db=pu
  bmed&dopt=Abstract&list_uids=11127574

- **Heparin in the irrigation solution during cataract surgery.**
  Author(s): Bayramlar H, Keskin UC.
  Source: Journal of Cataract and Refractive Surgery. 2002 December; 28(12): 2070-1.
  http://www.ncbi.nlm.nih.gov/entrez/query.fcgi?cmd=Retrieve&db=pu
  bmed&dopt=Abstract&list_uids=12498826

- **Heparinised intraocular infusion and bacterial contamination in cataract surgery.**
  Author(s): Manners TD, Turner DP, Galloway PH, Glenn AM.
  Source: The British Journal of Ophthalmology. 1997 November; 81(11): 949-52.
  http://www.ncbi.nlm.nih.gov/entrez/query.fcgi?cmd=Retrieve&db=pu
  bmed&dopt=Abstract&list_uids=9505816

- **Heparin-modified lenses for eyes at risk for breakdown of the blood-aqueous barrier during cataract surgery.**
  Author(s): Percival SP, Pai V.
  Source: Journal of Cataract and Refractive Surgery. 1993 November; 19(6): 760-5.
  http://www.ncbi.nlm.nih.gov/entrez/query.fcgi?cmd=Retrieve&db=pubmed&dopt=Abstract&list_uids=8271173

- **Heparin-surface-modified intraocular lenses in pediatric cataract surgery: prospective randomized study.**
  Author(s): Basti S, Aasuri MK, Reddy MK, Preetam P, Reddy S, Gupta S, Naduvilath TJ.
  Source: Journal of Cataract and Refractive Surgery. 1999 June; 25(6): 782-7.
  http://www.ncbi.nlm.nih.gov/entrez/query.fcgi?cmd=Retrieve&db=pubmed&dopt=Abstract&list_uids=10374157

- **Heterochromia after pediatric cataract surgery.**
  Author(s): Lenart TD, Drack AV, Tarnuzzer RW, Fernandes A, Lambert SR.
  Source: J Aapos. 2000 February; 4(1): 40-5.
  http://www.ncbi.nlm.nih.gov/entrez/query.fcgi?cmd=Retrieve&db=pubmed&dopt=Abstract&list_uids=10675870

- **High-resolution digital retroillumination imaging of the posterior -004 capsule after cataract surgery.**
  Author(s): Pande MV, Ursell PG, Spalton DJ, Heath G, Kundaiker S.
  Source: Journal of Cataract and Refractive Surgery. 1997 December; 23(10): 1521-7.
  http://www.ncbi.nlm.nih.gov/entrez/query.fcgi?cmd=Retrieve&db=pubmed&dopt=Abstract&list_uids=9456410

- **History of cataract surgery.**
  Author(s): Jaffe NS.
  Source: Ophthalmology. 1996 August; 103(8 Suppl): S5-16.
  http://www.ncbi.nlm.nih.gov/entrez/query.fcgi?cmd=Retrieve&db=pubmed&dopt=Abstract&list_uids=8764763

- **History of cataract surgery.**
  Author(s): Shugar JK.
  Source: Ophthalmology. 1997 February; 104(2): 173-4.
  http://www.ncbi.nlm.nih.gov/entrez/query.fcgi?cmd=Retrieve&db=pu
  bmed&dopt=Abstract&list_uids=9052617

- **Holistic impressions of an ophthalmologist having cataract surgery himself.**
  Author(s): Francis IC, Pettinger DF.
  Source: Clinical & Experimental Ophthalmology. 2002 August; 30(4): 311.
  http://www.ncbi.nlm.nih.gov/entrez/query.fcgi?cmd=Retrieve&db=pu
  bmed&dopt=Abstract&list_uids=12121378

- **Hormone replacement therapy, reproductive factors, and the incidence of cataract and cataract surgery: the Blue Mountains Eye Study.**
  Author(s): Younan C, Mitchell P, Cumming RG, Panchapakesan J, Rochtchina E, Hales AM.
  Source: American Journal of Epidemiology. 2002 June 1; 155(11): 997-1006.
  http://www.ncbi.nlm.nih.gov/entrez/query.fcgi?cmd=Retrieve&db=pu
  bmed&dopt=Abstract&list_uids=12034578

- **Hospital construction-associated outbreak of ocular aspergillosis after cataract surgery.**
  Author(s): Tabbara KF, al Jabarti AL.
  Source: Ophthalmology. 1998 March; 105(3): 522-6.
  http://www.ncbi.nlm.nih.gov/entrez/query.fcgi?cmd=Retrieve&db=pu
  bmed&dopt=Abstract&list_uids=9499785

- **How to calculate surgically induced astigmatism after cataract surgery?**
  Author(s): Goes FM Jr, Missotten L.
  Source: Bull Soc Belge Ophtalmol. 1998; 268: 35-40.
  http://www.ncbi.nlm.nih.gov/entrez/query.fcgi?cmd=Retrieve&db=pu
  bmed&dopt=Abstract&list_uids=9810082

- **Hyphema after peribulbar anesthesia for cataract surgery in Fuchs' heterochromic iridocyclitis.**
  Author(s): Belfort R Jr, Muccioli C.
  Source: Ocular Immunology and Inflammation. 1998 March; 6(1): 57-8.
  http://www.ncbi.nlm.nih.gov/entrez/query.fcgi?cmd=Retrieve&db=pu
  bmed&dopt=Abstract&list_uids=9798195

- **Iatrogenic retinal tear and vitreous haemorrhage with Rycroft cannula during phacoemulsification cataract surgery.**
  Author(s): Saha N, Price NC.
  Source: Eye (London, England). 2003 March; 17(2): 260-1.
  http://www.ncbi.nlm.nih.gov/entrez/query.fcgi?cmd=Retrieve&db=pu bmed&dopt=Abstract&list_uids=12640423

- **Impact of cataract surgery on self-reported visual difficulties: comparison with a no-surgery reference group.**
  Author(s): McGwin G Jr, Scilley K, Brown J, Owsley C.
  Source: Journal of Cataract and Refractive Surgery. 2003 May; 29(5): 941-8.
  http://www.ncbi.nlm.nih.gov/entrez/query.fcgi?cmd=Retrieve&db=pu bmed&dopt=Abstract&list_uids=12781280

- **Impact of cataract surgery on the visual ability of the very old.**
  Author(s): Monestam E, Wachmeister L.
  Source: American Journal of Ophthalmology. 2004 January; 137(1): 145-55.
  http://www.ncbi.nlm.nih.gov/entrez/query.fcgi?cmd=Retrieve&db=pu bmed&dopt=Abstract&list_uids=14700658

- **Incremental cost-effectiveness of initial cataract surgery.**
  Author(s): Busbee BG, Brown MM, Brown GC, Sharma S.
  Source: Ophthalmology. 2002 March; 109(3): 606-12; Discussion 612-3.
  http://www.ncbi.nlm.nih.gov/entrez/query.fcgi?cmd=Retrieve&db=pu bmed&dopt=Abstract&list_uids=11874769

- **Influence of cataract surgery with implantation of different intraocular lenses on scanning laser tomography and polarimetry.**
  Author(s): Kremmer S, Garway-Heath DF, De Cilla S, Steuhl KP, Selbach JM.
  Source: American Journal of Ophthalmology. 2003 December; 136(6): 1016-21.
  http://www.ncbi.nlm.nih.gov/entrez/query.fcgi?cmd=Retrieve&db=pu bmed&dopt=Abstract&list_uids=14644211

- **Influence of operator experience on the performance of ultrasound biometry compared to optical biometry before cataract surgery.**
  Author(s): Findl O, Kriechbaum K, Sacu S, Kiss B, Polak K, Nepp J, Schild G, Rainer G, Maca S, Petternel V, Lackner B, Drexler W.
  Source: Journal of Cataract and Refractive Surgery. 2003 October; 29(10): 1950-5.
  http://www.ncbi.nlm.nih.gov/entrez/query.fcgi?cmd=Retrieve&db=pubmed&dopt=Abstract&list_uids=14604716

- **Informed consent for cataract surgery: what patients do and do not understand.**
  Author(s): Scanlan D, Siddiqui F, Perry G, Hutnik CM.
  Source: Journal of Cataract and Refractive Surgery. 2003 October; 29(10): 1904-12.
  http://www.ncbi.nlm.nih.gov/entrez/query.fcgi?cmd=Retrieve&db=pubmed&dopt=Abstract&list_uids=14604709

- **Insight into cataract surgery. Improved implanted lenses boost benefits from cataract surgery.**
  Author(s): Monica ML.
  Source: Health News. 2003 September; 9(9): 3. No Abstract Available.
  http://www.ncbi.nlm.nih.gov/entrez/query.fcgi?cmd=Retrieve&db=pubmed&dopt=Abstract&list_uids=14584466

- **Intracameral heparin in pediatric cataract surgery.**
  Author(s): Dada T.
  Source: Journal of Cataract and Refractive Surgery. 2003 June; 29(6): 1056.
  http://www.ncbi.nlm.nih.gov/entrez/query.fcgi?cmd=Retrieve&db=pubmed&dopt=Abstract&list_uids=12842660

- **Intracameral mydriatics in phacoemulsification cataract surgery.**
  Author(s): Lundberg B, Behndig A.
  Source: Journal of Cataract and Refractive Surgery. 2003 December; 29(12): 2366-71.
  http://www.ncbi.nlm.nih.gov/entrez/query.fcgi?cmd=Retrieve&db=pubmed&dopt=Abstract&list_uids=14709298

- **Intraocular inflammation after cataract surgery.**
  Author(s): Kuchle M, Naumann GO.
  Source: Ophthalmology. 2003 June; 110(6): 1269-70.
  http://www.ncbi.nlm.nih.gov/entrez/query.fcgi?cmd=Retrieve&db=pubmed&dopt=Abstract&list_uids=12799271

- **Intraocular inflammation after cataract surgery.**
  Author(s): Kuchle M, Naumann GO.
  Source: Ophthalmology. 2003 April; 110(4): 632-3. Corrected and Republished In:
  http://www.ncbi.nlm.nih.gov/entrez/query.fcgi?cmd=Retrieve&db=pu bmed&dopt=Abstract&list_uids=12689877

- **Intraocular lens power calculation for cataract surgery after photorefractive keratectomy.**
  Author(s): Odenthal MT, Eggink CA, Melles G, Pameyer JH, Geerards AJ, Beekhuis WH.
  Source: Archives of Ophthalmology. 2003 July; 121(7): 1071.
  http://www.ncbi.nlm.nih.gov/entrez/query.fcgi?cmd=Retrieve&db=pu bmed&dopt=Abstract&list_uids=12860831

- **Intraocular ointment after small-incision cataract surgery causing chronic uveitis and secondary glaucoma.**
  Author(s): Riedl M, Maca S, Amon M, Nennadal T, Kruger A, Barisani T.
  Source: Journal of Cataract and Refractive Surgery. 2003 May; 29(5): 1022-5.
  http://www.ncbi.nlm.nih.gov/entrez/query.fcgi?cmd=Retrieve&db=pu bmed&dopt=Abstract&list_uids=12781294

- **Intraocular pressure after bilateral cataract surgery using Healon, Healon5, and Healon GV.**
  Author(s): Arshinoff SA, Albiani DA, Taylor-Laporte J.
  Source: Journal of Cataract and Refractive Surgery. 2002 April; 28(4): 617-25.
  http://www.ncbi.nlm.nih.gov/entrez/query.fcgi?cmd=Retrieve&db=pu bmed&dopt=Abstract&list_uids=11955901

- **Intraoperative light toxicity: a possible explanation for the association between cataract surgery and age-related macular degeneration.**
  Author(s): Libre PE.
  Source: American Journal of Ophthalmology. 2003 November; 136(5): 961.
  http://www.ncbi.nlm.nih.gov/entrez/query.fcgi?cmd=Retrieve&db=pu bmed&dopt=Abstract&list_uids=14597070

- **Intravitreal triamcinolone acetonide for cataract surgery with iris neovascularization.**
  Author(s): Jonas JB, Sofker A.
  Source: Journal of Cataract and Refractive Surgery. 2002 November; 28(11): 2040-1.
  http://www.ncbi.nlm.nih.gov/entrez/query.fcgi?cmd=Retrieve&db=pubmed&dopt=Abstract&list_uids=12457682

- **Iris prolapse in small incision cataract surgery.**
  Author(s): Taguri AH, Sanders R.
  Source: Ophthalmic Surgery and Lasers. 2002 January-February; 33(1): 66-70.
  http://www.ncbi.nlm.nih.gov/entrez/query.fcgi?cmd=Retrieve&db=pubmed&dopt=Abstract&list_uids=11820667

- **Is manual small incision cataract surgery affordable in the developing countries? A cost comparison with extracapsular cataract extraction.**
  Author(s): Gogate PM, Deshpande M, Wormald RP.
  Source: The British Journal of Ophthalmology. 2003 July; 87(7): 843-6.
  http://www.ncbi.nlm.nih.gov/entrez/query.fcgi?cmd=Retrieve&db=pubmed&dopt=Abstract&list_uids=12812880

- **Is there an association between cataract surgery and age-related macular degeneration? Data from three population-based studies.**
  Author(s): Freeman EE, Munoz B, West SK, Tielsch JM, Schein OD.
  Source: American Journal of Ophthalmology. 2003 June; 135(6): 849-56.
  http://www.ncbi.nlm.nih.gov/entrez/query.fcgi?cmd=Retrieve&db=pubmed&dopt=Abstract&list_uids=12788126

- **Keratolenticuloplasty: arcuate keratotomy for cataract surgery and astigmatism.**
  Author(s): Kershner RM.
  Source: Journal of Cataract and Refractive Surgery. 1995 May; 21(3): 274-7.
  http://www.ncbi.nlm.nih.gov/entrez/query.fcgi?cmd=Retrieve&db=pubmed&dopt=Abstract&list_uids=7674161

- **Keratome for sutureless cataract surgery.**
  Author(s): Laurence EP, Epstein RL, Ernest PH.
  Source: Journal of Cataract and Refractive Surgery. 1993 July; 19(4): 558-9.
  http://www.ncbi.nlm.nih.gov/entrez/query.fcgi?cmd=Retrieve&db=pubmed&dopt=Abstract&list_uids=8355169

- **Keratometric astigmatism after cataract surgery using small self-sealing scleral incision.**
  Author(s): Chen YC, Wu S.
  Source: Chang Gung Med J. 2001 January; 24(1): 19-26.
  http://www.ncbi.nlm.nih.gov/entrez/query.fcgi?cmd=Retrieve&db=pubmed&dopt=Abstract&list_uids=11299973

- **Keratomycosis after cataract surgery.**
  Author(s): Mendicute J, Orbegozo J, Ruiz M, Saiz A, Eder F, Aramberri J.
  Source: Journal of Cataract and Refractive Surgery. 2000 November; 26(11): 1660-6.
  http://www.ncbi.nlm.nih.gov/entrez/query.fcgi?cmd=Retrieve&db=pubmed&dopt=Abstract&list_uids=11084276

- **Ketorolac tromethamine 0.5% ophthalmic solution in the treatment of moderate to severe ocular inflammation after cataract surgery: a randomized, vehicle-controlled clinical trial.**
  Author(s): Akpek EK, Karadayi K.
  Source: American Journal of Ophthalmology. 1999 November; 128(5): 662-3.
  http://www.ncbi.nlm.nih.gov/entrez/query.fcgi?cmd=Retrieve&db=pubmed&dopt=Abstract&list_uids=10577550

- **Ketorolac tromethamine 0.5% ophthalmic solution in the treatment of moderate to severe ocular inflammation after cataract surgery: a randomized, vehicle-controlled clinical trial.**
  Author(s): Heier J, Cheetham JK, Degryse R, Dirks MS, Caldwell DR, Silverstone DE, Rosenthal A.
  Source: American Journal of Ophthalmology. 1999 March; 127(3): 253-9.
  http://www.ncbi.nlm.nih.gov/entrez/query.fcgi?cmd=Retrieve&db=pubmed&dopt=Abstract&list_uids=10088733

- **Knife for performing the initial groove for sutureless cataract surgery.**
  Author(s): John ME.
  Source: Journal of Cataract and Refractive Surgery. 1993 July; 19(4): 557-8.
  http://www.ncbi.nlm.nih.gov/entrez/query.fcgi?cmd=Retrieve&db=pubmed&dopt=Abstract&list_uids=8355168

- **Landmarks in the evolution of cataract surgery.**
  Author(s): Teichmann KD.
  Source: Survey of Ophthalmology. 2000 May-June; 44(6): 541.
  http://www.ncbi.nlm.nih.gov/entrez/query.fcgi?cmd=Retrieve&db=pubmed&dopt=Abstract&list_uids=10914522

- **Laser cataract surgery : A prospective clinical evaluation of 1000 consecutive laser cataract procedures using the Dodick photolysis Nd:YAG system.**
  Author(s): Kanellopoulos AJ; Photolysis Investigative Group.
  Source: Ophthalmology. 2001 April; 108(4): 649-54; Discussion 654-5.
  http://www.ncbi.nlm.nih.gov/entrez/query.fcgi?cmd=Retrieve&db=pubmed&dopt=Abstract&list_uids=11297476

- **Laser cataract surgery.**
  Author(s): Aasuri MK, Basti S.
  Source: Current Opinion in Ophthalmology. 1999 February; 10(1): 53-8. Review.
  http://www.ncbi.nlm.nih.gov/entrez/query.fcgi?cmd=Retrieve&db=pubmed&dopt=Abstract&list_uids=10387321

- **Laser cataract surgery: past, present, and evolving technologies.**
  Author(s): Gardiner MF, Pineda R, Dana MR.
  Source: International Ophthalmology Clinics. 2004 Winter; 44(1): 113-21. Review.
  http://www.ncbi.nlm.nih.gov/entrez/query.fcgi?cmd=Retrieve&db=pubmed&dopt=Abstract&list_uids=14704526

- **Laser in situ keratomileusis for correction of induced astigmatism from cataract surgery.**
  Author(s): Norouzi H, Rahmati-Kamel M.
  Source: Journal of Refractive Surgery (Thorofare, N.J. : 1995). 2003 July-August; 19(4): 416-24.
  http://www.ncbi.nlm.nih.gov/entrez/query.fcgi?cmd=Retrieve&db=pubmed&dopt=Abstract&list_uids=12899472

- **Laser in situ keratomileusis to correct residual myopia after cataract surgery.**
  Author(s): Ayala MJ, Perez-Santonja JJ, Artola A, Claramonte P, Alio JL.
  Source: Journal of Refractive Surgery (Thorofare, N.J. : 1995). 2001 January-February; 17(1): 12-6.
  http://www.ncbi.nlm.nih.gov/entrez/query.fcgi?cmd=Retrieve&db=pu bmed&dopt=Abstract&list_uids=11201772

- **Lens epithelial cell death after cataract surgery.**
  Author(s): Saika S, Miyamoto T, Ishida I, Ohnishi Y, Ooshima A.
  Source: Journal of Cataract and Refractive Surgery. 2002 August; 28(8): 1452-6.
  http://www.ncbi.nlm.nih.gov/entrez/query.fcgi?cmd=Retrieve&db=pu bmed&dopt=Abstract&list_uids=12160819

- **Lens particle glaucoma occurring 15 years after cataract surgery.**
  Author(s): Kee C, Lee S.
  Source: Korean J Ophthalmol. 2001 December; 15(2): 137-9.
  http://www.ncbi.nlm.nih.gov/entrez/query.fcgi?cmd=Retrieve&db=pu bmed&dopt=Abstract&list_uids=11811582

- **Lidocaine 2% gel versus lidocaine 4% unpreserved drops for topical anesthesia in cataract surgery: a randomized controlled trial.**
  Author(s): Bardocci A, Lofoco G, Perdicaro S, Ciucci F, Manna L.
  Source: Ophthalmology. 2003 January; 110(1): 144-9.
  http://www.ncbi.nlm.nih.gov/entrez/query.fcgi?cmd=Retrieve&db=pu bmed&dopt=Abstract&list_uids=12511360

- **Lidocaine versus ropivacaine for topical anesthesia in cataract surgery(1).**
  Author(s): Martini E, Cavallini GM, Campi L, Lugli N, Neri G, Molinari P.
  Source: Journal of Cataract and Refractive Surgery. 2002 June; 28(6): 1018-22.
  http://www.ncbi.nlm.nih.gov/entrez/query.fcgi?cmd=Retrieve&db=pu bmed&dopt=Abstract&list_uids=12036647

- **Lidocaine-clonidine retrobulbar block for cataract surgery in the elderly.**
  Author(s): Mjahed K, el Harrar N, Hamdani M, Amraoui M, Benaguida M.
  Source: Reg Anesth. 1996 November-December; 21(6): 569-75.
  http://www.ncbi.nlm.nih.gov/entrez/query.fcgi?cmd=Retrieve&db=pubmed&dopt=Abstract&list_uids=8956395

- **Limbal relaxing incisions for primary mixed astigmatism and mixed astigmatism after cataract surgery.**
  Author(s): Ophthalmology. 2003 Jun;110(6):1269-70
  Source: Journal of Cataract and Refractive Surgery. 2003 April; 29(4): 723-8.
  http://www.ncbi.nlm.nih.gov/entrez/query.fcgi?cmd=Retrieve&db=pubmed&dopt=Abstract&list_uids=12799271

- **Local or general anaesthesia for cataract surgery.**
  Author(s): Denha RF, Wraight WJ.
  Source: Anaesthesia. 1996 December; 51(12): 1191-2.
  http://www.ncbi.nlm.nih.gov/entrez/query.fcgi?cmd=Retrieve&db=pubmed&dopt=Abstract&list_uids=9038483

- **Long term clinical outcome of a randomised controlled trial of anterior chamber lenses after high volume intracapsular cataract surgery.**
  Author(s): Hennig A, Johnson GJ, Evans JR, Lagnado R, Poulson A, Pradhan D, Foster A, Wormald RP.
  Source: The British Journal of Ophthalmology. 2001 January; 85(1): 11-7.
  http://www.ncbi.nlm.nih.gov/entrez/query.fcgi?cmd=Retrieve&db=pubmed&dopt=Abstract&list_uids=11133704

- **Long-term disorders of the blood-aqueous barrier after small-incision cataract surgery.**
  Author(s): Schauersberger J, Kruger A, Mullner-Eidenbock A, Petternel V, Abela C, Svolba G, Amon M.
  Source: Eye (London, England). 2000 February; 14 (Pt 1): 61-3.
  http://www.ncbi.nlm.nih.gov/entrez/query.fcgi?cmd=Retrieve&db=pubmed&dopt=Abstract&list_uids=10755102

- **Long-term effect of cataract surgery on intraocular pressure after trabeculectomy: extracapsular extraction versus phacoemulsification.**
  Author(s): Casson RJ, Riddell CE, Rahman R, Byles D, Salmon JF.
  Source: Journal of Cataract and Refractive Surgery. 2002 December; 28(12): 2159-64.
  http://www.ncbi.nlm.nih.gov/entrez/query.fcgi?cmd=Retrieve&db=pubmed&dopt=Abstract&list_uids=12498852

- **Long-term endothelial changes after implantation of anterior chamber intraocular lenses in cataract surgery.**
  Author(s): Ravalico G, Botteri E, Baccara F.
  Source: Journal of Cataract and Refractive Surgery. 2003 October; 29(10): 1918-23.
  http://www.ncbi.nlm.nih.gov/entrez/query.fcgi?cmd=Retrieve&db=pubmed&dopt=Abstract&list_uids=14604711

- **Long-term follow-up of eye growth in pediatric patients after unilateral cataract surgery with intraocular lens implantation.**
  Author(s): Inatomi M, Kora Y, Kinohira Y, Yaguchi S.
  Source: J Aapos. 2004 February; 8(1): 50-5.
  http://www.ncbi.nlm.nih.gov/entrez/query.fcgi?cmd=Retrieve&db=pubmed&dopt=Abstract&list_uids=14970800

- **Long-term results of cataract surgery combined with trabeculotomy.**
  Author(s): Hoffmann E, Schwenn O, Karallus M, Krummenauer F, Grehn F, Pfeiffer N.
  Source: Graefe's Archive for Clinical and Experimental Ophthalmology = Albrecht Von Graefes Archiv Fur Klinische Und Experimentelle Ophthalmologie. 2002 January; 240(1): 2-6.
  http://www.ncbi.nlm.nih.gov/entrez/query.fcgi?cmd=Retrieve&db=pubmed&dopt=Abstract&list_uids=11954776

- **Long-term visual results in congenital cataract surgery associated with preoperative nystagmus.**
  Author(s): Garza-Reyes M, Rodriguez-Almaraz M, Ramirez-Ortiz MA.
  Source: Archives of Medical Research. 2000 September-October; 31(5): 500-4.
  http://www.ncbi.nlm.nih.gov/entrez/query.fcgi?cmd=Retrieve&db=pubmed&dopt=Abstract&list_uids=11179585

- **Management of the small pupil for clear corneal cataract surgery.**
  Author(s): Kershner RM.
  Source: Journal of Cataract and Refractive Surgery. 2002 October; 28(10): 1826-31.
  http://www.ncbi.nlm.nih.gov/entrez/query.fcgi?cmd=Retrieve&db=pubmed&dopt=Abstract&list_uids=12388036

- **Management of vitreous loss during cataract surgery under topical anesthesia with transconjunctival vitrectomy system.**
  Author(s): Shah VA, Gupta SK, Chalam KV.
  Source: Eur J Ophthalmol. 2003 October; 13(8): 693-6.
  http://www.ncbi.nlm.nih.gov/entrez/query.fcgi?cmd=Retrieve&db=pubmed&dopt=Abstract&list_uids=14620173

- **Managing cystoid macular edema after cataract surgery.**
  Author(s): Nelson ML, Martidis A.
  Source: Current Opinion in Ophthalmology. 2003 February; 14(1): 39-43. Review.
  http://www.ncbi.nlm.nih.gov/entrez/query.fcgi?cmd=Retrieve&db=pubmed&dopt=Abstract&list_uids=12544809

- **Managing intraoperative complications in cataract surgery.**
  Author(s): Arbisser LB.
  Source: Current Opinion in Ophthalmology. 2004 February; 15(1): 33-9. Review.
  http://www.ncbi.nlm.nih.gov/entrez/query.fcgi?cmd=Retrieve&db=pubmed&dopt=Abstract&list_uids=14743017

- **Meeting the challenge of glaucoma after paediatric cataract surgery.**
  Author(s): Papadopoulos M, Khaw PT.
  Source: Eye (London, England). 2003 January; 17(1): 1-2.
  http://www.ncbi.nlm.nih.gov/entrez/query.fcgi?cmd=Retrieve&db=pubmed&dopt=Abstract&list_uids=12579159

- **Microscope-induced retinal phototoxicity in cataract surgery of short duration.**
  Author(s): Kleinmann G, Hoffman P, Schechtman E, Pollack A.
  Source: Ophthalmology. 2002 February; 109(2): 334-8.
  http://www.ncbi.nlm.nih.gov/entrez/query.fcgi?cmd=Retrieve&db=pubmed&dopt=Abstract&list_uids=11825820

- **Midterm visual outcome and progression of diabetic retinopathy following cataract surgery. Midterm outcome of cataract surgery in diabetes.**
  Author(s): Schrey S, Krepler K, Biowski R, Wedrich A.
  Source: Ophthalmologica. Journal International D'ophtalmologie. International Journal of Ophthalmology. Zeitschrift Fur Augenheilkunde. 2002 September-October; 216(5): 337-40.
  http://www.ncbi.nlm.nih.gov/entrez/query.fcgi?cmd=Retrieve&db=pubmed&dopt=Abstract&list_uids=12424399

- **Modified technique using flexible iris retractors in clear corneal cataract surgery.**
  Author(s): Oetting TA, Omphroy LC.
  Source: Journal of Cataract and Refractive Surgery. 2002 April; 28(4): 596-8.
  http://www.ncbi.nlm.nih.gov/entrez/query.fcgi?cmd=Retrieve&db=pubmed&dopt=Abstract&list_uids=11955897

- **Monitoring visual outcome of cataract surgery in India.**
  Author(s): Limburg H, Foster A, Vaidyanathan K, Murthy GV.
  Source: Bulletin of the World Health Organization. 1999; 77(6): 455-60.
  http://www.ncbi.nlm.nih.gov/entrez/query.fcgi?cmd=Retrieve&db=pubmed&dopt=Abstract&list_uids=10427929

- **Multifocal versus monofocal intraocular lenses in cataract surgery: a systematic review.**
  Author(s): Leyland M, Zinicola E.
  Source: Ophthalmology. 2003 September; 110(9): 1789-98. Review.
  http://www.ncbi.nlm.nih.gov/entrez/query.fcgi?cmd=Retrieve&db=pubmed&dopt=Abstract&list_uids=13129879

- **Myopia and incident cataract and cataract surgery: the blue mountains eye study.**
  Author(s): Younan C, Mitchell P, Cumming RG, Rochtchina E, Wang JJ.
  Source: Investigative Ophthalmology & Visual Science. 2002 December; 43(12): 3625-32.
  http://www.ncbi.nlm.nih.gov/entrez/query.fcgi?cmd=Retrieve&db=pubmed&dopt=Abstract&list_uids=12454028

- **National cataract surgery survey 1997-8: a report of the results of the clinical outcomes.**
  Author(s): Desai P, Minassian DC, Reidy A.
  Source: The British Journal of Ophthalmology. 1999 December; 83(12): 1336-40.
  http://www.ncbi.nlm.nih.gov/entrez/query.fcgi?cmd=Retrieve&db=pubmed&dopt=Abstract&list_uids=10574810

- **Necessity of the Honan intraocular pressure reducer in cataract surgery using topical anesthesia.**
  Author(s): Black EH, Cohen KL, Tripoli NK, Winslow PA 3rd.
  Source: Journal of Cataract and Refractive Surgery. 1999 February; 25(2): 223-6.
  http://www.ncbi.nlm.nih.gov/entrez/query.fcgi?cmd=Retrieve&db=pubmed&dopt=Abstract&list_uids=9951668

- **Necrotizing sclerokeratitis following uncomplicated cataract surgery.**
  Author(s): Beatty S, Chawdhary S.
  Source: Acta Ophthalmologica Scandinavica. 1998 June; 76(3): 382-3.
  http://www.ncbi.nlm.nih.gov/entrez/query.fcgi?cmd=Retrieve&db=pubmed&dopt=Abstract&list_uids=9686862

- **Needle local anaesthesia for cataract surgery: a chip off the old block?**
  Author(s): Smerdon D.
  Source: Eye (London, England). 2001 August; 15(Pt 4): 439-40.
  http://www.ncbi.nlm.nih.gov/entrez/query.fcgi?cmd=Retrieve&db=pubmed&dopt=Abstract&list_uids=11767015

- **Neodymium: YAG laser membranotomy after extracapsular cataract surgery in diabetic patient.**
  Author(s): Parodi MB, Saviano S, Iustulin D, Gioulis D, Ravalico G.
  Source: Journal of Cataract and Refractive Surgery. 2001 August; 27(8): 1149-50.
  http://www.ncbi.nlm.nih.gov/entrez/query.fcgi?cmd=Retrieve&db=pubmed&dopt=Abstract&list_uids=11530791

- **Neovascular glaucoma developing after uncomplicated cataract surgery for heavily irradiated eyes.**
  Author(s): Kwok SK, Leung SF, Ho PC, Gandhi S, Chen IN, Michon JJ, Lam DS, Lai JS.
  Source: Ophthalmology. 1997 July; 104(7): 1112-5.
  http://www.ncbi.nlm.nih.gov/entrez/query.fcgi?cmd=Retrieve&db=pu bmed&dopt=Abstract&list_uids=9224462

- **Neuro-ophthalmologic complications of cataract surgery.**
  Author(s): Lee MS, Rizzo JF 3rd, Lessell S.
  Source: Seminars in Ophthalmology. 2002 September-December; 17(3-4): 149-52. Review.
  http://www.ncbi.nlm.nih.gov/entrez/query.fcgi?cmd=Retrieve&db=pu bmed&dopt=Abstract&list_uids=12759844

- **New caliper for small incision cataract surgery.**
  Author(s): Kohnen T.
  Source: Journal of Cataract and Refractive Surgery. 1997 November; 23(9): 1298-300.
  http://www.ncbi.nlm.nih.gov/entrez/query.fcgi?cmd=Retrieve&db=pu bmed&dopt=Abstract&list_uids=9423899

- **New perspectives in cataract surgery.**
  Author(s): Bahr RL.
  Source: Medicine and Health, Rhode Island. 1999 February; 82(2): 41-5. Review.
  http://www.ncbi.nlm.nih.gov/entrez/query.fcgi?cmd=Retrieve&db=pu bmed&dopt=Abstract&list_uids=10030113

- **New techniques for cataract surgery.**
  Author(s): Koch PS.
  Source: Current Opinion in Ophthalmology. 1995 February; 6(1): 41-5. Review.
  http://www.ncbi.nlm.nih.gov/entrez/query.fcgi?cmd=Retrieve&db=pu bmed&dopt=Abstract&list_uids=10150843

- **Occlusive scrub suits in operating theaters during cataract surgery: effect on airborne contamination.**
  Author(s): Andersen BM, Solheim N.
  Source: Infection Control and Hospital Epidemiology : the Official Journal of the Society of Hospital Epidemiologists of America. 2002 April; 23(4): 218-20.
  http://www.ncbi.nlm.nih.gov/entrez/query.fcgi?cmd=Retrieve&db=pubmed&dopt=Abstract&list_uids=12002238

- **Occurrence and progression of diabetic retinopathy after phacoemulsification cataract surgery.**
  Author(s): Hauser D, Katz H, Pokroy R, Bukelman A, Shechtman E, Pollack A.
  Source: Journal of Cataract and Refractive Surgery. 2004 February; 30(2): 428-32.
  http://www.ncbi.nlm.nih.gov/entrez/query.fcgi?cmd=Retrieve&db=pubmed&dopt=Abstract&list_uids=15030836

- **Occurrence of pigment precipitates after small incision cataract surgery.**
  Author(s): Ernest PH, Lavery KT, Hazariwala K.
  Source: Journal of Cataract and Refractive Surgery. 1998 January; 24(1): 91-7.
  http://www.ncbi.nlm.nih.gov/entrez/query.fcgi?cmd=Retrieve&db=pubmed&dopt=Abstract&list_uids=9494905

- **Ocular hypertension after cataract surgery: a comparison of three surgical techniques and two viscoelastics.**
  Author(s): Jurgens I, Matheu A, Castilla M.
  Source: Ophthalmic Surgery and Lasers. 1997 January; 28(1): 30-6.
  http://www.ncbi.nlm.nih.gov/entrez/query.fcgi?cmd=Retrieve&db=pubmed&dopt=Abstract&list_uids=9031302

- **Optic neuropathy secondary to sub-tenon anesthetic injection in cataract surgery.**
  Author(s): Kim SK, Andreoli CM, Rizzo JF 3rd, Golden MA, Bradbury MJ.
  Source: Archives of Ophthalmology. 2003 June; 121(6): 907-9.
  http://www.ncbi.nlm.nih.gov/entrez/query.fcgi?cmd=Retrieve&db=pubmed&dopt=Abstract&list_uids=12796271

- **Optical biometry in cataract surgery.**
  Author(s): Findl O, Drexler W, Menapace R, Kiss B, Hitzenberger CK, Fercher AF.
  Source: Dev Ophthalmol. 2002; 34: 131-40. No Abstract Available.
  http://www.ncbi.nlm.nih.gov/entrez/query.fcgi?cmd=Retrieve&db=pu
  bmed&dopt=Abstract&list_uids=12520609

- **Orbital abscess following uncomplicated phacoemulsification cataract surgery.**
  Author(s): Irvine F, McNab AA.
  Source: Clinical & Experimental Ophthalmology. 2002 December; 30(6): 430-1.
  http://www.ncbi.nlm.nih.gov/entrez/query.fcgi?cmd=Retrieve&db=pu
  bmed&dopt=Abstract&list_uids=12427235

- **Orbital cellulitis after peribulbar anaesthesia for cataract surgery.**
  Author(s): Varma D, Metcalfe TW.
  Source: Eye (London, England). 2003 January; 17(1): 105-6.
  http://www.ncbi.nlm.nih.gov/entrez/query.fcgi?cmd=Retrieve&db=pu
  bmed&dopt=Abstract&list_uids=12579185

- **Outcomes of cataract surgery in Bangladesh: results from a population based nationwide survey.**
  Author(s): Bourne RR, Dineen BP, Ali SM, Huq DM, Johnson GJ.
  Source: The British Journal of Ophthalmology. 2003 July; 87(7): 813-9.
  http://www.ncbi.nlm.nih.gov/entrez/query.fcgi?cmd=Retrieve&db=pu
  bmed&dopt=Abstract&list_uids=12812874

- **Outcomes of sulcus implantation of Array multifocal intraocular lenses in second-eye cataract surgery complicated by vitreous loss.**
  Author(s): Aralikatti AK, Tu KL, Kamath GG, Phillips RP, Prasad S.
  Source: Journal of Cataract and Refractive Surgery. 2004 January; 30(1): 155-60.
  http://www.ncbi.nlm.nih.gov/entrez/query.fcgi?cmd=Retrieve&db=pu
  bmed&dopt=Abstract&list_uids=14967284

- **Patient communication during cataract surgery.**
  Author(s): Mokashi A, Leatherbarrow B, Kincey J, Slater R, Hillier V, Mayer S.
  Source: Eye (London, England). 2004 February; 18(2): 147-51.
  http://www.ncbi.nlm.nih.gov/entrez/query.fcgi?cmd=Retrieve&db=pu
  bmed&dopt=Abstract&list_uids=14762406

- **Patient preferences for anaesthesia management during cataract surgery.**
  Author(s): Friedman DS, Reeves SW, Bass EB, Lubomski LH, Fleisher LA, Schein OD.
  Source: The British Journal of Ophthalmology. 2004 March; 88(3): 333-5.
  http://www.ncbi.nlm.nih.gov/entrez/query.fcgi?cmd=Retrieve&db=pu
  bmed&dopt=Abstract&list_uids=14977763

- **Persistent vertical binocular diplopia after cataract surgery.**
  Author(s): Hagan JC 3rd.
  Source: American Journal of Ophthalmology. 2002 June; 133(6): 860; Author Reply 860-1.
  http://www.ncbi.nlm.nih.gov/entrez/query.fcgi?cmd=Retrieve&db=pu
  bmed&dopt=Abstract&list_uids=12036698

- **Phacoemulsification cataract surgery and unplanned anterior vitrectomy--is it bad news?**
  Author(s): Tan JH, Karwatowski WS.
  Source: Eye (London, England). 2002 March; 16(2): 117-20.
  http://www.ncbi.nlm.nih.gov/entrez/query.fcgi?cmd=Retrieve&db=pu
  bmed&dopt=Abstract&list_uids=11988808

- **Pharmacologic considerations for cataract surgery.**
  Author(s): Tipperman R.
  Source: Current Opinion in Ophthalmology. 2004 February; 15(1): 51-5. Review.
  http://www.ncbi.nlm.nih.gov/entrez/query.fcgi?cmd=Retrieve&db=pu
  bmed&dopt=Abstract&list_uids=14743020

- **Phototoxic maculopathy following uneventful cataract surgery in a predisposed patient.**
  Author(s): Manzouri B, Egan CA, Hykin PG.
  Source: The British Journal of Ophthalmology. 2002 June; 86(6): 705-6.
  http://www.ncbi.nlm.nih.gov/entrez/query.fcgi?cmd=Retrieve&db=pu
  bmed&dopt=Abstract&list_uids=12034700

- **Predicting the refractive outcome after cataract surgery: the comparison of different IOLs and SRK-II v SRK-T.**
  Author(s): Elder MJ.
  Source: The British Journal of Ophthalmology. 2002 June; 86(6): 620-2.
  http://www.ncbi.nlm.nih.gov/entrez/query.fcgi?cmd=Retrieve&db=pubmed&dopt=Abstract&list_uids=12034681

- **Prednisolone and flurbiprofen drops to maintain mydriasis during phacoemulsification cataract surgery.**
  Author(s): Shaikh MY, Mars JS, Heaven CJ.
  Source: Journal of Cataract and Refractive Surgery. 2003 December; 29(12): 2372-7.
  http://www.ncbi.nlm.nih.gov/entrez/query.fcgi?cmd=Retrieve&db=pubmed&dopt=Abstract&list_uids=14709299

- **Prophylactic intracameral cefuroxime. Efficacy in preventing endophthalmitis after cataract surgery.**
  Author(s): Montan PG, Wejde G, Koranyi G, Rylander M.
  Source: Journal of Cataract and Refractive Surgery. 2002 June; 28(6): 977-81.
  http://www.ncbi.nlm.nih.gov/entrez/query.fcgi?cmd=Retrieve&db=pubmed&dopt=Abstract&list_uids=12036639

- **Prophylactic intracameral cefuroxime. Evaluation of safety and kinetics in cataract surgery.**
  Author(s): Montan PG, Wejde G, Setterquist H, Rylander M, Zetterstrom C.
  Source: Journal of Cataract and Refractive Surgery. 2002 June; 28(6): 982-7.
  http://www.ncbi.nlm.nih.gov/entrez/query.fcgi?cmd=Retrieve&db=pubmed&dopt=Abstract&list_uids=12036640

- **Quality of care in cataract surgery cases experiencing post-operative complications with co-managed care.**
  Author(s): Revicki DA, Poe ML.
  Source: J Am Optom Assoc. 1995 May; 66(5): 268-73.
  http://www.ncbi.nlm.nih.gov/entrez/query.fcgi?cmd=Retrieve&db=pubmed&dopt=Abstract&list_uids=7629366

- **Quality of cataract surgery.**
  Author(s): Haaskjold E.
  Source: Acta Ophthalmologica Scandinavica. 2001 August; 79(4): 335.
  http://www.ncbi.nlm.nih.gov/entrez/query.fcgi?cmd=Retrieve&db=pubmed&dopt=Abstract&list_uids=11453849

- **Quality of life after first- and second-eye cataract surgery: five-year data collected by the Swedish National Cataract Register.**
  Author(s): Lundstrom M, Stenevi U, Thorburn W.
  Source: Journal of Cataract and Refractive Surgery. 2001 October; 27(10): 1553-9.
  http://www.ncbi.nlm.nih.gov/entrez/query.fcgi?cmd=Retrieve&db=pubmed&dopt=Abstract&list_uids=11687351

- **Quality of life and cataracts: a review of patient-centered studies of cataract surgery outcomes.**
  Author(s): Legro MW.
  Source: Ophthalmic Surg. 1991 August; 22(8): 431-43. Review.
  http://www.ncbi.nlm.nih.gov/entrez/query.fcgi?cmd=Retrieve&db=pubmed&dopt=Abstract&list_uids=1923293

- **Quantification of posterior capsular opacification in digital images after cataract surgery.**
  Author(s): Barman SA, Hollick EJ, Boyce JF, Spalton DJ, Uyyanonvara B, Sanguinetti G, Meacock W.
  Source: Investigative Ophthalmology & Visual Science. 2000 November; 41(12): 3882-92.
  http://www.ncbi.nlm.nih.gov/entrez/query.fcgi?cmd=Retrieve&db=pubmed&dopt=Abstract&list_uids=11053290

- **Quantification of the reduction of glare disability after standard extracapsular cataract surgery.**
  Author(s): Cink DE, Sutphin JE.
  Source: Journal of Cataract and Refractive Surgery. 1992 July; 18(4): 385-90.
  http://www.ncbi.nlm.nih.gov/entrez/query.fcgi?cmd=Retrieve&db=pubmed&dopt=Abstract&list_uids=1501093

- **Questions use of nasal cannula for oxygen supplementation during cataract surgery.**
  Author(s): Livingston M.
  Source: Anesthesiology. 1999 October; 91(4): 1176.
  http://www.ncbi.nlm.nih.gov/entrez/query.fcgi?cmd=Retrieve&db=pubmed&dopt=Abstract&list_uids=10519522

- **Randomized, clinical trial of multiquadrant hydrodissection in pediatric cataract surgery.**
  Author(s): Vasavada AR, Trivedi RH, Apple DJ, Ram J, Werner L.
  Source: American Journal of Ophthalmology. 2003 January; 135(1): 84-8.
  http://www.ncbi.nlm.nih.gov/entrez/query.fcgi?cmd=Retrieve&db=pubmed&dopt=Abstract&list_uids=12504702

- **Reasons for poor cataract surgery uptake - a qualitative study in rural South Africa.**
  Author(s): Rotchford AP, Rotchford KM, Mthethwa LP, Johnson GJ.
  Source: Tropical Medicine & International Health : Tm & Ih. 2002 March; 7(3): 288-92.
  http://www.ncbi.nlm.nih.gov/entrez/query.fcgi?cmd=Retrieve&db=pubmed&dopt=Abstract&list_uids=11903992

- **Recent advances in customising cataract surgery.**
  Author(s): Woodcock M, Shah S, Smith RJ.
  Source: Bmj (Clinical Research Ed.). 2004 January 10; 328(7431): 92-6. Review.
  http://www.ncbi.nlm.nih.gov/entrez/query.fcgi?cmd=Retrieve&db=pubmed&dopt=Abstract&list_uids=14715604

- **Refractive changes following cataract surgery: the Blue Mountains Eye Study.**
  Author(s): Guzowski M, Rochtchina E, Wang JJ, Mitchell P.
  Source: Clinical & Experimental Ophthalmology. 2002 June; 30(3): 159-62.
  http://www.ncbi.nlm.nih.gov/entrez/query.fcgi?cmd=Retrieve&db=pubmed&dopt=Abstract&list_uids=12010205

- **Refractive outcome of cataract surgery using partial coherence interferometry and ultrasound biometry: clinical feasibility study of a commercial prototype II.**
  Author(s): Kiss B, Findl O, Menapace R, Wirtitsch M, Petternel V, Drexler W, Rainer G, Georgopoulos M, Hitzenberger CK, Fercher AF.
  Source: Journal of Cataract and Refractive Surgery. 2002 February; 28(2): 230-4.
  http://www.ncbi.nlm.nih.gov/entrez/query.fcgi?cmd=Retrieve&db=pubmed&dopt=Abstract&list_uids=11821201

- **Results of cataract surgery in previously vitrectomized eyes.**
  Author(s): Biro Z, Kovacs B.
  Source: Journal of Cataract and Refractive Surgery. 2002 June; 28(6): 1003-6.
  http://www.ncbi.nlm.nih.gov/entrez/query.fcgi?cmd=Retrieve&db=pubmed&dopt=Abstract&list_uids=12036644

- **Results of cataract surgery in renal transplantation patients.**
  Author(s): Akbulut A, Tayanc E, Cetinkaya A, Akman A, Yilmaz G, Oto S, Akova Y, Aydin P, Haberal M.
  Source: Eye (London, England). 2003 April; 17(3): 346-9.
  http://www.ncbi.nlm.nih.gov/entrez/query.fcgi?cmd=Retrieve&db=pubmed&dopt=Abstract&list_uids=12724697

- **Risks and benefits of anticoagulant and antiplatelet medication use before cataract surgery.**
  Author(s): Katz J, Feldman MA, Bass EB, Lubomski LH, Tielsch JM, Petty BG, Fleisher LA, Schein OD; Study of Medical Testing for Cataract Surgery Team.
  Source: Ophthalmology. 2003 September; 110(9): 1784-8. Erratum In: Ophthalmology. 2003 December; 110(12): 2309.
  http://www.ncbi.nlm.nih.gov/entrez/query.fcgi?cmd=Retrieve&db=pubmed&dopt=Abstract&list_uids=13129878

- **Role of posterior capsulotomy with vitrectomy and intraocular lens design and material in reducing posterior capsule opacification after pediatric cataract surgery.**
  Author(s): Ram J, Brar GS, Kaushik S, Gupta A, Gupta A.
  Source: Journal of Cataract and Refractive Surgery. 2003 August; 29(8): 1579-84.
  http://www.ncbi.nlm.nih.gov/entrez/query.fcgi?cmd=Retrieve&db=pubmed&dopt=Abstract&list_uids=12954310

- **Ropivacaine-lidocaine versus bupivacaine-lidocaine for retrobulbar anesthesia in cataract surgery.**
  Author(s): Uy HS, de Jesus AA, Paray AA, Flores JD, Felizar LB.
  Source: Journal of Cataract and Refractive Surgery. 2002 June; 28(6): 1023-6.

  http://www.ncbi.nlm.nih.gov/entrez/query.fcgi?cmd=Retrieve&db=pubmed&dopt=Abstract&list_uids=12036648

- **Selective and specific targeting of lens epithelial cells during cataract surgery using sealed- capsule irrigation.**
  Author(s): Maloof A, Neilson G, Milverton EJ, Pandey SK.
  Source: Journal of Cataract and Refractive Surgery. 2003 August; 29(8): 1566-8.

  http://www.ncbi.nlm.nih.gov/entrez/query.fcgi?cmd=Retrieve&db=pubmed&dopt=Abstract&list_uids=12954307

- **Selective argon laser suturelysis versus needle suturelysis to treat induced corneal astigmatism after cataract surgery.**
  Author(s): Yip CC, Lee HM, Nah G, Yong V, Au Eong KG.
  Source: Journal of Cataract and Refractive Surgery. 2002 April; 28(4): 689-91.

  http://www.ncbi.nlm.nih.gov/entrez/query.fcgi?cmd=Retrieve&db=pubmed&dopt=Abstract&list_uids=11955912

- **Socioeconomic status and incident cataract surgery: the Blue Mountains Eye Study.**
  Author(s): Younan C, Mitchell P, Cumming R, Rochtchina E.
  Source: Clinical & Experimental Ophthalmology. 2002 June; 30(3): 163-7.
  http://www.ncbi.nlm.nih.gov/entrez/query.fcgi?cmd=Retrieve&db=pubmed&dopt=Abstract&list_uids=12010206

- **Spectrum and clinical profile of post cataract surgery endophthalmitis in north India.**
  Author(s): Gupta A, Gupta V, Gupta A, Dogra MR, Pandav SS, Ray P, Chakraborty A.
  Source: Indian J Ophthalmol. 2003 June; 51(2): 139-45.
  http://www.ncbi.nlm.nih.gov/entrez/query.fcgi?cmd=Retrieve&db=pubmed&dopt=Abstract&list_uids=12831144

- **Sterile corneal melting and necrotizing scleritis after cataract surgery in patients with rheumatoid arthritis and collagen vascular disease.**
  Author(s): Perez VL, Azar DT, Foster CS.
  Source: Seminars in Ophthalmology. 2002 September-December; 17(3-4): 124-30. Review.
  http://www.ncbi.nlm.nih.gov/entrez/query.fcgi?cmd=Retrieve&db=pubmed&dopt=Abstract&list_uids=12759840

- **Strategy to reduce the number of patients perceiving impaired visual function after cataract surgery.**
  Author(s): Lundstrom M, Brege KG, Floren I, Stenevi U, Thorburn W.
  Source: Journal of Cataract and Refractive Surgery. 2002 June; 28(6): 971-6.
  http://www.ncbi.nlm.nih.gov/entrez/query.fcgi?cmd=Retrieve&db=pubmed&dopt=Abstract&list_uids=12036638

- **Subjective visual experience during phacoemulsification cataract surgery under sub-Tenon's block.**
  Author(s): Prasad N, Kumar CM, Patil BB, Dowd TC.
  Source: Eye (London, England). 2003 April; 17(3): 407-9.
  http://www.ncbi.nlm.nih.gov/entrez/query.fcgi?cmd=Retrieve&db=pubmed&dopt=Abstract&list_uids=12724704

- **Suprachoroidal haemorrhage complicating cataract surgery in the UK: a case control study of risk factors.**
  Author(s): Ling R, Kamalarajah S, Cole M, James C, Shaw S.
  Source: The British Journal of Ophthalmology. 2004 April; 88(4): 474-7.
  http://www.ncbi.nlm.nih.gov/entrez/query.fcgi?cmd=Retrieve&db=pubmed&dopt=Abstract&list_uids=15031158

- **Suprachoroidal haemorrhage complicating cataract surgery in the UK: epidemiology, clinical features, management, and outcomes.**
  Author(s): Ling R, Cole M, James C, Kamalarajah S, Foot B, Shaw S.
  Source: The British Journal of Ophthalmology. 2004 April; 88(4): 478-80.
  http://www.ncbi.nlm.nih.gov/entrez/query.fcgi?cmd=Retrieve&db=pubmed&dopt=Abstract&list_uids=15031159

- **Surodex in paediatric cataract surgery.**
  Author(s): Lee SY, Chee SP, Balakrishnan V, Farzavandi S, Tan DT.
  Source: The British Journal of Ophthalmology. 2003 November; 87(11): 1424-6.
  http://www.ncbi.nlm.nih.gov/entrez/query.fcgi?cmd=Retrieve&db=pubmed&dopt=Abstract&list_uids=14609850

- **The development and demise of a cataract surgery database.**
  Author(s): Lum F, Schachat AP, Jampel HD.
  Source: Jt Comm J Qual Improv. 2002 March; 28(3): 108-14.
  http://www.ncbi.nlm.nih.gov/entrez/query.fcgi?cmd=Retrieve&db=pubmed&dopt=Abstract&list_uids=11902025

- **The epidemiology of acute endophthalmitis after cataract surgery in an Asian population.**
  Author(s): Wong TY, Chee SP.
  Source: Ophthalmology. 2004 April; 111(4): 699-705.
  http://www.ncbi.nlm.nih.gov/entrez/query.fcgi?cmd=Retrieve&db=pubmed&dopt=Abstract&list_uids=15051201

- **The immediate approach anterior capsulorhexis (IAAC) in cataract surgery: contribution to safety and efficacy.**
  Author(s): van Setten G, Al Ahmary AM.
  Source: Acta Ophthalmologica Scandinavica. 2003 December; 81(6): 661-2.
  http://www.ncbi.nlm.nih.gov/entrez/query.fcgi?cmd=Retrieve&db=pubmed&dopt=Abstract&list_uids=14641274

- **The risk of a new retinal break or detachment following cataract surgery in eyes that had undergone repair of phakic break or detachment: a hypothesis of a causal relationship to cataract surgery.**
  Author(s): Grand MG.
  Source: Trans Am Ophthalmol Soc. 2003; 101: 335-69.
  http://www.ncbi.nlm.nih.gov/entrez/query.fcgi?cmd=Retrieve&db=pubmed&dopt=Abstract&list_uids=14971585

- **The Royal College of Ophthalmologists cataract surgery guidelines: what can patients see with their operated eye during cataract surgery?**
  Author(s): Au Eong KG.
  Source: Eye (London, England). 2002 January; 16(1): 109-10. Review.
  http://www.ncbi.nlm.nih.gov/entrez/query.fcgi?cmd=Retrieve&db=pubmed&dopt=Abstract&list_uids=11915874

- **Topical anesthesia is the technique of choice for routine cataract surgery.**
  Author(s): Sosis MB.
  Source: Anesthesiology. 2004 January; 100(1): 197; Author Reply 197.
  http://www.ncbi.nlm.nih.gov/entrez/query.fcgi?cmd=Retrieve&db=pubmed&dopt=Abstract&list_uids=14695750

- **Topical antibiotics before cataract surgery.**
  Author(s): Sauer S.
  Source: Jama : the Journal of the American Medical Association. 2003 December 10; 290(22): 2937-8; Author Reply 2937-8.
  http://www.ncbi.nlm.nih.gov/entrez/query.fcgi?cmd=Retrieve&db=pubmed&dopt=Abstract&list_uids=14665647

- **Topical ketorolac tromethamine 0.5% versus diclofenac sodium 0.1% to inhibit miosis during cataract surgery.**
  Author(s): Srinivasan R, Madhavaranga.
  Source: Journal of Cataract and Refractive Surgery. 2002 March; 28(3): 517-20.
  http://www.ncbi.nlm.nih.gov/entrez/query.fcgi?cmd=Retrieve&db=pubmed&dopt=Abstract&list_uids=11973101

- **Topical naproxen sodium for inhibition of miosis during cataract surgery. Prospective, randomized clinical trials.**
  Author(s): Papa V, Russo S, Russo P, Di Bella A, Santocono M, Milazzo G; Naproxen Study Group.
  Source: Eye (London, England). 2002 May; 16(3): 292-6.
  http://www.ncbi.nlm.nih.gov/entrez/query.fcgi?cmd=Retrieve&db=pubmed&dopt=Abstract&list_uids=12032720

- **Two-incision push-pull capsulorhexis for pediatric cataract surgery.**
  Author(s): Nischal KK.
  Source: Journal of Cataract and Refractive Surgery. 2002 April; 28(4): 593-5.
  http://www.ncbi.nlm.nih.gov/entrez/query.fcgi?cmd=Retrieve&db=pubmed&dopt=Abstract&list_uids=11955896

- **Ultrasound biomicroscopy of the anterior segment after congenital cataract surgery.**
  Author(s): Nishijima K, Takahashi K, Yamakawa R.
  Source: American Journal of Ophthalmology. 2000 October; 130(4): 483-9.
  http://www.ncbi.nlm.nih.gov/entrez/query.fcgi?cmd=Retrieve&db=pu bmed&dopt=Abstract&list_uids=11024421

- **Underestimation of intraocular lens power for cataract surgery after myopic photorefractive keratectomy.**
  Author(s): Seitz B, Langenbucher A, Nguyen NX, Kus MM, Kuchle M.
  Source: Ophthalmology. 1999 April; 106(4): 693-702.
  http://www.ncbi.nlm.nih.gov/entrez/query.fcgi?cmd=Retrieve&db=pu bmed&dopt=Abstract&list_uids=10201589

- **Underestimation of intraocular lens power for cataract surgery after myopic PRK.**
  Author(s): Coulibaly R.
  Source: Ophthalmology. 2000 February; 107(2): 222-3.
  http://www.ncbi.nlm.nih.gov/entrez/query.fcgi?cmd=Retrieve&db=pu bmed&dopt=Abstract&list_uids=10690809

- **Unilateral endophthalmitis after simultaneous bilateral cataract surgery.**
  Author(s): Bayramlar H, Keskin UC.
  Source: Journal of Cataract and Refractive Surgery. 2002 September; 28(9): 1502.
  http://www.ncbi.nlm.nih.gov/entrez/query.fcgi?cmd=Retrieve&db=pu bmed&dopt=Abstract&list_uids=12231296

- **Update on a long-term, prospective study of capsulotomy and retinal detachment rates after cataract surgery.**
  Author(s): Olsen G, Olson RJ.
  Source: Journal of Cataract and Refractive Surgery. 2000 July; 26(7): 1017-21.
  http://www.ncbi.nlm.nih.gov/entrez/query.fcgi?cmd=Retrieve&db=pu bmed&dopt=Abstract&list_uids=10946193

- **Use of a wick to deliver preoperative mydriatics for cataract surgery.**
  Author(s): Ong-Tone L.
  Source: Journal of Cataract and Refractive Surgery. 2003 November; 29(11): 2060-2.
  http://www.ncbi.nlm.nih.gov/entrez/query.fcgi?cmd=Retrieve&db=pubmed&dopt=Abstract&list_uids=14670412

- **Use of clonidine as a component of the peribulbar block in patients undergoing cataract surgery.**
  Author(s): Connelly NR, Camerlenghi G, Bilodeau M, Hall S, Reuben SS, Papale J.
  Source: Regional Anesthesia and Pain Medicine. 1999 September-October; 24(5): 426-9.
  http://www.ncbi.nlm.nih.gov/entrez/query.fcgi?cmd=Retrieve&db=pubmed&dopt=Abstract&list_uids=10499754

- **Use of piritramide for analgesia and sedation during peribulbar nerve block for cataract surgery.**
  Author(s): Reinhardt S, Burkhardt U, Nestler A, Wiedemann R.
  Source: Ophthalmologica. Journal International D'ophtalmologie. International Journal of Ophthalmology. Zeitschrift Fur Augenheilkunde. 2002 July-August; 216(4): 256-60.
  http://www.ncbi.nlm.nih.gov/entrez/query.fcgi?cmd=Retrieve&db=pubmed&dopt=Abstract&list_uids=12207128

- **Use of vision tests in clinical decision making about cataract surgery: results of a national survey.**
  Author(s): Frost NA, Sparrow JM.
  Source: The British Journal of Ophthalmology. 2000 April; 84(4): 432-4. Erratum In: Br J Ophthalmol 2000 September; 84(9): 1085.
  http://www.ncbi.nlm.nih.gov/entrez/query.fcgi?cmd=Retrieve&db=pubmed&dopt=Abstract&list_uids=10729305

- **Uveal effusion after cataract surgery: an echographic study.**
  Author(s): Sabti K, Lindley SK, Mansour M, Discepola M.
  Source: Ophthalmology. 2001 January; 108(1): 100-3.
  http://www.ncbi.nlm.nih.gov/entrez/query.fcgi?cmd=Retrieve&db=pubmed&dopt=Abstract&list_uids=11150272

- **Validity of a personal and family history of cataract and cataract surgery in genetic studies.**
  Author(s): Bowie H, Congdon NG, Lai H, West SK.
  Source: Investigative Ophthalmology & Visual Science. 2003 July; 44(7): 2905-8.
  http://www.ncbi.nlm.nih.gov/entrez/query.fcgi?cmd=Retrieve&db=pubmed&dopt=Abstract&list_uids=12824230

- **Variation in coronary artery bypass grafting, angioplasty, cataract surgery, and hip replacement rates among primary care groups in London: association with population and practice characteristics.**
  Author(s): Majeed A, Eliahoo J, Bardsley M, Morgan D, Bindman AB.
  Source: Journal of Public Health Medicine. 2002 March; 24(1): 21-6.
  http://www.ncbi.nlm.nih.gov/entrez/query.fcgi?cmd=Retrieve&db=pubmed&dopt=Abstract&list_uids=11939378

- **Views of older people on cataract surgery options: an assessment of preferences by conjoint analysis.**
  Author(s): Ross MA, Avery AJ, Foss AJ.
  Source: Quality & Safety in Health Care. 2003 February; 12(1): 13-7.
  http://www.ncbi.nlm.nih.gov/entrez/query.fcgi?cmd=Retrieve&db=pubmed&dopt=Abstract&list_uids=12571339

- **Visual function and outcomes after cataract surgery in a Singapore population.**
  Author(s): Saw SM, Tseng P, Chan WK, Chan TK, Ong SG, Tan D.
  Source: Journal of Cataract and Refractive Surgery. 2002 March; 28(3): 445-53.
  http://www.ncbi.nlm.nih.gov/entrez/query.fcgi?cmd=Retrieve&db=pubmed&dopt=Abstract&list_uids=11973091

- **Visual functional outcomes of cataract surgery in the United States, Canada, Denmark, and Spain: report of the International Cataract Surgery Outcomes Study.**
  Author(s): Norregaard JC, Bernth-Petersen P, Alonso J, Andersen TF, Anderson GF.
  Source: Journal of Cataract and Refractive Surgery. 2003 November; 29(11): 2135-42.
  http://www.ncbi.nlm.nih.gov/entrez/query.fcgi?cmd=Retrieve&db=pubmed&dopt=Abstract&list_uids=14670422

- **Visual outcome after high volume cataract surgery in Pakistan.**
  Author(s): Malik AR, Qazi ZA, Gilbert C.
  Source: The British Journal of Ophthalmology. 2003 August; 87(8): 937-40.
  http://www.ncbi.nlm.nih.gov/entrez/query.fcgi?cmd=Retrieve&db=pu
  bmed&dopt=Abstract&list_uids=12881328

- **Visual outcome of cataract surgery in children with congenital rubella syndrome.**
  Author(s): Vijayalakshmi P, Srivastava KK, Poornima B, Nirmalan P.
  Source: J Aapos. 2003 April; 7(2): 91-5.
  http://www.ncbi.nlm.nih.gov/entrez/query.fcgi?cmd=Retrieve&db=pu
  bmed&dopt=Abstract&list_uids=12736620

- **Visual outcomes after vitreous loss during cataract surgery performed by residents.**
  Author(s): Blomquist PH, Rugwani RM.
  Source: Journal of Cataract and Refractive Surgery. 2002 May; 28(5): 847-52.
  http://www.ncbi.nlm.nih.gov/entrez/query.fcgi?cmd=Retrieve&db=pu
  bmed&dopt=Abstract&list_uids=11978467

- **Visual perception during phacoemulsification cataract surgery under subtenons anaesthesia.**
  Author(s): Wickremasinghe SS, Tranos PG, Sinclair N, Andreou PS, Harris ML, Little BC.
  Source: Eye (London, England). 2003 May; 17(4): 501-5.
  http://www.ncbi.nlm.nih.gov/entrez/query.fcgi?cmd=Retrieve&db=pu
  bmed&dopt=Abstract&list_uids=12802351

- **Visual perception during phacoemulsification cataract surgery under topical and regional anaesthesia.**
  Author(s): Tranos PG, Wickremasinghe SS, Sinclair N, Foster PJ, Asaria R, Harris ML, Little BC.
  Source: Acta Ophthalmologica Scandinavica. 2003 April; 81(2): 118-22.
  http://www.ncbi.nlm.nih.gov/entrez/query.fcgi?cmd=Retrieve&db=pu
  bmed&dopt=Abstract&list_uids=12752048

- **Waiting in the dark: cataract surgery in older people.**
  Author(s): Gray CS, Crabtree HL, O'Connell JE, Allen ED.
  Source: Bmj (Clinical Research Ed.). 1999 May 22; 318(7195): 1367-8.
  http://www.ncbi.nlm.nih.gov/entrez/query.fcgi?cmd=Retrieve&db=pu
  bmed&dopt=Abstract&list_uids=10334727

- **Warfarin therapy and cataract surgery.**
  Author(s): Morris A, Elder MJ.
  Source: Clinical & Experimental Ophthalmology. 2000 December; 28(6): 419-22.
  http://www.ncbi.nlm.nih.gov/entrez/query.fcgi?cmd=Retrieve&db=pubmed&dopt=Abstract&list_uids=11202464

- **Warm balanced salt solution for clearing tear film precipitation during cataract surgery.**
  Author(s): Otto CS, McMann MA, Parmley VC, Dahlhauser KF, Bushley DM, Carroll RB.
  Source: Journal of Cataract and Refractive Surgery. 2002 August; 28(8): 1318-9.
  http://www.ncbi.nlm.nih.gov/entrez/query.fcgi?cmd=Retrieve&db=pubmed&dopt=Abstract&list_uids=12160797

- **Water modulation of lens epithelial cells during cataract surgery.**
  Author(s): Crowston JG, Maloof A, Healey PR, Neilson G, Milverton EJ.
  Source: Journal of Cataract and Refractive Surgery. 2003 December; 29(12): 2464-5.
  http://www.ncbi.nlm.nih.gov/entrez/query.fcgi?cmd=Retrieve&db=pubmed&dopt=Abstract&list_uids=14709318

- **Wavefront technology in cataract surgery.**
  Author(s): Packer M, Fine IH, Hoffman RS.
  Source: Current Opinion in Ophthalmology. 2004 February; 15(1): 56-60. Review.
  http://www.ncbi.nlm.nih.gov/entrez/query.fcgi?cmd=Retrieve&db=pubmed&dopt=Abstract&list_uids=14743021

- **What is the risk of complications from cataract surgery in patients taking anticoagulants?**
  Author(s): Langston RH.
  Source: Cleve Clin J Med. 2001 February; 68(2): 97-8. No Abstract Available.
  http://www.ncbi.nlm.nih.gov/entrez/query.fcgi?cmd=Retrieve&db=pubmed&dopt=Abstract&list_uids=11220461

- **What patients want to know before they have cataract surgery.**
  Author(s): Elder MJ, Suter A.
  Source: The British Journal of Ophthalmology. 2004 March; 88(3): 331-2.
  http://www.ncbi.nlm.nih.gov/entrez/query.fcgi?cmd=Retrieve&db=pu
  bmed&dopt=Abstract&list_uids=14977762

- **Willingness to pay for cataract surgery in Kathmandu valley.**
  Author(s): Shrestha MK, Thakur J, Gurung CK, Joshi AB, Pokhrel S, Ruit S.
  Source: The British Journal of Ophthalmology. 2004 March; 88(3): 319-20.
  http://www.ncbi.nlm.nih.gov/entrez/query.fcgi?cmd=Retrieve&db=pu
  bmed&dopt=Abstract&list_uids=14977759

- **Wound complications associated with incision enlargement for foldable intraocular lens implantation during cataract surgery.**
  Author(s): Kumar R, Reeves DL, Olson RJ.
  Source: Journal of Cataract and Refractive Surgery. 2001 February; 27(2): 224-6.
  http://www.ncbi.nlm.nih.gov/entrez/query.fcgi?cmd=Retrieve&db=pu
  bmed&dopt=Abstract&list_uids=11226786

- **Wound complications following cataract surgery. A case-control study.**
  Author(s): Arango JL, Margo CE.
  Source: Archives of Ophthalmology. 1998 August; 116(8): 1021-4.
  http://www.ncbi.nlm.nih.gov/entrez/query.fcgi?cmd=Retrieve&db=pu
  bmed&dopt=Abstract&list_uids=9715681

Vocabulary Builder

Abscess: A localized, circumscribed collection of pus. [NIH]

Adjustment: The dynamic process wherein the thoughts, feelings, behavior, and biophysiological mechanisms of the individual continually change to adjust to the environment. [NIH]

Antibiotic: A substance usually produced by vegetal micro-organisms capable of inhibiting the growth of or killing bacteria. [NIH]

Applicability: A list of the commodities to which the candidate method can be applied as presented or with minor modifications. [NIH]

Breakdown: A physical, metal, or nervous collapse. [NIH]

Catheters: A small, flexible tube that may be inserted into various parts of the body to inject or remove liquids. [NIH]

Consumption: Pulmonary tuberculosis. [NIH]

Cystoid: Like a bladder or a cyst. [NIH]

Cytokine: Small but highly potent protein that modulates the activity of many cell types, including T and B cells. [NIH]

Density: The logarithm to the base 10 of the opacity of an exposed and processed film. [NIH]

Diaphragm: Contraceptive intra-uterine device. [NIH]

Dissection: Cutting up of an organism for study. [NIH]

Duke: A lamp which produces ultraviolet radiations for certain ophthalmologic therapy. [NIH]

Effector: It is often an enzyme that converts an inactive precursor molecule into an active second messenger. [NIH]

Enhancer: Transcriptional element in the virus genome. [NIH]

Epstein: Failure of the upper eyelid to move downward on downward movement of the eye, occurring in premature and nervous infants. [NIH]

Grafting: The operation of transfer of tissue from one site to another. [NIH]

Growth: The progressive development of a living being or part of an organism from its earliest stage to maturity. [NIH]

Host: Any animal that receives a transplanted graft. [NIH]

Hyaluronidase: An enzyme that splits hyaluronic acid and thus lowers the viscosity of the acid and facilitates the spreading of fluids through tissues either advantageously or disadvantageously. [NIH]

Infections: The illnesses caused by an organism that usually does not cause disease in a person with a normal immune system. [NIH]

Insight: The capacity to understand one's own motives, to be aware of one's own psychodynamics, to appreciate the meaning of symbolic behavior. [NIH]

Jefferson: A fracture produced by a compressive downward force that is transmitted evenly through occipital condyles to superior articular surfaces of the lateral masses of C1. [NIH]

Koch: It was an early form of tuberculin of low specificity, devised by Robert Koch and made by heat concentration of a broth culture of Mycobacterium tuberculosis. [NIH]

Linkage: The tendency of two or more genes in the same chromosome to remain together from one generation to the next more frequently than expected according to the law of independent assortment. [NIH]

Microsurgery: Surgical procedures on the cellular level; a light microscope and miniaturized instruments are used. [NIH]

Migration: The systematic movement of genes between populations of the same species, geographic race, or variety. [NIH]

Morphological: Relating to the configuration or the structure of live organs. [NIH]

Neutrophil: A motile, short-lived polymorphonuclear leucocyte with a multilobed nucleus and a cytoplasm filled with numerous minute granules, which is primarily responsible for maintaining normal host defenses against invading microorganisms. [NIH]

Nystagmus: Rhythmical oscillation of the eyeballs, either pendular or jerky. [NIH]

Opacity: Degree of density (area most dense taken for reading). [NIH]

Pathologies: The study of abnormality, especially the study of diseases. [NIH]

Pharmacokinetic: The mathematical analysis of the time courses of absorption, distribution, and elimination of drugs. [NIH]

Phosphorylated: Attached to a phosphate group. [NIH]

Protocol: The detailed plan for a clinical trial that states the trial's rationale, purpose, drug or vaccine dosages, length of study, routes of administration, who may participate, and other aspects of trial design. [NIH]

Psychoactive: Those drugs which alter sensation, mood, consciousness or other psychological or behavioral functions. [NIH]

Reassurance: A procedure in psychotherapy that seeks to give the client confidence in a favorable outcome. It makes use of suggestion, of the prestige of the therapist. [NIH]

Reliability: Used technically, in a statistical sense, of consistency of a test with itself, i. e. the extent to which we can assume that it will yield the same result if repeated a second time. [NIH]

Restoration: Broad term applied to any inlay, crown, bridge or complete denture which restores or replaces loss of teeth or oral tissues. [NIH]

Retractor: An instrument designed for pulling aside tissues to improve exposure at operation; an instrument for drawing back the edge of a wound. [NIH]

Sensor: A device designed to respond to physical stimuli such as temperature, light, magnetism or movement and transmit resulting impulses for interpretation, recording, movement, or operating control. [NIH]

Sinclair: A special glue for applying extension in fractures. [NIH]

Snellen: Congestion of the ear from stimulating of the cut end of the great auricular nerve. [NIH]

Spike: The activation of synapses causes changes in the permeability of the dendritic membrane leading to changes in the membrane potential. This difference of the potential travels along the axon of the neuron and is called spike. [NIH]

Streptococci: A genus of spherical Gram-positive bacteria occurring in chains or pairs. They are widely distributed in nature, being important pathogens but often found as normal commensals in the mouth, skin, and intestine of humans and other animals. [NIH]

Temporal: One of the two irregular bones forming part of the lateral surfaces and base of the skull, and containing the organs of hearing. [NIH]

Threshold: For a specified sensory modality (e. g. light, sound, vibration), the lowest level (absolute threshold) or smallest difference (difference threshold, difference limen) or intensity of the stimulus discernible in prescribed conditions of stimulation. [NIH]

Thrush: A disease due to infection with species of fungi of the genus Candida. [NIH]

Ubiquitin: A highly conserved 76 amino acid-protein found in all eukaryotic cells. [NIH]

Vitreoretinal: A rare familial condition characterized by a clear vitreous, except for preretinal filaments and veils which have been loosened from the retina, a dense hyaloid membrane which is perforated and detached, and masses of peripheral retinal pigmentation inters. [NIH]

Vitro: Descriptive of an event or enzyme reaction under experimental investigation occurring outside a living organism. Parts of an organism or microorganism are used together with artificial substrates and/or conditions. [NIH]

Vivo: Outside of or removed from the body of a living organism. [NIH]

Wound: Any interruption, by violence or by surgery, in the continuity of the external surface of the body or of the surface of any internal organ. [NIH]

CHAPTER 4. PATENTS ON CATARACT SURGERY

Overview

You can learn about innovations relating to cataract surgery by reading recent patents and patent applications. Patents can be physical innovations (e.g. chemicals, pharmaceuticals, medical equipment) or processes (e.g. treatments or diagnostic procedures). The United States Patent and Trademark Office defines a patent as a grant of a property right to the inventor, issued by the Patent and Trademark Office.[18] Patents, therefore, are intellectual property. For the United States, the term of a new patent is 20 years from the date when the patent application was filed. If the inventor wishes to receive economic benefits, it is likely that the invention will become commercially available to patients within 20 years of the initial filing. It is important to understand, therefore, that an inventor's patent does not indicate that a product or service is or will be commercially available to patients. The patent implies only that the inventor has "the right to exclude others from making, using, offering for sale, or selling" the invention in the United States. While this relates to U.S. patents, similar rules govern foreign patents.

In this chapter, we show you how to locate information on patents and their inventors. If you find a patent that is particularly interesting to you, contact the inventor or the assignee for further information.

---

[18]Adapted from The U. S. Patent and Trademark Office: **http://www.uspto.gov/web/offices/pac/doc/general/whatis.htm.**

Patents on Cataract Surgery

By performing a patent search focusing on cataract surgery, you can obtain information such as the title of the invention, the names of the inventor(s), the assignee(s) or the company that owns or controls the patent, a short abstract that summarizes the patent, and a few excerpts from the description of the patent. The abstract of a patent tends to be more technical in nature, while the description is often written for the public. Full patent descriptions contain much more information than is presented here (e.g. claims, references, figures, diagrams, etc.). We will tell you how to obtain this information later in the chapter. The following is an example of the type of information that you can expect to obtain from a patent search on cataract surgery:

- **Accommodative intraocular lens system**

  Inventor(s): Preussner; Paul Rolf (Am Linsenberg 18, D-55131 Mainz, DE)

  Assignee(s): None Reported

  Patent Number: 6,645,245

  Date filed: June 29, 2001

  Abstract: Disclosed is an implant for implantation in the human eye, which enables natural adjustment of the eye to different distances (accommodation) after **cataract surgery** (lens opacity). Permanent magnets (inner magnets) rest on the periphery of the intraocular lens located inside the capsular sack. Two additional permanent magnets that are fixed to the sclera (outer magnets) are located opposite to said inner magnets and slightly staggered to the back. The inner and outer magnets are polarized and geometrically disposed in such a way that they repel one another. Said repulsion effects a forward movement of the capsular sack and the lens located therein when the ciliary muscle contracts. Before placing the outer magnets, a measurement can be conducted with the aid of electromagnets whose strength can be regulated, whereby accommodation is determined as a function of the strength of the outer magnets. On the basis of the data obtained during said measurement, the strength, number, geometry and position of the outer (permanent) magnets can be selected.

  Excerpt(s): The invention is an intraocular lens with accompanying auxiliary devices by means of which a patient once again gains the capability of optical near vision (accommodation) through and after an operation on the natural lens.... Intraocular lenses which are in accordance with the state of technology normally only allow sharp vision at exactly one distance. In addition, for some years, intraocular lenses have been known which have two or more focal distances ("multifocal lenses") and thus allow sharp vision at several distances. As several images are hereby superimposed indistinctly, the contrast with these lenses is markedly worse than with a monofocal lens. Also, it is only possible to see sharply at certain distances, the intermediate area is markedly more indistinct. Vision, as in the case of natural accommodation, can thus not be attained with these lenses.... Systems in which the refractive power of the intraocular implant can be adjusted by external measures represent an intermediate notional step towards accommodation. The optical elements can here be shifted on the optical axis by changing the posture of the head, by means of gravity or by magnetic forces (US5326347A, US5593437A). In the latter case, a magnetic layer is applied to the intraocular lens and the lens is moved by an adjustable magnet which is positioned in front of the eye in a kind of spectacles. In US5800533A, the shift on the optical axis is induced by means of a screw thread, whereby the screwing process is carried out by means of magnetic tools from outside of the eye.

Web site: http://www.delphion.com/details?pn=US06645245__

- **Anterior capsular punch with deformable cutting member**

Inventor(s): Lehmer; Lara (3301 S. Sepulveda Blvd., No. 13, Los Angeles, CA 90034)

Assignee(s): None Reported

Patent Number: 5,135,530

Date filed: November 12, 1991

Abstract: The present invention is an anterior capsular incising apparatus having a pair of crisscrossing arms hinged at a crisscross joint and each having a forward portion and a rearward portion and a deformable circular cutting ring having a sharp bottom circular cutting edge detachably mounted onto and between the forward portions of the pair of crisscross arms, such that the deformable circular cutting ring can be compressed into a narrow elliptical shape by squeezing the rearward portions of the pair of crisscrossing arms. The present invention anterior capsular incising method utilizes the deformable circular cutting ring in **cataract surgery** and includes compressing the deformable circular cutting ring into a narrow elliptical shape, inserting it into the anterior chamber of an eye through a narrow wound cut on the corneoscleral tissue of the eye, allowing it to fully return to its original configuration once inside the anterior chamber, cutting an incision on the anterior lens capsule of the eye, compressing it into the narrow elliptical shape again, and withdrawing it from the anterior chamber through the narrow wound on the corneoscleral tissue.

Excerpt(s): The present invention relates to the field of apparatus for ophthalmic surgery. More particularly, the present invention relates to the field of apparatus for **cataract surgery...** In many types of ophthalmic surgery, it is often necessary to incise the anterior lens capsule of the crystalline lens of an eye to provide an opening on the anterior lens capsule so that the cataractous opaque lens can be removed. However, the anterior lens capsule of the eye is shielded by the corneal tissue. Therefore, before any cataract surgical apparatus can reach the anterior lens capsule of the eye, a passage wound has to be cut in the corneal tissue. After the **cataract surgery,** the corneal wound is closed with sutures.... The following prior art patents are found to be related to the field of surgical apparatus used in cataract surgeries.

Web site: http://www.delphion.com/details?pn=US05135530__

- **Antipyretic and analgesic methods using optically pure R-ketorolac**

Inventor(s): Barberich; Timothy J. (Concord, MA), Matson; Stephen L. (Harvard, MA), Wechter; William J. (Redlands, CA)

Assignee(s): Sepracor Inc. (marlborough, Ma)

Patent Number: 5,382,591

Date filed: September 8, 1993

Abstract: Methods are disclosed utilizing optically pure R-ketorolac for the treatment of pain, including but not limited to pain associated with toothaches, headaches, sprains, joint pain and surgical pain, for example dental pain (e.g., after periodontal surgery) and ophthalmic pain (e.g., after cataract surgery) while avoiding adverse effects which are associated with the administration of the racemic mixture of ketorolac. The optically pure R-ketorolac is also useful in treating pyrexia while avoiding the adverse effects associated with the administration of the racemic mixture of ketorolac.

Excerpt(s): This invention relates to novel compositions of matter containing optically pure R-ketorolac. These compositions possess potent activity in treating pain, including but not limited to pain associated with toothaches, headaches, sprains, joint pain and surgical pain, for example dental pain (e.g., after periodontal surgery) and ophthalmic pain (e.g., after cataract surgery) while avoiding adverse effects including but not limited to gastrointestinal, renal and hepatic toxicities, which are associated with the administration of the racemic mixture of ketorolac.

Additionally, these novel compositions of matter containing optically pure R-ketorolac are useful in treating or preventing pyrexia while avoiding the adverse effects associated with the administration of the racemic mixture of ketorolac. Also disclosed are methods for treating the above-described conditions in a human while avoiding the adverse effects that are associated with the racemic mixture of ketorolac, by administering the R-isomer of ketorolac to said human.... The active compound of these compositions and methods is an optical isomer of ketorolac. This compound is described in U.S. Pat. No. 4,089,969. Chemically, the active compound is the R-isomer of 5-benzoyl-1,2-dihydro-3H-pyrrolo[1,2-a]pyrrole-1-carboxylic acid, hereinafter referred to as R-ketorolac. The terms "R-isomer of ketorolac" and "R-ketorolac" encompass both the optically pure and the substantially optically pure compositions.... Ketorolac is available commercially only as the 1:1 racemic mixture. That is, it is available only as a mixture of optical isomers, called enantiomers.

Web site: http://www.delphion.com/details?pn=US05382591__

- **Apparatus for folding flexible intraocular lenses**

Inventor(s): Tunis; Scott W. (2000 NE 49th St., Ft. Lauderdale, FL)

Assignee(s): None Reported

Patent Number: 5,549,614

Date filed: December 27, 1994

Abstract: Apparatus for and methods of preparing and inserting flexible intraocular lenses, through incisions in ocular tissue made during phacoemulsification **cataract surgery.** The incisions are preferably no longer than 3 mm. The intraocular lens is placed on a template which facilitates multiple folding of the intraocular lens. Multiple folds in the lens are then accomplished with the template providing necessary and proper orientation, stabilization, and positioning of the lens. The intraocular lens folded using the template is held with a lens-insertion forceps and is inserted and released inside the eye, whereupon the lens unfolds in its proper position and configuration inside the eye. An intraocular lens having both plate haptics and J-style or C-style haptics is provided.

Excerpt(s): The present invention relates to the methods of and apparatus for preparing and inserting flexible intraocular lenses used in the field of ophthalmology wherein flexible intraocular lenses made of silicone and/or other deformable materials are inserted into the eye to replace natural lenses during **cataract surgery,** and to a configuration for flexible intraocular lenses. More particularly, the invention relates to methods, apparatus and lenses used in the field of ophthalmology wherein flexible intraocular lenses made of silicone and/or other deformable materials are inserted into the eye to replace the natural lens during **cataract surgery...** In **cataract surgery,** a cataractous human lens is removed through a 3 mm or larger incision by phacoemulsification. A prosthetic intraocular lens is then substituted for the human lens. The intraocular lens obviates the patient's need for a high dioptric power spectacle correction after surgery, which would otherwise be necessary.... Intraocular lenses may be made of flexible materials such as silicone. Although lenses made of these materials have dimensions in their uncompressed state which are larger than 3 mm, such lenses may be folded in various configurations and inserted through 3 mm or slightly larger incisions. When using flexible intraocular lenses, surgical incisions necessary for performing **cataract surgery** need not be enlarged following phacoemulsification. Accordingly, surgically induced trauma is minimized, healing and convalescence time are reduced, visual recovery for the patient is expedited, and the chance of intraoperative and postoperative complications relative to the wound are minimized.

Web site: http://www.delphion.com/details?pn=US05549614__

- **Buffer-containing devices for preventing clouding of posterior capsule after extracapsular cataract eye surgery and method of performing cataract surgery**

Inventor(s): Dubroff; Seymour (3806 Thornapple St., Chevy Chase, MD 20815)

Assignee(s): None Reported

Patent Number: 5,188,590

Date filed: March 26, 1991

Abstract: The present invention relates to devices for killing undifferentiated epithelial cells during **cataract surgery** on an eye to prevent posterior capsule clouding after the surgery and to a method for performing **cataract surgery** on an eye including injecting a cell-killing substance between the anterior capsule and the natural lens prior to removing the natural lens from the eye. The cell-killing substance is preferably an acid or base adjusted, aqueous, buffer-containing a solution having a pH in the range between about 1.0 to below 6.5 or about above 7.5 to 14.0 or a buffer-containing hypotonic solution having a salinity less than 0.06%. The devices of the present invention optionally incorporate a viscoelastic material, a dye or a mixture thereof, in combination with the cell-killing substance.

Excerpt(s): The present invention pertains to **cataract surgery** and, more particularly, to the prevention of clouding of the posterior capsule after extracapsular **cataract extraction**..... Clouding of the posterior capsule after extracapsular **cataract extraction,** with or without the implant of an intraocular lens, has been a principal, later occurring, complication of such extracapsular **cataract surgery.** During **cataract surgery,** it is preferable to extract the natural lens while leaving the posterior portion of the lens capsule intact in front of the vitreous cavity of the eye to provide a barrier to prevent anterior movement or loss of the vitreous which fills the cavity and to also provide a support for an intraocular lens implanted in the posterior chamber. If the natural lens is removed intact with the capsule, referred to as intracapsular **cataract extraction,** the vitreous can move through the pupil causing vitreous loss and increasing the chances of complications, such as glaucoma, corneal opacity, displacement of an intraocular lens, retinal hemorrhage, holes, breaks and detachment, and cystoid macula edema.... In many cases after extracapsular **cataract extraction,** with or without the implant of an intraocular lens, the posterior capsule becomes opacified or clouded due to migration of proliferating undifferentiated epithelial cells into the optical zone which, clustered, form Elschnig's pearls. Along with Elschnig's pearls, visual acuity is also reduced by invading fibroblasts through metaplasia developing into myoepithelial fibers, lens fibers, collagen, fibrosis and Sommering rings. This opacification or clouding of the posterior capsule, referred to as secondary cataract, occurs in a large percentage of extracapsular cataract extractions and is a primary cause of post operative complications.

Web site: http://www.delphion.com/details?pn=US05188590__

- **Capsular adhesion preventing ring**

  Inventor(s): Nagamoto; Toshiyuki (2-29-23 Nozawa Setagaya, Tokyo 154, JP)

  Assignee(s): None Reported

  Patent Number: 6,063,118

  Date filed: April 9, 1998

  Abstract: The capsular adhesion preventing ring includes a wristband-like member having a diameter larger than that of an anterior capsular opening. The ring has multiple engaging holes and multiple guide slots formed through the circumferential wall of the ring, and each guide slot extends from the lower or upper rims of the ring to a corresponding engaging hole. In this ring, each guide slot may have a slant angle to the rim of the ring, be opened to a corresponding engaging hole along a cutting line of the hole, and an engaging protrusion may be formed between the guide slot and engaging hole. The direction of the engaging holes and guide slots from inside to outside of the wall may be almost parallel to the direction of a corresponding part of the loops of the intraocular lens that is inserted into the capsular bag before the insertion of the ring. This ring prevents adhesion of the capsular bag, which is adopted to prevent adhesion of the anterior and posterior lens capsules at the incised edge of the anterior capsule after **cataract surgery,** and also prevents lens regeneration, so as to prevent secondary cataracts.

Excerpt(s): The present invention relates to a ring for preventing adhesion of the capsular bag of the crystalline lens, which contributes to prevent secondary cataracts that is a postoperative complication after **cataract surgery**... When visual function or acuity is declined because of cataract, a general method to improve the impaired vision is a surgery. In the current cataract surgeries, an intraocular lens is inserted into the capsular bag after removal of the central anterior lens capsule, lens nucleus and cortex, so as to substitute for the refractive function of the crystalline lens.... As one of the postoperative problems, opacification frequently occurs along the capsular bag, and visual function or acuity is impaired if the opacity reaches the pupillary area. This is called secondary cataracts or after-cataracts. The reduction of visual function due to the secondary cataracts has been a serious problem in the medical field though there have been no effective preventions for surely avoiding occurrence of the secondary cataract.

Web site: http://www.delphion.com/details?pn=US06063118__

- **Cataract disassembly**

  Inventor(s): Steinert; Roger F. (83 Sandra La., North Andover, MA 01845)

  Assignee(s): None Reported

  Patent Number: 5,451,230

  Date filed: October 11, 1994

  Abstract: An instrument to facilitate nuclear disassembly during **cataract surgery** includes a proximal handle, a shaft portion axially aligned with the proximal handle, an intermediate portion constructed to traverse the cortex of the eye, and a hook-form distal end. An inner region of the hook-form has a leading edge defined by diverging surfaces. The diverging surfaces lie at an acute splitting angle to one another selected to have a wedging effect when the leading edge is drawn along a cleavage plane of the nucleus. The diverging surfaces define a relatively bulky back portion that imparts desired stiffness to the leading edge. The hook-form is shaped to facilitate maintaining contact with the nucleus while the leading edge is drawn along the cleavage plane. A method of performing nuclear disassembly during **cataract surgery** utilizing the instrument is also described.

Excerpt(s): This invention relates in general to instruments and methods of removing a cataractous lens. More particularly, it relates to an instrument and method for cataract disassembly.... Clouding of the natural crystalline lens of the eye is termed "cataract formation". To restore vision, the cataractous lens must be removed. It has been known to perform **cataract surgery** using a technique which "disassembles" the hard central nucleus of the lens into a number of fragments to be removed progressively from the eye. The nucleus is disassembled using a bent wire hook made out of round stiff surgical wire material and the resulting pieces of the lens nucleus are aspirated. Typically the lens is stabilized by a phacoemulsifier while the hook is drawn across the nucleus. The hook has typically been of approximate "L" shape, with a portion extending at substantially a right angle to the shaft of the instrument.... In order to disassemble the appropriate size nuclear fragments without encountering difficulties in containing the nuclear fragments within the posterior capsular sac away from the corneal endothelium, it has been known to create a central trough or crater in the nucleus using the phacoemulsifier alone or in combination with the hook, followed by splitting the nucleus into two halves with the hook. These two large nuclear pieces, due to their bulk, remain stable within the posterior capsular sac. The hook is drawn across the nuclear pieces following the natural cleavage planes progressively splitting off only small wedges in a circumferential direction. Although the technique as described has had a modicum of success, difficulties have been encountered in that the hook has tended to slip and lose contact with the nucleus during the drawing motion.

Web site: http://www.delphion.com/details?pn=US05451230__

- **Device for testing vision potential**

  Inventor(s): Hofeldt; Albert J. (200 E. 57th St., New York, NY 10022)

  Assignee(s): None Reported

  Patent Number: 5,398,085

  Date filed: May 14, 1993

Abstract: A device for testing vision potential of humans comprises an enclosure containing two transparent areas through one surface, two pairs of rollers, means for turning one of the rollers, a length of material fitted around the two pairs of rollers in snug engagement therewith so that by operating the means for turning one of the rollers the material moves around the two pairs of rollers, said material having a series of vision testing lines of indicia sized to test visual acuity from 20/20 to 20/200, each of said lines being visible in one area and each of said lines having on the material and visible through the other area markings from 20/20 to 20/200. Two sources of illumination are disposed within the enclosure, one illumination source being disposed in a position to illuminate the line of indicia and the other being positioned to illuminate the series of numbers from 20/20 to 20/200. Means for providing sufficient energy to the illumination means to enable them to provide illumination and means for positioning the person to be tested at the desired from the device are provided. The device has particular applicability for determining the vision potential of humans having a cataract in one or both eyes which through utilizing a device with a pinhole through which the person to be tested views the lines of indicia one can accurately determine the visual acuity which will be achieved following **cataract surgery.**

Excerpt(s): The present invention is concerned with a device for accurately testing vision and has particular applicability for testing vision potential following **cataract surgery** for people having cataracts in one or both eyes prior to the surgery.... When there is a vision loss, determining the vision potential after surgery is an important goal of all eye care specialists. Cataracts are a common and correctable cause of vision loss. A cataract is the result of opacification of the lens of the eye. Accurate prediction of the vision potential of patients considered for **cataract surgery** is a challenge to the ophthalmic surgeon. According to Sadun and Libondi (Amer. J. Ophthalmology 110:710-712, 1990), cataracts can reduce 90% of the light from being transmitted through the lens of the eye. If a sufficient quantity of focused light penetrates the cataract an accurate measurement of the visual ability of the retina is possible.... The present invention is based on the provision of a device which contains a brightly illuminated series of lines of indicia which are capable of determining visual acuity from 20/20 to 20/200. When vision loss is due to a mild or moderate opacification in the ocular media, viewing the brightly illuminated indicia in my device can accurately predict the visual potential of the eye being tested after surgery has been performed. In patients with more severe clouding of the ocular media, a device having a pinhole placed in the line of sight can improve focusing while viewing the illuminated lines of indicia. In general, the stenopaeic hole (pinhole) greatly improves visual defects due to refractive anomalies, to a less extent than those due to abnormalities in the media, but does not ameliorate and may even aggravate those due to faulty perception (Duke-Elder, Textbook of Ophthalmology, Vol. IV). The pinhole places the eye in an almost universal depth of focus and allows the near point to be brought close while maintaining image clarity. As the distance of the image decreases the magnification of the retinal image increases (Lebensohn, Amer. J. Ophthalmology 33:1612-1614, 1950). To avoid image magnification that would overestimate the potential visual ability, the working distance for near vision testing must be maintained at a standard distance. While the pinhole improves the focusing, the small aperture of the pinhole reduces the illumination and must be compensated by supplemental lighting of the lines of indicia to ensure the fullest utilization of the pinhole acuity.

Web site: http://www.delphion.com/details?pn=US05398085__

- **Device for treating bodily substances**

  Inventor(s): Donitzky; Christof (Eckental, DE), Pribbernow; Arnold (Simmelsdorf, DE)

  Assignee(s): Wavelight Laser Technologies Gmbh (erlangen, De)

  Patent Number: 6,328,732

  Date filed: June 10, 1999

  Abstract: A device for treating bodily substances, in particular for intraocular **cataract surgery,** said device comprising a laser beam source, for example, an erbium YAG laser, which produces pulsed laser radiation at wavelengths in the infrared range. A control device comprises a first arrangement (38, 48) by means of which an acceptable range for the pulse energy and/or pulse length and/or pulse frequency can be predetermined before an operation, and a second arrangement (34, 36, 40, 42) by means of which the pulse energy and/or pulse length and/or pulse frequency can be adjusted to a given value or values within the predetermined range during the operation.

  Excerpt(s): The invention relates to a device for treating bodily substances, comprising a laser beam source which produces pulsed laser radiation at wavelengths particularly in the infrared range, an arrangement for guiding the laser radiation to the location of treatment, and further comprising a control device by means of which the pulse energy and/or pulse length and/or pulse frequency can be adjusted.... Quite generally, the invention is suitable for treating bodily substances, i.e. producing an effect on bodily substances in many different ways. The term "treatment" may either refer to changing the conditions of these substances, or to removing these substances from the body, or to changing the position of the substances in the body. The bodily substances can be manifold, for example diseased tissue, or a substance generated in diseased form, or tissue which is sound per se but is to be removed for medical reasons. The following is a description of the invention with regard to what is known as intraocular **cataract surgery**... A cataract is a change of the lens of the human eye, resulting in loss of transparency of the visible optical range of the lens. The region of the lens becomes cloudy. Loss of transparency causes impairment of vision.

Web site: http://www.delphion.com/details?pn=US06328732__

- **Fiber optic sleeve for surgical instruments**

Inventor(s): Reynard; Michael (1301 20th St., #260, Santa Monica, CA 90404)

Assignee(s): None Reported

Patent Number: 5,651,783

Date filed: December 20, 1995

Abstract: A fiber optic integrated phacoemulsification system is disclosed comprising surgical handpieces for **cataract surgery** which incorporate fiber optic bundles that transmit visible light to enhance visualization by intraocular illumination. Patient safety is improved by the oblique lighting to the retina, thereby reducing the necessity of direct coaxial light from the surgical microscope. The fiber optic bundles enable the application of laser energy or visible light and permit endoscope visualization of intraocular structures either through the surgical handpiece or through an end piece attachment.

Excerpt(s): This invention relates to surgical devices and, more particularly, to devices for effecting the transmission of light for endoillumination, intraocular endoscopy, or laser application to intraocular tissue.... The most widely accepted prior art means for performing intraocular surgery in the anterior segment of the eye comprise a variety of instruments designed for irrigation, ablation, cutting and removal of tissue. Separate instruments for irrigation, illumination and laser application are known, but they have the disadvantage of requiring multiple surgical openings in the eye and may be cumbersome to operate for the surgeon. Multiple surgical openings in the eye and multiple surgical instruments add to the risk of complications and increase the difficulty of the surgical procedure. Surgical instruments that combine water infusion, suction and light conducting elements in a single probe have been described, but they have the inherent physical limitations imposed by side-by-side conducting channels. Another problem that arises in the use of complex multiple-element surgical instruments is the cost and labor of repeated sterilization.... Examples of ophthalmic instruments of the type described are commercially available from Grieshaber & Co., Inc., 3000 Cabot Boulevard West, Langhorne, Pa. 19047. These are shown in company brochures under the title "The Grieshaber Light Source and Family of Accessories".

Web site: http://www.delphion.com/details?pn=US05651783__

- **Handpiece for cataract surgery**

Inventor(s): Malinowski; Igor (955 Deep Valley Dr., Box No. 2981, Palos Verdes Estates, CA 90274)

Assignee(s): None Reported

Patent Number: 5,453,087

Date filed: November 26, 1993

Abstract: An ultrasonic handpiece for **cataract surgery** comprises a driver assembly (10), a housing (11), a nose part (13, 113) and an end or rear manifold (20) of one-piece construction. Housing (11) includes tubular parts (12, 12' and 14), which are concentrically assembled and attached to and between nose part (13, 113) and rear or end manifold (20). Nose part (13, 113) is provided with a plurality of integral front irrigation holes (19) and end manifold (20) with a plurality of integral irrigation holes (36a, 36b and 36c). The number and inclinations of the irrigation holes permit and maintain a uniform, gradual and substantially unimpeded and high volume flow of irrigation fluid from an irrigation luer fitting (2) into the annular space between tubular parts (12, 12' and 14), resulting in a fluid flow concentric with driver assembly (10) and inside housing (11), thus eliminating any need for external irrigation tubes of conventional handpieces. In one embodiment, outer tube (12, 12') is also capable of being completely removed from the unit comprising nose part (113), inner tube (14) and rear manifold (20) and this unit's internally sealed driver assembly (10), to permit full cleansing of the outer surface of inner tube (14) and the inner surface of outer tube (12, 12') while maintaining the fluid-tight integrity of driver assembly (10).

Excerpt(s): The present invention relates in general to handpieces for **cataract surgery** and, in particular, to ultrasonic handpieces which can be easily cleaned and provide improved and more efficient routing of fluids through irrigation and aspiration channels to and from a patient's eye.... A typical ultrasonic handpiece used in ophthalmic surgery includes a housing, an ultrasonic driver assembly centered within the housing, a rear part or cap at one end of the housing, a front part with a cataract needle at the other end of the housing, and an irrigation conduit extending between the front and the rear parts.... The rear part furnishes irrigating fluid to the front part for supply to the eye, receives the fluid after being flushed through the eye, and seals about an electrical connection between the driver assembly and an exterior source of power. The front part with a cataract needle is adapted to penetrate the patient's eye for supplying ultrasonic vibrations thereto and for channelling the fluid into and out of the eye.

Web site: http://www.delphion.com/details?pn=US05453087___

- **Instrument for fixating the eye during cataract surgery**

Inventor(s): Stamler; John (540 E. Jefferson St., Iowa City, IA 52245)

Assignee(s): None Reported

Patent Number: 6,299,617

Date filed: March 30, 1998

Abstract: A method and apparatus for fixating an eye during ocular surgery, including inserting a two-pronged tool through an incision in the cornea into the anterior chamber. The two prongs prohibit movement of the eye in all directions. An alternate embodiment provides for use of two such two-pronged tools which are coupled together and each of the two-pronged tools is inserted in the incision and help to prohibit movement of the eye.

Excerpt(s): The present invention pertains to instruments for fixating the eye during ocular surgery such as **cataract extraction** by the small incision technique, commonly known as Phacoemulsification or Phaco technique and other operations of the anterior segment of the eye that are performed under local anesthesia.... In recent years, two surgical techniques for removing a cataract from the eye are employed. The large incision technique and the small incision or Phaco technique.... In the large incision technique, an incision (approximately 8-10 mm), almost half of the circumference of the cornea is made, and the cataract is expressed or squeezed out of the eye manually. The advantage with this technique is that it is much easier to perform. The disadvantages are the longer time to recuperate, and it produces more astigmatism.

Web site: http://www.delphion.com/details?pn=US06299617___

- **Instrument for protecting corneal endothelium during cataract surgery**

  Inventor(s): Tan; Ben G. (20924 Kelly Rd., Eastpointe, MI 48021)

  Assignee(s): None Reported

  Patent Number: 5,320,113

  Date filed: April 1, 1993

  Abstract: An instrument and method for protecting the corneal endothelium during **cataract removal** surgery are described. The instrument includes wire legs having curved shielding sections held extending across the endothelium to prevent contact of the cataract nucleus during its removal. An angled tip formed by a wire loop connecting the legs contacts the endothelium and holds the shielding section away. The legs are compressed by squeezing together a pair of leg extensions having pads at the ends to be inserted in a small corneal incision, and a locating section of each leg contacts the cornea surface to position and hold the instrument in position when the legs are released.

  Excerpt(s): The present invention pertains to an instrument for protecting the corneal endothelium of the eye during **cataract extraction** by the small incision technique, commonly known as the Phacoemulsification or Phaco technique.... In recent years, two surgical techniques for removing a cataract from the eye are employed. The large incision technique and the small incision or Phaco technique.... In the large incision technique, a large incision (approximately 8-10 mm) almost half the circumference of the cornea is made, and the cataract is expressed or squeezed out of the eye manually. The advantage with this technique is that it is much easier to perform. The disadvantages are the longer time to recuperate and it also creates more astigmatism.

  Web site: http://www.delphion.com/details?pn=US05320113__

- **Intraocular implants**

  Inventor(s): Cumming; J. Stuart (#201 - 1211 W. La Palma Ave., Anaheim, CA 92801)

  Assignee(s): None Reported

  Patent Number: 5,326,347

  Date filed: August 12, 1991

  Abstract: An intraocular implant for use in a human eye following cataract, refractive or other eye surgery. The implant has a holder and imaging optics which may be folded to a compact configuration, inserted into the eye separately, and then assembled by the surgeon in the eye by mounting the optics on the holder after the holder has been implanted in the eye. These optics include a lens which is adjustable within the eye relative to the holder by the surgeon during surgery to focus the optics on the retina of the eye and are adjustable postoperatively by the implantee to near and distant focus positions by movement of the implantee's head and by magnetic action. The disclosed implants are inserted into the capsular bag of an eye from which the nucleus and cortex have been removed and retain the bag in substantially its natural shape and volume in a manner which inhibits opacification of the posterior capsule of the bag, prevents the vitreous volume from increasing postoperatively, and thereby prevents many complications which often attend **cataract surgery.**

Excerpt(s): This invention relates generally to intraocular correction of human vision disorders and more particularly to novel intraocular implants and methods for this purpose.... The human eye is commonly regarded as comprising an outer anterior transparent cornea, an iris behind the cornea which contains the pupil and forms with the cornea an intervening anterior chamber, a lens behind the iris which forms with the iris an intervening posterior chamber, and a retina at the rear of the eye on which entering light rays are focussed by the lens and which forms with the lens an intervening vitreous chamber containing vitreous. The natural lens of the eye comprises a transparent envelope, called a capsular bag, which contains a crystalline structure and is suspended by zonules from the surrounding ciliary body. The front and rear walls of the capsular bag are known as anterior and posterior capsules, respectively.... One of the eye abnormalities or disorders that seriously affects vision is a cataract which is a condition of the natural lens of the human eye characterized by progressive opacification of the lens. A cataractous eye condition is corrected or cured by surgical removal of the cataractous lens material through an incision in the cornea. In the early days, **cataract surgery** involved removal of the entire cataractous lens, i.e. both the inner lens structure and the outer capsulary bag. The artificial lenses used to replace the removed human lens were thick external "cataract lenses" worn as glasses.

Web site: http://www.delphion.com/details?pn=US05326347__

- **Intraocular lens apparatus with haptics of varying cross-sectional areas**

Inventor(s): Kraff; Manus C. (5600 W. Addison, Chicago, IL 60634)

Assignee(s): None Reported

Patent Number: 4,990,159

Date filed: December 2, 1988

Abstract: An intraocular lens apparatus for replacement of the natural lens following the extraction of the natural lens in **cataract surgery.** One or more resilient haptics, having one or both ends affixed to the lens body, are provided with alternating regions of varying transverse cross-sectional area along their length, so as to combine a relatively narrow insertion profile with great flexibility and stability once implanted within the eye.

Excerpt(s): In **cataract surgery,** the clouded natural lens is normally removed. An artificial lens known as an intraocular lens, or IOL, is implanted within either the posterior chamber or the anterior chamber of the eye. The IOL comprises an optic lens portion and a portion to retain and support the lens within the eye. The supporting and retaining portion usually employs one or more elongated strands, referred to as loops or haptics, which are resiliently deformable to facilitate insertion of the IOL into the eye, and expansion of the portion bearing against the interior surface of the eye, once implanted. The present invention relates in general to such an intraocular lens apparatus, and in particular, to a posterior chamber intraocular lens apparatus having loop-shaped haptics having areas of varying transverse cross-sectional area, so as to minimize the effective maximum width dimension or transverse profile of the IOL upon insertion through the smallest possible incision, and maximize the region of contact by the haptics with the interior surface of the eye upon implantation for greater stability.... In order to effectively utilize an intraocular lens within the eye, the clouded natural lens must first be removed prior to insertion of the IOL. Such removal can be achieved by a number of different processes. One such process is phacoemulsification, wherein a micro-needle is vibrated approximately forty thousand times per second so as to effectively liquify the nucleus of the natural lens for facilitated removal. Once this occurs, the remainder of the natural lens is removed from the eye by a finely regulated suction process.... Historically, conventional IOLs have been of either the C-loop type or the J-loop type.

Web site: http://www.delphion.com/details?pn=US04990159__

- **Intraocular lens implant and method of making same**

Inventor(s): Sambursky; Daniel Louis. (5 Riverside Dr., Apt. 806, Binghamton, NY 13905)

Assignee(s): None Reported

Patent Number: 5,919,230

Date filed: March 18, 1997

Abstract: An intraocular lens implant including a lens optic portion, a haptic portion and a support structure formed with the lens implant. The support structure extending longitudinally along at least a portion of the implant. The intraocular lens can be implanted in the capsular bag or placed in the ciliary sulcus after **cataract surgery.**

Excerpt(s): The invention relates generally to an intraocular lens and more particularly to an intraocular lens for implantation in the capsular bag or ciliary sulcus after removal of the human lens with **cataract surgery**... Cataract surgery involves the replacement of an opacified crystalline human lens with an intraocular lens implant. A technique for removing the human lens, phacoemulsification, removes the nucleus and cortex of the opacified lens while leaving the thin transparent membrane known as the capsular bag virtually intact. Generally, a scleral or corneal incision is made and the nucleus of the cataract is emulsified preserving the capsular bag. The remaining cortex of the lens is then removed using irrigation and aspiration. Next, an intraocular lens is implanted in the capsular bag and the incision is closed. In patients where the posterior capsule has been compromised during surgery, an intraocular lens may also be positioned in the cillary silcus located in front of the anterior capsule and behind the iris portion of the eye.... The lens used for either capsular bag or cillary silcus implantation may be a hard lens, typically made from glass or plastic materials, or a foldable lens typically formed from silicone, acrylic, hydrogel or other soft materials. The size of the incision is proportional to the type of lens to be implanted. For example, if a hard lens is to be implanted in the capsular bag, usually a scleral incision is used and the incision size typically ranges from 5.5 mm to 7.0 mm. Implantation of a hard lens in the cillary silcus requires an incision size of approximately 6.0 mm. However, a hard lens is incapable of being folded or otherwise manipulated for insertion through a relatively small incision as compared with the incision size required for a foldable lens. Generally, a smaller incision is preferred because of the advantages associated therewith which include greater wound stability, decreased induced astigmatism, more rapid visual and physical rehabilitation as well as reduction of associated medical and surgical expenses.

Web site: http://www.delphion.com/details?pn=US05919230__

- **Intraocular lens with multiple-fulcrum haptic**

Inventor(s): Kelman; Charles D. (269 Grand Central Pkwy., Floral Park, NY 11005)

Assignee(s): None Reported

Patent Number: 4,863,465

Date filed: February 10, 1987

Abstract: An intraocular lens for implantation within an eye after **cataract surgery.** The intraocular lens has a haptic having an elongated gently curving seating portion having a free end and a weakened portion about which such seating portion pivots. The weakened portion is spaced from the fulcrum formed at the location at which the haptic is anchored to the lens body such that the free end of the seating portion moves toward the lens body in response to compression of the seating portion toward the lens body for facilitating seating thereof, while minimizing the risk of injury to the delicate membranes in the eye by outwardly extending distal portions of the haptics. The construction of the lens being such that except for the weakened portion of the haptic, the entire haptic, including the seating portion, would pivot about the point of connection of the haptic to the lens body with the result that the free end portion would move away from, or at least not toward, the lens body, in response to such compression of the seating portion.

Excerpt(s): In opthalmic surgery, following removal of the natural lens of the eye, an intraocular lens is implanted to take the place of the lens removed. Lenses designed to be placed in the posterior chamber may be implanted in either the ciliary sulcus or the capsular bag of the eye. Various types of such lenses have been proposed and are in use. For example, U.S. Pat. No. 4,159,546 discloses an intraocular lens supported by a plurality of flexible strands secured to the lens body. Another lens design is the so called "Simcoe Posterior Chamber Lens" sold by Cilco Inc. as their "S2" posterior chamber lens. The latter has long strands which gently curve from the point of connection to the free ends thereof.... Each support strand of such prior art structure generally pivots about the point at which such support strand is anchored to the lens body, i.e., typically a point "P" on, or close to, the periphery of the lens body. Thus, generally radial pressure on the elongated seating portion of the support strands, such as is typically applied for manipulating the lens through the pupil and seating it in the posterior chamber, causes the free ends of the strands to move away from, or at least not toward, the lens body. Consequently, increased intraocular manipulation is required to move the lens, having these outwardly extending free ends of the haptics, into the posterior chamber without damaging the delicate membranes within the eye and it is particularly difficult to safely manipulate these outwardly extending free ends into the capsular bag.... U.S. Pat. No. 4,624,670, issued to Bechert on Nov. 25, 1986, discloses an intraocular lens having a pair of loops which extend from opposite sides of the lens body. Each of the loops includes a notch disposed generally mid-way along the curved seating portion of the loop in question. The notches are said to divide the seating portions so as to simulate a four-point fixation in the eye and at the same time facilitate insertion by reducing the possibility of slippage of the inserting instrument. The Bechert lens is shown to have haptics which pivot generally about their point of connection to the lens body, in response to compression of the haptic preparatory to seating thereof. The free ends of the haptics of Bechert, therefore, will move outwardly rather than inwardly with respect to the lens body in response to such compression.

Web site: http://www.delphion.com/details?pn=US04863465__

- **Intra-ocular pressure apparatus**

Inventor(s): Morrison; David P. (875 N. Easton Rd., Doylestown, PA 18901)

Assignee(s): None Reported

Patent Number: 4,909,783

Date filed: October 14, 1987

Abstract: An apparatus for maintaining intra-ocular pressure while simultaneously removing and replacing fluid in a patient's eye, for example, during **cataract surgery,** includes a pair of cooperating expansible bodies connected via fluid conduits to the eye. The expansible bodies may be piston/cylinder assemblies such as syringes. The plungers and/or the barrels of the syringes are mechanically linked together for equal and opposite operation of the two syringes, whereby input and output flow are precisely equal. The syringes are preferably placed back to back along a common axis. The barrels are rigidly spaced and a drive means is applied between the spaced barrels and the endwise-connected plungers.

Excerpt(s): This invention relates to an aspiration/infusion apparatus for body cavities, and in particular to a precision apparatus adapted for maintaining the pressure within an eye cavity during simultaneous removal and replacement of fluid therein, for example, during opthalmic surgery for removal of cataracts.... A variety of devices are known in the art for control of intra-ocular pressure. Such devices are sometimes combined with hand-held tools adapted for removal and aspiration of intra-ocular material or infusion of fluid to replace the aspirated material. The need to precisely control pressure is known, but in general, the currently available devices are complicated and expensive.... Surgical procedures for removal of cataracts now conventionally involve surgery on a normally pressurized eye. Instruments are passed through small incisions at the edges of the cornea in order to access and remove opaque cataract material clouding the lens, located immediately behind the anterior aqueous chamber of the eye. Cataracts in the lens are broken up by cutting apparatus or vibratory apparatus, and the broken-up material is aspirated together with a quantity of the aqueous fluid in the chamber. In order to maintain normal pressure within the eye, the aqueous fluid is simultaneously replaced by means of a gravity-powered infusion of a balanced salt solution supplied through a needle inserted in the anterior chamber or through a passage in the incision or aspiration instrument. Accordingly, the conventional means of pressure regulation during endophthalmic surgery is to ignore the extent of fluid flow and any variations thereof, and to employ a pressure regulation technique only. In other words, an indefinite quantity of fluid is supplied so long as intra-ocular pressure is less than a predetermined reference pressure.

Web site: http://www.delphion.com/details?pn=US04909783__

- **Irrigation and aspiration apparatus**

Inventor(s): Horiguchi; Masayuki (Ichinomiya, JP), Oda; Hideo (Gamagori, JP)

Assignee(s): Nidek Co., Ltd. (aichi, Jp)

Patent Number: 5,328,456

Date filed: April 23, 1993

Abstract: An irrigation and aspiration apparatus for **cataract surgery** or the like, which is particularly suitable for aspiration and removal of the cortex lentis during the surgical operation. As for the structure, the irrigation and aspiration apparatus of the present application includes a selector coupling to which ends of a plurality of aspiration tubes are connected, while the other ends of the aspiration tubes are respectively connected to handpieces which can perform aspiration, so that one of the handpieces for aspirating irrigating fluid and the like from a diseased eye of a patient can be chosen by switching the selector coupling. With this structure, aspiration and removal of the residual cortex after removal of the lens nucleus in the surgery of the crystalline lens can be accomplished easily and reliably, thereby relieving the doctor and the patient from the stress and load of the surgical operation.

Excerpt(s): The present invention relates to an irrigation and aspiration apparatus for **cataract surgery** and, more particularly, to an apparatus suitable for aspiration and removal of the cortex lentis.... In the field of ophthalmology, there has been known an irrigation and aspiration apparatus for removing, out of an eye, the residual cortex lentis after removal of the lens nucleus, and tissue particles emulsified by an ultrasonic probe in a method called the phacoemulsification. More specifically, it is an apparatus by which irrigating fluid is supplied to a patient's eye, and the cortex and tissue particles, along with the irrigating fluid, are discharged out of the eye while controlling the suction pressure to be maintained within a predetermined range. Conventionally, only one type of handpiece for irrigation and aspiration is connected to this kind of apparatus, and the operator inevitably needs to use this only one handpiece (aspiration port) to aspirate and remove all the residual cortex in the lens capsule, or to reconnect a different handpiece to the apparatus. Furthermore, in case of using two handpieces for irrigation-aspiration and phacoemulsification, it is necessary to reconnect each handpiece to an irrigation tube and an aspiration tube.... Such a conventional apparatus involves the following problems taking an example of aspirating and removing the cortex lentis. FIGS. 6A and 6B are simplified explanatory views illustrating a method of surgical operation for removing the residual cortex lentis. The operator stands on the head top side of a patient's eye. (Hereinafter, this position will be expressed as the "twelve-o'clock position", and positions at angles of 90, 180 and 270 degrees clockwise from here are respectively referred to as the "three-, six- and nine-o'clock positions".) Usually, as shown in the drawings, a portion of the patient's eye in the twelve-o'clock position is incised, and from this incision, the handpiece for irrigation and aspiration is inserted into the lens capsule so as to perform the surgical operation. As clearly understood from the drawings, however, it is extremely difficult to aspirate and remove the residual cortex within the capsule in the twelve-o'clock position in the vicinity of the incision because the iris and the anterior capsule become obstacles. Unless the cortex of the anterior capsule is completely aspirated, it is highly probable that the anterior capsular opacification will be caused after the surgery. Taking the post-operative progress into consideration, it is unfavorable to form another incision for inserting the handpiece in the three-, six- or nine-o'clock position. Then, if the distal end of the aspiration port is forcibly approached toward the capsule in the twelve-o'clock position, there is a risk that the incision and the corneal endothelium will be damaged.

Further, due to such operational difficulty, time for the operation will be extended, resulting in a problem that the operator and the patient will be fatigued to an increased degree.

Web site: http://www.delphion.com/details?pn=US05328456__

- **Medical forceps instrument for implanting intraocular lenses**

Inventor(s): Dusek; Jarmila (6210 Lake Washington Blvd., Renton, WA 98056), Dusek; Vaclav (6210 Lake Washington Blvd., Renton, WA 98056)

Assignee(s): None Reported

Patent Number: 5,176,701

Date filed: May 17, 1991

Abstract: Elongated generally horizontal blades are spaced apart vertically and have proximate handle end portions and distal grasping end portions. By manipulation of the handle end portions, the grasping end portions can be brought together into clamping engagement. The lower grasping end portion is return bent and includes a marginal portion offset laterally from the remainder of the lower blade. The upper grasping end portion is movable downward alongside the lower blade so as to engage against such laterally offset marginal portion of the lower grasping end portion. The composite forceps-type instrument is useful for implanting intraocular lenses during **cataract surgery,** particularly for positioning the superior haptic of an intraocular lens in a lens capsule.

Excerpt(s): The present invention relates to a forceps-type medical instrument used during **cataract surgery** for insertion of an artificial lens in an otherwise natural eye.... Moving from the exterior toward the center, a human eye includes the cornea, anterior chamber behind the cornea, iris, posterior chamber behind the iris and vitreous body which encompasses the major portion of the volume of the eyeball. The lens is located in the posterior chamber between the iris and the vitreous and consists of a relatively hard central nucleus surrounded by the softer cortex enclosed in a membrane called the capsule. The capsule and lens structure are held in position centered behind the iris by fibers called zonules that extend between the lens capsule and the periphery of the posterior chamber.... In modern **cataract surgery,** a short incision is made along the margin of the cornea for access to the lens through the central opening of the iris (pupil). The lens capsule is opened adjacent to the iris and the cloudy natural lens is removed. Preferably, the posterior portion of the lens capsule is left intact so that the posterior chamber remains isolated from the vitreous. Also, the zonules are not disturbed so that the opened lens capsule continues to be supported in the posterior chamber.

Web site: http://www.delphion.com/details?pn=US05176701__

- **Method and a system for performing cataract surgery**

Inventor(s): Nun; Yehoshua Ben (Doar Vitkin, IL)

Assignee(s): Itos Innovative Technology in Ocular Surgery, Ltd. (ra'anana, Il)

Patent Number: 6,328,747

Date filed: September 18, 1998

Abstract: A cataract removing device (CRD) in a system for surgically removing a cataract from an eye includes a cryomanipulator having a body and a manipulator head with a cryogenic tip for selectively freeze-gripping a region of contact of the cataract and for manipulating it within the eye. The cryomanipulator may also include a surgical tip and a heating device. The cryomanipulator may further include a sleeve having an aperture associated with a supply of liquid for providing irrigation of the eye. The sleeve may be also associated with a vacuum suction device for producing suction at the aperture. The CRD is designed for breaking up the cataract while it is at least partially frozen by the cryomanipulator. The CRD includes a drilling unit for breaking the cataract and a handle for manipulating the drilling unit within the eye. The drilling unit includes a housing having a hollow member having an aperture therein for aspiring irrigation fluid from the eye and a drill bit rotatably disposed within the hollow member. The drill bit includes a drill shaft and a drill blade for breaking the cataract. The drill bit is rotatably couplable to a motor. The housing may also include a second hollow member surrounding the first hollow member for providing irrigation fluid to the eye and for aspiring excess irrigation fluid and fragments of the broken cataract. The housing may also include a guard lip. The drilling unit may be disposable.

Excerpt(s): The present invention relates to the field of devices for eye surgery in general and to the field of devices for **cataract surgery** in particular.... Surgical removal of cataract is well known in the art. In **cataract surgery,** the content of the eye lens is completely removed leaving only the posterior lens capsule, in which an artificial lens may be subsequently installed. It is appreciated that one of the main risks in **cataract surgery** is a potential damage, e.g. rupture, of the lens capsule. In the past, it was common practice to "freeze" the entire lens using appropriate means and then, to remove the lens in its entirety via a large opening which is formed in the cornea, specifically, along the Cornea Limbus. This procedure resulted in damage to the lens capsule and to the vitreous body and is, therefore, no longer in use.... The soft tissue in cortex layer 26 is typically removed gradually using a vacuum suction device and/or a "scooping" device (not shown in the drawings). To remove nucleus 28, the hard tissue is typically, first, broken into small fragments and/or dissolved using appropriate instruments and/or solutions and, then, removed gradually by suction and/or "scooping" as described above. Alternatively, the entire nucleus can be removed in one piece, however, this requires cutting a large opening in the cornea.

Web site: http://www.delphion.com/details?pn=US06328747__

- **Method for enhancing or accelerating re-epithelialization or re-endothelialization of a tissue**

Inventor(s): Araneo; Barbara A. (Salt Lake City, UT)

Assignee(s): University of Utah Research Foundation (salt Lake City, Ut)

Patent Number: 5,922,701

Date filed: July 28, 1997

Abstract: The present invention is related to a method for enhancing or accelerating re-epithelialization or re-endothelialization of a tissue. Examples of re-epithelialization in which the invention is particularly suited include, but are not limited to, re-epithelialization of (a) skin following surgical wounds, (b) skin abrasions caused by mechanical trauma, caustic agents or burns, (c) cornea following **cataract surgery** or corneal transplants, (d) mucosal epithelium (respiratory, gastrointestinal, genitourinary, mammary, oral cavity, ocular tissue, liver and kidney) following infection, nonpathological etiologies or drug therapy, (e) skin following grafting and (f) renal tubule following acute tubular necrosis. Examples of re-endothelialization in which the invention is particularly suited include, but are not limited to, re-endothelialization (or regrowth of endothelium) in blood vessels following angioplasty, and the lysis of fibrin clots or lysis or mechanical disruption of thrombi in coronary arteries. In accordance with the present invention, the time to complete re-epithelialization or re-endothelialization is enhanced or accelerated by administering a dehydroepiandrosterone (DHEA) derivative.

Excerpt(s): The publications and other materials used herein to illuminate the background of the invention and in particular cases, to provide additional details respecting the practice, are incorporated by reference, and for convenience are nuinerically referenced in the following text and respectively grouped in the appended bibliography.... After a lesion occurs in the epidermis, it becomes critical to survival that access of the environment to the dermis is blocked without delay. In this event, the body effects wound closure in two temporally related steps: within minutes by the formation of a blood clot, which reestablishes a temporary barrier, and then within hours to days by the movement of residual epithelium below the clot and over the underlying dermis - - - the process of re-epithelialization.

Web site: http://www.delphion.com/details?pn=US05922701__

- **Nuclear hydrolysis cannula**

Inventor(s): Koch; Paul S. (15 Red Oak Rd., East Greenwich, RI 02818)

Assignee(s): None Reported

Patent Number: 5,284,476

Date filed: March 20, 1992

Abstract: A cannula for use in **cataract surgery** during the phases of hydrodissection and hydrodelamination/hydrodelineation/hydrodemarcation is described. The cannula has a hub for mating with a syringe and a needle originating from the distal end of the hub. The needle comprises a first section, second section, and truncated surface. The first section originates from the distal end of the hub and extends forward in a plane delineating the central longitudinal axis of the cannula. The second section originates from the distal end of the first section and is flattened and curved away from the central longitudinal axis of the hub. The truncated surface of the needle forms a rounded tip with beveled surfaces. The intersection of the bevel and sides of the cannula are sharpened to provide a cutting edge.

Excerpt(s): This invention relates generally to cannulas and relates more particularly to cannulas for use in removing cataracts during the surgical phases of hydrodissection and hydrodelamination/hydrodelineation/hydrodemarcation....
Embryologically, the human lens forms with a fetal nucleus which, after development, becomes the center of the crystalline lens. The inner side of the anterior capsule of the lens contain epithelial cells which migrate peripherally and posteriorly to lay down concentric lamellae of nuclear tissue. An adult nucleus next forms around the fetal nucleus and concentrically disposed lamellae, and the lens takes shape.... Throughout life, the epithelial cells continue to migrate and lay down lamellae of nuclear tissue. However, because the lens is now enclosed by the adult nucleus, the area of lens growth is confined causing the layers to become compressed and tightly packed. This increased compression and packing causes the lens to become stiff and firm, and by the age of 40 the ability of the lens to flex and focus is greatly reduced. As successive layers continue

to be deposited, the lens becomes so dense that it begins to change color and the clarity is lost. At this point, the successively deposited layers of lamellae are referred to as a cataract. The inner nucleus of the cataract consists of a firm, dense material while the outer nucleus consists of a less dense material. The material surrounding the nucleus of a cataractous lens is known as the cortex.

Web site: http://www.delphion.com/details?pn=US05284476__

- **Ophthalmic composition**

  Inventor(s): Fergeus; Susanna (Bjorklinge, SE), Lundberg; Kerstin (Uppsala, SE), Wik; Ove (Uppsala, SE)

  Assignee(s): Pharmacia & Upjohn AB (stockholm, Se)

  Patent Number: 6,086,597

  Date filed: March 25, 1997

  Abstract: Ophthalmic composition for use in ocular surgery includes an aqueous solution of sodium hyaluronate with a concentration within the range of 18-40 mg sodium hyaluronate/ml solution and the molecular mass of sodium hyaluronate being in the range of 1.times.10.sup.6 - 10.times.10.sup.6 <M>.sub.r,M. In a method for conducting ocular surgery, the composition is introduced into the eye as a surgical aid. The composition may be used in a method for conducting **cataract surgery.**

  Excerpt(s): The present invention relates to an ophthalmic composition for use in ocular surgery and a method for conducting ocular surgery. In particular the invention relates to a composition of sodium hyaluronate with a specifically defined molecular mass and concentration, for use in ocular surgery.... Intraocular lens implantation has today become routine surgery. A major tool to accomplish this was the introduction of Healon.RTM. (1980), the high molecular mass, viscoelastic, noninflammatory preparation of sodium hyaluronate. Since then, the **cataract surgery** has undergone a tremendous progress and many viscoelastic products have been developed. Typically these products are aqueous solutions containing a polysaccharide such as sodium hyaluronate, sodium chondroitin sulfate and hydroxypropylmethylcellulose, at concentrations varying from 10-70 mg/ml. The molecular mass (expressed as mass average relative molecular mass,<M>.sub.r,M) varies from about 20,000 (chondroitin sulfate) to about 5,000,000 (sodium hyaluronate).... A **cataract surgery** of today can be divided into several steps. The first step is pupil dilatation and local anaesthesia. The operation starts by making an incision into the anterior chamber of the eye. When the eye is punctured, the aqueous humour leaks out and the anterior chamber becomes shallow. A viscoelastic product is injected into the anterior chamber, which then regains its former shape and depth. The viscoelastic product maintains the anterior chamber and protects the vulnerable tissues, especially the endothelial cells on the cornea.

Web site: http://www.delphion.com/details?pn=US06086597__

- **Ophthalmic instrument for cataract surgery**

  Inventor(s): Anschutz; Till Rainer (Alte Wein Str. 5, 76593 Gersbach, DE)

  Assignee(s): None Reported

  Patent Number: 5,860,985

  Date filed: October 18, 1996

  Abstract: An ophthalmic instrument for removal of the natural cataractogenious lens includes a distal end portion configured to be received through a small incision into the anterior capsule of the eye. This distal end portion includes a pair of opposed jaw portions movable by manual manipulation of a pair of handle portions defined on a proximal portion of the instrument. One of the opposed jaw portions is perforate to more effectively fracture the cataractogenious lens. One of the opposed jaws may include a conduit allowing irrigation liquid to be supplied into the eye, while the other opposed jaw may include a conduit allowing aspiration of irrigation liquid and fractured particles of the lens. Because the small incision may fit relatively tightly around the instrument, fluid loss from the eye is minimized.

  Excerpt(s): The present invention relates to ophthalmic instruments for use in **cataract surgery.** More particularly, the invention relates to an instrument which is usable to remove the natural lens from the eye, and which may also provide irrigation to the eye and aspiration of irrigation liquid and fragments of the fractured natural lens during surgery.... During ophthalmic surgery, it is often necessary to perform various functions within the eye. For example, during **cataract surgery,** these functions include breaking up of the natural lens of the eye, irrigating the eye and aspirating the natural lens particles and irrigation liquid from the eye.... A conventional device for breaking up the natural cataractogenious lens is a phacoemulsifier. This device uses a tubular cutting tip vibrated by ultrasonic energy and centrally provided with vacuum aspiration to remove the natural lens in fragments. However, the conventional phacoemulsifier has a significant risk of damage to surrounding eye tissues because of the vigor of its action.

Web site: http://www.delphion.com/details?pn=US05860985__

- **Phacoemulsification, irrigation and aspiration method and apparatus**

Inventor(s): Shearing; Steven P. (P.O. Box 27212, Las Vegas, NV 89126)

Assignee(s): None Reported

Patent Number: 5,154,696

Date filed: April 8, 1991

Abstract: In a method and apparatus for phacoemulsification **cataract surgery,** a primary handpiece operable for phacoemulsification, irrigation and aspiration is inserted through a first incision in the limbus of an eye at a 12 o'clock position. An auxiliary handpiece for aspiration is inserted during the phacoemulsification, irrigation and aspiration operative procedure through a smaller second incision at approximately a three o'clock position. Both handpieces are fluidly connected to a power source aspiration from either the primary or auxiliary handpieces by rotation of the valve.

Excerpt(s): This invention relates to a method and apparatus for surgically removing a cataractous lens from a human eye. More specifically, this invention is directed to a safe and efficient method and apparatus of small incision, phacoemulsification, irrigation and aspiration of a cataract lens.... Through trauma, age, etc., a human natural crystalline lens may become opaque or cloudy and thus ceases to clearly transmit and focus light. This condition is referred to as a cataract or cataractous lens and is a leading cause of blindness in humans throughout the world.... In the last forty years or so techniques have been developed to surgically remove the cataract lens and replace it with an artificial or intraocular lens.

Web site: http://www.delphion.com/details?pn=US05154696__

- **Prevention of posterior capsular opacification**

Inventor(s): Okada; Kiyoshi (30-304, Ichigaya Yakuoji-cho, Shinjuku-ku, Tokyo 162-0063, JP)

Assignee(s): None Reported

Patent Number: 6,186,148

Date filed: August 12, 1999

Abstract: Posterior capsular opacification can be prevented by modulating focal contacts, which mediate adhesion between lens epithelial cells and the lens capsule, using a treating solution containing a focal contact-modulating substance or a proenzyme, such as Lys-plasminogen, which is introduced into the lens capsular bag during **cataract surgery.** To secure the passage of a treating solution between the lens epithelial cells, a calcium chelating agent, such as ethylenediamine tetraacetic acid CEDTA), is included in a treating solution. To limit the effect of the treating solution to lens epithelial cells prior to, during, and/or after capsulotomy, an inhibitor, such as.omega.-amino acid, can be introduced into the anterior chamber before the treating solution as a mixture with a viscoelastic material, such as sodium hyaluronate, or into the lens capsular bag without a viscoelastic material during capsulotomy.

Excerpt(s): The present invention relates to **cataract surgery,** specifically to compositions and methods for preventing proliferation of remnant lens epithelial cells occurring after **cataract surgery.** More specifically, the invention relates to the use of a combination for prevention of posterior capular opacification, particularly for surgically difficult cases.... A natural lens is enveloped in a structure called the lens capsule, which is the basement membrane of lens epithelial cells, and held behind the iris and in front of the vitreous by a suspensory ligament called the zonules. The inside of the lens capsule consists of lens epithelial cells and lens fibers. Lens epithelial cells form a monolayer underlying the lens capsule from the anterior pole to the equator of the lens. Lens fibers occupy the rest of the inside of the lens capsule. Lens epithelial cells become elongated in the equator of the lens and turn into lens fibers. As well as the morphological change, lens epithelial cells show the alteration in biochemical features. That is, protein synthesis of lens epithelial cells greatly changes toward the lens equator. These morphological and biochemical changes are called differentiation. In an area between the anterior pole and the lens equator, lens epithelial cells continue to undergo cell mitosis throughout life. This area is called germinate zone. Lens epithelial cells that underwent cell mitosis in the germinate zone gradually move toward the lens equator and differentiate into lens fibers.... Lens fibers are divided into two parts; the lens cortex and the lens nucleus. The lens cortex is a relatively soft tissue that consists of young lens fibers located near the lens equator. These fibers accumulate throughout life and gradually lose their intracellular organelles moving toward the center of the lens forming a hard, closely packed lamellar structure called the lens nucleus.

Web site: http://www.delphion.com/details?pn=US06186148__

- **Sarfarazi method of closing a corneal incision**

Inventor(s): Sarfarazi; Faezeh (25 Wiswall Rd., Newton Center, MA 02159)

Assignee(s): None Reported

Patent Number: 5,190,057

Date filed: December 13, 1991

Abstract: A method of sealing the corneal incision resulting from **cataract surgery** is presented. The edges of the incision are maneuvered under a keratoscope until an undistorted corneal surface is obtained. Biological glue is then applied to the maneuvered incision. The seal provides for greatly reduced postoperative astigmatism.

Excerpt(s): This invention relates to closing ophthalmic incisions to prevent astigmatism and wound leakage.... Cataract extraction is the most common ophthalmic surgical procedure performed in the in the United States. During **cataract extraction,** an incision is made at the edge, of cornea followed by capsulorhexis and removal of the nucleus and lens material by aspiration and irrigation or phacoemulsification techniques. For a decade, replacement of the natural lens with an intraocular lens has allowed for improved postoperative vision. However, subsequent closure of the corneal incision by suturing results in surgically induced astigmatism, compromising the improved vision. The suturing procedure requires surgical skill and is time consuming. The surgically induced astigmatism is between one and eight diopters depending on the surgeon's skill, the size of the incisions and the type of suture used. Presently the amount of time required for suturing is between 15 minutes to 1 hour depending on the skill of the surgeon and technique. Surgically induced astigmatism is not limited to **cataract surgery,** it also occurs in corneal graft. It has been observed that the tightest sutures produce the greatest amount of astigmatism. The astigmatism requires correction by glasses or contact lenses, otherwise the patient cannot have perfect vision even with the best surgical techniques.... Previous methods of managing the surgically induced astigmatism have included selective suture removal, an adjustable running suture technique, external corrective lenses and addition of compressional sutures.

Web site: http://www.delphion.com/details?pn=US05190057__

- ## Spare parts for use in ophthalmic surgical procedures

Inventor(s): Langerman; David W. (99 Dutch Hill Plz., Orangeburg, NY 10962)

Assignee(s): None Reported

Patent Number: 5,628,795

Date filed: March 15, 1995

Abstract: Ophthalmic "spare parts" which are made of biocompatible material and may be implanted by a surgeon in either the ciliary sulcus or the residual natural capsular bag of a patient's eye following **cataract surgery** so as to serve as a receptacle for an IOL or other optical or mechanical device, may have the form of an either anteriorly incomplete and posteriorly complete capsular bag-like structure with a generally toroidal equatorial region, or the form of a both anteriorly and posteriorly incomplete generally toroidally ring-shaped capsular bag-like structure, the interior space of the toroidal part of the structure between the anterior and posterior walls constituting a compartment, which may be divided into two subcompartments by an interior circumferential rib, into which an optical or other device may be inserted. The capsular bag-like structures can also serve to provide an enhanced capability of inhibiting posterior capsular opacification in the residual natural capsular bag, can have a circumferentially resiliently compressible split washer-like configuration, and can have visually perceptible features on the anterior and/or posterior walls to facilitate manipulation and/or orientation of those structures and the optical or other devices being inserted therein.

Excerpt(s): This invention relates to the art of ophthalmic surgical procedures, and in particular to a class of novel "spare parts" which are adapted for use by ophthalmic surgeons in the course of those surgical procedures which involve the removal of a cataract from a human eye.... As is well known, human beings, especially elderly persons, tend to develop a degree of opacity or clouding of the lens fibers surrounding the inert nucleus. The condition where this opacity spreads into the center of the lens in the region behind the pupil so as to impair vision, is designated cataract. When the opacity has progressed sufficiently to cause the loss of useful functional vision, the cataract is said to be mature, and the only currently available treatment for that condition is the removal of the cataract by extraction of the lens from the eye. Such a **cataract removal,** which is a very delicate operation but probably one of the most common and widely performed ophthalmic surgical procedures these days, may involve either an intracapsular or an extracapsular extraction of the lens.... In an extracapsular **cataract extraction** (ECCE), by way of contrast, first a major portion of the anterior capsule is cut away, leaving in place only that part of the natural or endogenous capsular bag which consists of the posterior capsule and the remaining, generally annular, anterior capsular flap. Then the lens nucleus is extracted from the capsular bag by any well-known type of expression or by phacoemulsification, and finally the cortex is removed by irrigation and aspiration. In such a case, the current practice is to follow up the removal procedure by the implantation of an IOL into the posterior chamber of the eye, with the haptics or position fixation elements being received either in the ciliary sulcus, where the residual portion of the endogenous capsular bag constitutes the means for preventing the IOL from falling into the vitreous humor, or in the residual capsular bag itself at the equatorial region thereof, i.e., where the anterior capsular flap adjoins the posterior capsule.

Web site: http://www.delphion.com/details?pn=US05628795__

- **Surgical blade and method for ocular surgery**

Inventor(s): Fugo; Richard J. (1507 Plymouth Blvd., Norristown, PA 19401)

Assignee(s): None Reported

Patent Number: 5,411,510

Date filed: July 6, 1993

Abstract: A surgical blade and method incorporating the surgical blade which ensure uniform incision depth and angulation, and the creation of self sealing surgical wounds during **cataract surgery.**

Excerpt(s): This invention relates to ocular surgical instruments and methods, specifically to surgical blades and methods employed in creating incisions during ocular surgery.... Opthalmologists currently performing **cataract surgery** by employing self sealing, no-stitch incisions are faced with the dilemma of creating precise surgical wounds with techniques and instrumentation which defy precision. Ideally, self sealing surgical incisions used in **cataract surgery** are trifaceted. The first facet is a vertical incision into the outer wall of the sclera, setting the depth for the second facet, the scleral tunnel, which is an incision extending horizontally from the base of the vertical scleral incision into the clear cornea. The third facet is an incision which theoretically extends perpendicularly from the corneal base of the scleral tunnel, downward through the underlying cornea and into the anterior chamber of the eye.... Cataract surgeons refer to the vertical scleral incision as penetrating half of the thickness of the sclera. However, scleral thickness varies from patient to patient and surgeons rely on subjective, imprecise techniques to determine whether the depth of the scleral tunnel is appropriate. Once the vertical scleral incision is made, the depth of which is a product of the surgeon's subjective judgment, a common method for determining appropriate scleral tunnel depth is for the surgeon to attempt to keep the blade used to create the incision in sight through the scleral tissue until the horizontal scleral tunnel incision is completed.

Web site: http://www.delphion.com/details?pn=US05411510__

- **Surgical knife blade and method of performing cataract surgery utilizing a surgical knife blade**

Inventor(s): Wishinsky; David H. (Rincon, PR)

Assignee(s): Medical Sterile Products, Inc. (rincon, Pr)

Patent Number: 5,217,476

Date filed: October 1, 1991

Abstract: A surgical knife blade for forming an incision of predetermined length in bodily tissue includes indicia disposed adjacent opposing portions of a cutting edge such that alignment of the opposing indicia with the tissue during insertion of the knife blade in the tissue produces an incision of the predetermined length. A method of performing **cataract surgery** utilizes the surgical knife blade to precisely form a smaller incision for lens removal and a larger incision for implant of the intraocular lens.

Excerpt(s): The present invention pertains to surgical knife blades and, more particularly, to a surgical knife blade for precisely forming incisions of predetermined lengths (sometimes referred to as incision widths) in bodily tissue and to a method of performing **cataract surgery** utilizing the surgical knife blade.... In **cataract surgery** and other microsurgical procedures, the lengths of incisions must be very small; and, when forming incisions that are small in length, a knife blade having a known size, or maximum width, as close as possible to the length of incision desired is usually inserted in tissue in a direction normal thereto in the manner of a plunge cut to form an incision in the tissue surface extending lengthwise between the lateral sides of the blade. In other words, an incision having an end-to-end length corresponding to the known width of the blade is formed in the tissue surface when the blade is inserted deep enough to penetrate the tissue surface to the known blade width. Because individual knife blades are conventionally sized to reflect a single, known blade width, an individual blade can precisely form only a single incision of a predetermined width. The lengths of incisions that can be precisely formed utilizing conventional surgical knife blades are limited due to the knife blades being manufactured in a limited number of sizes, or widths. Consequently, in many cases the actual lengths of incisions made with surgical knife blades must be subjectively estimated during incision formation to approximate the optimal incision length, and the actual length of an incision thusly formed is not known absent the use of extraneous measuring devices.... In **cataract surgery,** the length of an incision made in the sclera or adjacent tissue must be large enough to provide access for lens removal yet no larger than necessary to avoid distortion of the curvature of the eye, or astigmatism, when the incision is closed. In lens removal and replacement surgery of the eye, an incision is made in the eye to be only large enough in length to permit removal of the natural lens due to a blindness causing condition, such as cataract. The optimal length for the incision is very small, i.e. approximately 3 mm, and a surgical knife blade having a known size, close to 3 mm is selected for forming the incision or a thin blade is used with a lateral cutting movement. With a surgeon manipulating the blade via the handle thereon, the tip of the blade is utilized to initially penetrate the sclera, and the blade is inserted while calipers set to 3 mm are held adjacent the incision to compare actual incision length with the calibrated length. If the length of the incision is smaller than desired, the blade is manipulated and incision length measurements are repeated until the proper length incision has been obtained. Once the incision is determined to be accurately formed, the blade is removed, and a surgical instrument is introduced through the incision to remove the natural lens in accordance with a procedure selected for lens removal, such as phacoemulsification. After the natural lens has been removed, a lens implant selected to replace the natural lens is inserted through the incision; and, in most cases, the initial incision must be lengthened to accommodate the implant. Usually, the length of the initial incision must be enlarged to at least 4 mm and, more typically, to approximately 5 mm. A second blade with a known size, as close as possible to the minimum length incision required to accommodate the implant is inserted in the initial incision in a direction normal to the sclera or the incision is enlarged with a smaller blade. As with the initial incision, calipers set to the desired length for the final incision are employed to compare the enlarged incision length with the desired length. Once the desired incision length if formed, the implant is inserted through the incision into the eye. The need for multiple blades having known sizes closely matching desired incision lengths and for measuring instruments to ascertain actual incision length significantly complicates and protracts the surgical procedure while the use of a blade smaller than the desired incision leads to inaccurate incision lengths.

Web site: http://www.delphion.com/details?pn=US05217476__

- **Treating ophthalmic fibrosis using interferon-.alpha.**

Inventor(s): Gillies; Mark Cedric (Randwick, AU), Morlet; Nigel (Watsons Bay, AU), Sarossy; Marc George (Narrabundah, AU)

Assignee(s): Spruson & Ferguson (sydney, Au)

Patent Number: 5,863,530

Date filed: October 4, 1996

Excerpt(s): The present invention relates to the use of topical interferon-.alpha. for the treatment of various forms of fibrosis in and around the eye arising from various ophthalmic diseases and procedures. Specifically the invention relates to alleviation of corneal scarring after laser photoablative refractive keratectomy (PRK). It also relates to the alleviation of posterior (lens) capsular opacification after extracapsular **cataract surgery** with lens implant; the alleviation of wound scarring following glaucoma filtration surgery. Interferon-.alpha. may also be used to coat the lens implant prior to or during implantation. It may also possibly be injected into the eye during eye surgery for inhibiting posterior capsule opacification after **cataract surgery** and in addition may be injected into the vitreous body to prevent retinal fibrosis and proliferative vitreo-retinopathy, and injected subconjunctivally to inhibit fibrosis and scarring following glaucoma filtration surgery.... In the field of ophthalmic surgery, it is known to use excimer laser photoablative refractive keratectomy to sculpt the cornea of the eye in order to relieve refractive errors (e.g. myopia) and a number of corneal conditions and diseases. Specifically, the 193 nm argon fluoride excimer laser is able to discretely remove corneal tissue by photoablation without thermal damage to surrounding tissue.... Of major concern is the activation of the stromal keratocytes when a wound is made to the stroma. As is well known, the basic response of wounded tissue is to repair the defect and therefore the ophthalmic surgeon when using this technique is confronted with alteration to the biochemistry, morphologic features and tissue function unpredictability brought about by the wound itself and the healing phenomenon.

Web site: http://www.delphion.com/details?pn=US05863530__

- **Trial frames, adjustable spectacles and associated lens systems**

Inventor(s): Sims; Clinton N. (3432 W. Riverside Dr., Ft. Myers, FL 33901)

Assignee(s): None Reported

Patent Number: 5,104,214

Date filed: October 27, 1989

Abstract: Trial frames including two independently rotatable cells alignable with each eye are disclosed. Each set of cells is designed to house a pair of either cylinder, polarized, prism, crossed cylinder or sphero-cylinder lenses as appropriate for correcting optical errors such as astigmatism, macular defects, or diplopia. Because the lenses associated with the cells are designed to rotate independently, no synchorinized gear mechanism is required. Moreover, because axes throughout the entire visual field may be generated using independent rotation of two lenses, the batteries of trial lenses used in connection with conventional trial frames need not be used. Adjustable spectacles and an alternative lens system also are disclosed. The adjustable spectacles are particularly useful for persons whose refractive error is changing relatively rapidly over a short period of time (such as persons recovering from cataract surgery) and who therefore cannot practically use conventional glasses or contact lenses. The lens systems may easily be adapted for use in the oculars of microscopes, telescopes, cameras, binoculars, kaleidoscopes, slit lamps, and other similar devices.

Excerpt(s): This invention relates to subjective devices and associated lens systems for measuring or correcting optical errors in the eyes of humans.... A variety of lens systems have been designed to produce variable crossed cylinder powers for measuring or correcting astigmatic errors through the use of refractors. One such lens structure, the Snellen-Stokes system, uses two counter-rotating cylinder lenses of equal power and opposite sign to produce variable crossed cylinder powers. A second system, disclosed by Humphrey in U.S. Pat. No. 3,822,932, utilizes two pairs of Snellen-Stokes lenses, with the combined lens axis of one pair offset 45.degree. from the combined lens axis of the other pair. The pairs are alternatively counter-rotated to produce a desired combined cylinder power at a desired angle. Finally, a novel system described in my patent application Ser. No. 07/310,334 teaches use of four rotatable cylinder lenses of equal power and sign and a stationary lens of double the power and opposite sign of each of the cylinder lenses, to produce variable crossed-cylinder powers at various angles.... Diplopic errors typically are measured using two pairs of Risley prisms, with one pair aligned with each eye. Each Risley prism pair consists of two equal power prism lenses and is counter-rotated until fusion is obtained. The amount of rotation for one of the pairs of Risley prisms is related to the amount of base up/down defect present in the patient's eyes, while the rotation of the other pair corresponds to the base in/out defect present.

Web site: http://www.delphion.com/details?pn=US05104214__

- **Universal port/seal device for ocular surgery**

Inventor(s): Grant; Kenneth W. (26 Haven St., Dover, MA 02030), Meade; John C. (6 Garfield St., Walpole, MA 02081), Skolik; Stephanie A. (706 Eleventh Ave., Huntington, WV 25701)

Assignee(s): None Reported

Patent Number: 5,817,099

Date filed: June 6, 1996

Abstract: A universal port/seal device is provided for ocular surgery, notably for **cataract surgery.** The device is inserted into an ocular incision and is adapted to serve as (1) a port for inserting, manipulating and withdrawing a surgical instrument, e.g., the tip of a phacoemulsification handpiece, so as to protect the surrounding tissue from mechanical and thermal injury, and (2) a seal to prevent leakage of fluid from the eye. The device comprises (1) a housing having an internal passageway that permits it to function as a cannula or port for a surgical instrument, (2) at least two jaws that are movable toward and away from one another and are shaped so as to (a) serve as a seal to prevent leakage from a surgical eye incision and (b) accommodate a surgical instrument or tool that is inserted between them via the housing's internal passageway, and (3) sealing member for preventing leakage of fluid via the housing's internal passageway while allowing relative movement of an inserted surgical device.

Excerpt(s): This invention relates to **cataract surgery** utilizing phacoemulsification and more particularly to a universal device for ocular surgery that is placed in the eye once an incision has been made and is adapted to serve as (1) an entry port for the tip of a phacoemulsification handpiece or another surgical device, (2) a seal to prevent leakage of fluid from the eye, and (3) an insulation device to help protect the wound from thermal and/or mechanical injury.... The human eye is divided by a normally transparent lens into anterior and posterior chambers. The transparent lens focuses light onto the retina lining the inner surface of the rear posterior chamber. For various reasons, including age and disease, the lens may become cloudy or otherwise deteriorate to the extent of failing to function normally. A typical age-related deterioration problem is the clouding phenomenon commonly known as a "cataract", which inhibits the transmission of visual light information through the lens to the retina. When this happens, the cloudy cataracteous lens material is usually removed if restoration of the maximum light transmission is desired. Thereafter the function of the removed lens material is performed by an intraocular lens ("IOL") implant or by using thick glasses or contact lenses.... A currently accepted practice for removing a cataract through a surgical incision involves a method known as phacoemulsification using ultrasonic energy. This method is preferred since the incision in the eye can be smaller than with some other **cataract removal** techniques. As currently practiced, the phacoemulsification technique involves use of an electrically-powered "phaco" handpiece or instrument that serves to provide phacoemulsification, irrigation and aspiration. A typical phaco handpiece comprises an acoustic wave-generating transducer that is adapted to conduct ultrasonic energy to the eye via a thin-walled (e.g., 0.250 mm) hollow metal needle or tip. The typical phaco needle is made of titanium and has a length in the order of 24 mm and an outside diameter (o.d.) of about 1 mm. The transducer converts electrical current into acoustic waves with a frequency well beyond the range of human hearing (normally 16,000 cps). Typically the transducer provides an ultrasonic output at a frequency of 28,000 to 50,000 cycles per second. This ultrasonic energy causes the phaco tip to vibrate. The ultrasonic vibrations transmitted to the tip cause the nearby cataracteous tissue to erode and fragment.

Web site: http://www.delphion.com/details?pn=US05817099__

- **Use of growth factor and antimetabolite combination to prevent or retard secondary cataract formation**

  Inventor(s): Nixon; Jon C. (Fort Worth, TX), Sams; Karen C. (Arlington, TX), York; Billie M. (Fort Worth, TX)

  Assignee(s): Alcon Laboratories, Inc. (fort Worth, Tx)

  Patent Number: 5,696,091

  Date filed: February 20, 1996

  Abstract: The intraocular use of combinations of lens epithelial cell growth stimulators (e.g., TGF-.beta.) and antimetabolites (e.g., mitomycin C) is described. The combination is applied to the capsular bag to prevent or retard the formation of secondary cataracts following **cataract surgery.** The lens epithelial cell stimulators activate DNA synthesis in dormant lens epithelial cells, and thereby make those cells susceptible to the anti-metabolites. This enables the antimetabolites to suppress the proliferation of lens epithelial cells to a much greater extent, relative to the proliferation observed when the metabolites alone are utilized. The increased suppression of the growth of lens epithelial cells results in a significant improvement in the ability to prevent or retard the formation of opacities on the lens capsule (i.e., secondary cataracts).

Excerpt(s): The present invention relates to the field of ophthalmology. More specifically, the invention relates to the field of **cataract surgery,** wherein the natural crystallin lens of the human eye is surgically removed and an artificial lens is implanted.... Modern **cataract surgery** typically involves implantation of an artificial lens, referred to as an "intraocular lens" or "IOL", in the posterior chamber of the eye. The preferred site of implantation is within the capsule which surrounds the natural crystallin lens. When the natural crystallin lens is surgically removed, a portion of the anterior face of the lens capsule is also removed. This provides an opening which allows the artificial lens to be placed within the remaining portion of the lens capsule, which is also referred to as the "capsular bag". The capsular bag is considered to be the ideal location for implantation of an intraocular lens. Unfortunately, there is a significant problem associated with implantation of intraocular lenses in the capsular bag.... The capsular bag is normally cleaned or "polished" by the ophthalmic surgeon to remove lens epithelial cells and other tissue remnants. This helps to ensure that deposits in the lens capsule do not impair the vision of the patient. However, it is generally not possible for the surgeon to remove all of the lens epithelial cells, particularly in the outer perimeter of the capsular bag. The remaining lens epithelial cells may eventually cause opacifications which impair the vision of the patient. Such impairment is referred to as "secondary cataract". The formation of a secondary cataract may require further medical treatment, such as use of a YAG laser to break up the opacifications, or further surgery.

Web site: http://www.delphion.com/details?pn=US05696091__

Patent Applications on Cataract Surgery

As of December 2000, U.S. patent applications are open to public viewing.[19] Applications are patent requests which have yet to be granted (the process to achieve a patent can take several years). The following patent applications have been filed since December 2000 relating to cataract surgery:

---

[19] This has been a common practice outside the United States prior to December 2000.

- **Cataract surgery devices and methods for using same**

Inventor(s): Ben-Nun, Joshua; (Moshav Beit Herut, IL)

Correspondence: Edward Langer; Shiboleth Yisraeli Roberts Zisman & CO; 60th Floor; 350 Fifth Avenue; New York; NY; 10118; US

Patent Application Number: 20030158567

Date filed: April 15, 2003

Abstract: There are disclosed methods and apparatus for surgical removal of encapsulated tissue, and in particular removal of cataracts from lens capsules. These methods involve accessing the tissue in the capsule and maintaining control on the capsule, by gripping the capsule with an apparatus, a portion of which has been cooled, this cooling providing chilling to the apparatus portion and capsule, such that the apparatus portion adheres to the capsule by freezing. The apparatus is also heated, to limit any backwards conduction of the cooling, toward the remainder of the apparatus, with this heating keeping the apparatus at temperatures within a biocompatible range.

Excerpt(s): This application claims priority from and is related to U.S. Provisional Patent Applications: 1) Serial No. 60/286,306, filed Apr. 25, 2001, entitled: **CATARACT SURGERY** DEVICES AND METHODS FOR USING SAME; and 2) Serial No. 60/205,554, filed May 22, 2000 and entitled: A METHOD AND A SYSTEM FOR PERFORMING **CATARACT SURGERY**. U.S. Provisional Patent Application S/No. 60/205,554 is related to U.S. patent application Ser. No. 09/156,982 filed Sep. 18, 1998 and entitled: A METHOD AND SYSTEM FOR PERFORMING CATATACT SURGERY, which is a continuation in part application of U.S. patent application Ser. No. 08/851,505, filed May 5, 1997 and entitled: A METHOD AND SYSTEM FOR PERFORMING CATATACT SURGERY, now U.S. Pat. No. 6,217,584. All four of these U.S. patent applications are incorporated by reference in their entirety herein.... The present invention relates to the field of devices for eye surgery in general and to the field of devices for **cataract surgery** in particular.... The soft tissue in cortex layer 26 is typically removed gradually using a vacuum suction device and/or a "scooping" device (not shown in the drawings). To remove nucleus 28, the hard tissue is typically, first, broken into small fragments and/or dissolved using appropriate instruments and/or solutions and is then removed gradually by suction and/or "scooping" as described above. Alternatively, the entire nucleus can be removed in one piece. However, this requires cutting a large opening in the cornea.

Web site: http://appft1.uspto.gov/netahtml/PTO/search-bool.html

- **Incising apparatus for use in cataract surgery**

Inventor(s): Feinsod, Matthew; (Great Neck, NY)

Correspondence: Frommer Lawrence & Haug; 745 Fifth Avenue- 10th Fl.; New York; NY; 10151; US

Patent Application Number: 20020091402

Date filed: March 19, 2002

Abstract: An incising apparatus for **cataract surgery** is provided. The incising apparatus includes a handle having a proximal end and a distal end. A circular cutting band is adapted to slide along the handle. At least one stopper element is provided in the vicinity of the proximal end of the handle. The at least one stopper element is positioned within the interior of the circular band so as to restrict the motion of the circular band relative to the handle.

Excerpt(s): The invention relates generally to an apparatus used in the field of ophthalmology and more particularly to an incising apparatus used in **cataract surgery**... The lens of a human eye is a transparent, biconvex crystalline structure located just behind the iris of the eye. The lens substance is contained within an elastic, transparent lens capsule, similar in structure to the substance of a grape being held inside its skin. This lens capsule has a relatively thin cross section, with an average thickness of between 14 microns to 21 microns at its anterior surface.... Cataracts occur when the lens substance opacifies, obscuring the passage of light therethrough and resulting in a decrease in the clarity of a patient's vision. **Cataract surgery** involves removing the opacified lens and typically replacing it with an artificial intraocular lens implant. The preferred method of routine **cataract surgery** is referred to as extracapsular **cataract extraction**.. In this procedure the lens is removed through an opening formed in the anterior lens capsule. The remaining portion of the-lens capsule is left in place to hold the lens implant that is to be introduced. More modem extracapsular cataract extractions involve the phacoemulsification technique, enabling a smaller surgical incision. The phacoemulsification instrument uses ultrasonic power to fragment the lens nucleus and aspirate the lens contents from the eye. This technique theoretically results in fewer complications, faster healing, and more rapid visual rehabilitation.

Web site: http://appft1.uspto.gov/netahtml/PTO/search-bool.html

- **Intraocular lens with photocatalytic coating**

Inventor(s): Cheng, Shen-Wen; (Hsinchu, TW), Kuo, Tsung-Nan; (Hsinchu, TW), Peng, Su-Chen; (Taipei, TW), Tsai, Ming-Ling; (Taipei, TW)

Correspondence: Ladas & Parry; 26 West 61st Street; New York; NY; 10023; US

Patent Application Number: 20040082996

Date filed: May 7, 2003

Abstract: The subject invention provides an intraocular lens comprising an optic lens body and a layer of a photocatalytic material coated on at least a portion of a surface of the optic lens body. The intraocular lens of the subject invention can eliminate endophthalmitis and inhibit after-cataracts following **cataract surgery.**

Excerpt(s): The subject invention relates to an intraocular lens (IOL) on which at least a portion of the lens surface is coated with a photocatalytic material to prevent and control the **cataract surgery** complications, such as endophthalmitis and after-cataract.... Cataract surgery is one of the most common ophthalmic operations in the world. Standard **cataract surgery** includes extracapsular lens extraction and intraocular lens implantation. However, several complications, such as endophthalmitis (intraocular infection) and after-cataract (posterior capsular opacity) following **cataract surgery,** may be occurred after **cataract surgery...** Endophthalmitis is a devastating complication of **cataract surgery** with 0.05% to 0.5% incidence rate; which is characterized by hypopyon and vitreous cavity pus formation. This devastating intraocular infection results from the introduction of microorganism into ocular anterior chamber during **cataract surgery.** The microorganisms of endophthalmitis commonly include Staphylococci aureus, Pseudomonus aeriginosa, and Escherichia coli. These microorganisms may arise from contaminated instruments or patient's periorbital region, such as eyelash and conjunctiva. The microorganisms existed in ocular anterior chamber may pass through pupil and lens front surface into vitreous cavity after **cataract surgery.** Once the organisms gain access to the vitreous cavity, severe inflammation may occur and eventually result in severe visual loss. However, Ciulla T A, et al., "Bacterial endophthalmitis prophylaxis for cataract surgery: an evidence-based update," Ophthalmology, 2002, January;109(1):13-24, reports that there is no effective method or procedure can prevent endophthalmitis such as pre-operative ocular irrigation, intra-operative antibiotic irrigation and post-operative antibiotic injection.

Web site: http://appft1.uspto.gov/netahtml/PTO/search-bool.html

- **Lenticular net instruments and methods of cataract surgery using a lenticular net**

Inventor(s): Sabet, Sina J.; (Alexandria, VA)

Correspondence: Karen M. Gerken; Epstein & Gerken; Suite 340; 1901 Research Blvd.; Rockville; MD; 20850; US

Patent Application Number: 20030135221

Date filed: December 18, 2002

Abstract: A lenticular net instrument comprises an elongate handle coupled with a lenticular net movable to contracted and expanded configurations via an actuator of the handle. The net in the contracted configuration has a narrow profile for insertion in and removal from a lens capsule through a small incision in the eye. The net is movable to the expanded configuration within the lens capsule between a cataractous nucleus and a ruptured capsular wall. The net has a plurality of openings therein of a size to prevent fragments of the cataractous nucleus produced by fragmentation with a fragmenting instrument from passing therethrough such that the fragments do not pass through the ruptured wall. A method of **cataract surgery** involves deploying a net between a cataractous nucleus and a ruptured capsular wall upon the occurrence of the rupture in the wall.

Excerpt(s): The subject patent application claims priority from prior provisional patent application Serial No. 60/340,480 filed Dec. 18, 2001, the entire disclosure of which is incorporated herein by reference.... The present invention relates generally to ocular medical instruments and, more specifically, to safety net instruments for use in **cataract surgery**... During their lifetimes, many people become afflicted with cataracts, i.e. lenticular opacities that interfere with vision. Indeed, cataracts may be considered the most prevalent visually disabling eye disease in the world. The cloudiness or opacity associated with cataract arises in the nucleus of the anatomical lens, which includes a lens capsule also known as the capsular bag, the nucleus within the lens capsule, and gelatinous cortical material between the nucleus and the lens capsule. Currently, the only effective treatment for cataract is surgical removal of the cataract from the eye.

Web site: http://appft1.uspto.gov/netahtml/PTO/search-bool.html

- **Method and instrument for cataract surgery**

Inventor(s): Anthone, Kenneth D.; (Clarence, NY)

Correspondence: James C. Simmons; the Law Office of James C. Simmons; 11 Falmouth Lane; Williamsville; NY; 14221; US

Patent Application Number: 20030093099

Date filed: November 8, 2002

Abstract: A method to provide an efficient, safe, and easy to use supracapsular method for removal of cataracts, wherein a groove is formed in the cataract nucleus, the nucleus is cracked along the groove into two halves and rotated approximately 90 degrees, force is applied to the proximal half to effect movement of the distal half into a stacked position relative to the proximal half, and the nucleus halves along with the remainder of the cataract are then emulsified and removed.In order to minimize the chances of trauma to the capsule while sweeping the lens capsule away from cataract portions as well as making a crack in the nucleus and for otherwise assisting in manipulation of nucleus portions, an instrument has a prongless cataract-engaging portion, preferably with a convex frontal edge.

Excerpt(s): Priority of U.S. provisional patent application serial No. 60/338,138, filed Nov. 9, 2001, the disclosure of which is hereby incorporated herein by reference, is hereby claimed.... The present invention relates generally to **cataract surgery.** More particularly, the present invention relates to a supracapsular method of cataract phacoemulsification and an instrument therefor.... A cataract refers to an area or portion of the crystalline lens of an eye that has become opaque. Usually, the cataract, which is contained within a lens capsule, comprises the hardened opaque or cloudy lens portion known as the cataract nucleus surrounded by the softer cortex. Treatment therefor involves removing a portion of the capsule to provide an opening (capsulorrhexis) and removal of the diseased lens through the opening and its replacement within the remaining portion of the capsule with an artificial lens. For the purposes of this specification and the claims, the term "cataract" refers to the entire diseased lens.

Web site: http://appft1.uspto.gov/netahtml/PTO/search-bool.html

- **Method for use in cataract surgery**

Inventor(s): Holmen, Jorgen; (Moholm, SE)

Correspondence: Jenkens & Gilchrist, PC; 1445 Ross Avenue; Suite 3200; Dallas; TX; 75202; US

Patent Application Number: 20020165522

Date filed: May 3, 2001

Abstract: A method for treatment of residual lens epithelial cells is disclosed. The method provides increased safety during local treatment in ocular surgery by improved administration of active agents. The method is particularly useful in treatment of proliferative events in ocular surgery, such as posterior capsular opacification.

Excerpt(s): The present invention relates to **cataract surgery,** specifically to a method for preventing proliferation of remaining lens epithelial cells after **cataract surgery...** The crystalline lens of the human eye is located in the posterior chamber between the posterior iris surface and the vitreous body. It is a biconvex transparent tissue without nerves and blood vessels, weighing approximately 0.2 g. The lens is enveloped in a capsule, a structureless, transparent and elastic membrane bag. Approximately 80 zonular fibres, extending between the capsule and the ciliary body, suspend the lens. The inside of the lens capsule consists of lens epithelial cells and lens fibres. The lens epithelial cells form a monolayer underlying the capsule from the anterior pole to the equator of the lens. These cells continue to undergo cell mitosis throughout life in the area located between the anterior pole and the lens equator. The lens epithelial cells that underwent cell mitosis gradually move toward the lens equator and differentiate into lens fibres. These cells make up the rest of the lens New layers of fibre cells are constantly formed on top of those previously formed. The older fibre cells become denser and during the 3.sup.rd decade of life a hard nucleus is formed in the middle of the human lens, consisting of old dehydrated fibre cells.... A cataract is defined as every form of opacity in the lens or its capsule; the lens becomes cloudy, resulting in a loss of visual ability. A cataract is a painless phenomenon, but decreases the quality of life if the lens is not surgically extracted and replaced by an artificial lens.

Web site: http://appft1.uspto.gov/netahtml/PTO/search-bool.html

- ### Method of using a small incision lens

Inventor(s): Callahan, Jeffery S.; (Blountville, TN), Callahan, Wayne B.; (Abingdon, VA)

Correspondence: Douglas W. Schelling, Ph.d.; Waddey & Patterson; Suite 2020; 414 Union Street; Nashville; TN; 37219; US

Patent Application Number: 20030033013

Date filed: July 16, 2002

Abstract: This patent represents a deformable artificial intraocular lens for implantation into the human eye. The lens is used for implantation after **cataract surgery.** The lens optic consists of one smooth optical surface. The second optical surface is a series of annular concentric rings. The rings allow the lens to have extremely thin edges, which reduce glare, halos, and distortion. The extremely thin lens optic along with the thin haptic can be rolled, folded, or squeezed to pass through a small incision (<1.5 millimeters) in the cornea or sclera of the human eye. This lens represents a breakthrough in removal of mass from the lens. The ultra thin lens and haptic design allows the lens to move in the eye providing accommodation for the patient. The lens and haptic design reduces the radial forces on the eye to the point where the naturally occurring pressures in the eye move the lens thus providing accommodation. In all current lens designs the haptics apply enough radial force to prevent the natural forces in the eye from moving the lens. The ultra thin lens and haptic design allows the lens to move in the eye providing accommodation for the patient.

Excerpt(s): The present invention relates generally to the area of intraocular lens and use thereof to correct visual problems. More particularly, this invention provides a lens and method of use thereof for the correction of a lack of accommodation. The lens can be inserted into a human eye through a 1.5 millimeter or smaller incision.... Doctors trained in ophthalmology routinely surgically extract cataract-impaired natural crystalline lenses from patients' eyes and subsequently implant artificial lenses to prevent blindness.... Using an intraocular lens for correction of visual problems is currently problematic. In order to insert an intraocular lens, an incision is made through the cornea or sclera. The new lens is passed through the incision into the anterior chamber of the eye. The inserted lens is then positioned over the pupil and anchored either anteriorly to or posteriorly from the iris, or other structure of the eye. Unfortunately, the making of the incision causes astigmatism of the cornea.

Web site: http://appft1.uspto.gov/netahtml/PTO/search-bool.html

- **Methods for reducing postoperative intraocular pressure**

Inventor(s): Soll, David B.; (Ambler, PA)

Correspondence: Akin, Gump, Strauss, Hauer & Feld, L.l.p.; One Commerce Square; 2005 Market Street, Suite 2200; Philadelphia; PA; 19103; US

Patent Application Number: 20020185139

Date filed: April 10, 2001

Abstract: Hyaluronic acid is commonly used as a spacer in eye surgeries such as **cataract surgery,** intraocular lens surgery, corneal transplant surgery and some types of glaucoma surgery. One common side effect of these surgical procedures is a postoperative rise in intraocular pressure which can be serious and can cause permanent loss of function of optic nerve fibers and, therefore, loss of visual field function as well as visual acuity function. Intraoperative and postoperative rises in intraocular pressure also occur in vitreous, retina and other posterior segment surgeries. Methods are provided for reducing the postoperative intraocular pressure in an eye to normal preoperative levels while maintaining the therapeutic effects of the hyaluronic acid. One method comprises anesthetizing the eye at the start of the surgical procedure, administering to the eye substantially concurrently amounts of hyaluronic acid and hyaluronidase and leaving the hyaluronic acid and hyaluronidase in the eye after the operative procedure.

Excerpt(s): Hyaluronic acid is a natural, high molecular weight, highly viscous polymer consisting of alternating acetylglycosamine and glucuronic acid units. This acid is found in the trabecular meshwork in the vitreous humor of the eye, as well as in other locations in the body. The polymeric structure of hyaluronic acid is broken down by the enzyme hyaluronidase which cleaves the glycosidic bonds.... Hyaluronic acid, a mucopolysaccharide, has been used in eye surgery for over twenty years. High molecular weight hyaluronic acid is used primarily as a spacer during cataract and intraocular lens surgical procedures. It is also used in other ocular surgical procedures such as glaucoma, vitreous and retina surgery and in corneal transplantation. Hyaluronic acid solutions are pseudoplastic and the cellular protective qualities of hyaluronic acid are primarily related to the fact that it keeps tissue apart and therefore prevents contact trauma.... A common side effect occurring in postoperative cataract patients is a significant early, and occasionally prolonged, rise in intraocular pressure. Such a condition is sometimes serious, especially in patients with glaucomatous optic disc changes.

Although the pressure increase tends to be more severe when visco-elastic agents such as hyaluronic acid are injected into the eye during surgery, the intraocular pressure can become elevated postoperatively even when such agents are not utilized. Furthermore, such a pressure increase can occur even when no additional medications are used during the surgical procedure. In some cases, it is advantageous to leave a viscoelastic agent in the eye, which often necessitates giving patients large doses of carbonic anhydrase inhibitors. These inhibitors lower the intraocular pressure by decreasing the formation of aqueous humor, a fluid that is normally secreted in the eye, by the ciliary body. Current methods for relieving postoperative pressure increases in the eye include various types of eyedrops such as beta-adrenergic blocking agents, sympathomimetic agents, miotics, alpha II selective agents, carbonic anhydrase inhibitors and prostaglandin agents. Tables listing some of these agents appeared in the Physician's Desk Reference for Ophthalmology 2000.

Web site: http://appft1.uspto.gov/netahtml/PTO/search-bool.html

- **Modular intraocular implant**

Inventor(s): Eggleston, Harry C.; (Creve Coeur, MO)

Correspondence: Paul M. Denk; 763 South New Ballas Road; St. Louis; MO; 63141; US

Patent Application Number: 20020128710

Date filed: May 10, 2002

Abstract: An adjustable ocular insert to be implanted during refractive **cataract surgery** and clear (human) crystalline lens refractive surgery and adjusted post-surgically. The implant comprises relatively soft but compressible and resilient base annulus designed to fit in the lens capsule and keep the lens capsule open. Alternatively the annulus may be placed in the anterior or posterior chamber. The annulus can include a pair of opposed haptics for secure positioning within the appropriate chamber. A rotatable annular lens member having external threads is threadedly engaged in the annulus. The lens member is rotated to move the lens forward or backward so to adjust and fine-tune the refractive power and focusing for hyperopia, myopia and astigmatism. The intraocular implant has a power range of approximately +3{square root}0.PI.-3 diopters.

Excerpt(s): This application is a continuation in part of application Ser. No. 09/372,493, filed Aug. 20, 1999, which is a continuation in part of application Ser. No. 08/764,501, filed Dec. 12, 1996, which is a continuation in part of application Ser. No. 08/617,183, filed Mar. 18,

1996, now U.S. Pat. No. 5,628,798.... This invention relates generally to ocular implants and more specifically to a modular intraocular implant with an adjustable and replaceable lens.... A cataract is a condition where a normally clear lens of the eye becomes progressively opaque. The opacification generally occurs over a period of time and the amount of light which passes through the lens decreases thereby decreasing vision. It is necessary, therefore, to surgically remove and replace the clouded lens. Often, there is a coexistent refractive defect such as myopia (short sightedness), hyperopia and astigmatism.

Web site: http://appft1.uspto.gov/netahtml/PTO/search-bool.html

- **Non-aspirating transitional viscoelastics for use in surgery**

Inventor(s): Brunstedt, Michael R.; (Cleveland, OH), Chan, Kwan Y.; (Fort Worth, TX), Jinkerson, David L.; (Benbrook, TX), Karakelle, Mutlu; (Fort Worth, TX), Patel, Anilbhai S.; (Arlington, TX)

Correspondence: Alcon Research, Ltd.; R&d Counsel, Q-148; 6201 South Freeway; Fort Worth; TX; 76134-2099; US

Patent Application Number: 20030060447

Date filed: April 24, 2002

Abstract: Non-aspirating viscoelastics, compositions and methods of use are disclosed. The non-aspirating, transitional viscoelastics possess sufficient viscosity to be useful in ophthalmic viscosurgery, but may be left in the eye with little or no resulting IOP spike. The compositions are particularly useful in cataract surgery

Excerpt(s): The present invention relates to the field of viscous and viscoelastic materials suitable for use in surgical procedures. In particular, non-aspirating viscoelastics, including transitional viscoelastics (having non-shear related variable viscosities), which may be left iii situ at the close of surgery are disclosed. Methods of using transitional viscoelastics in surgery, especially ophthalmic surgery are also disclosed.... Viscous or viscoelastic agents used in surgery may perform a number of different functions, including without limitation maintenance and support of soft tissue, tissue manipulation, lubrication, tissue protection, and adhesion prevention. It is recognized that the differing rheological properties of these agents will necessarily impact their ability to perform these functions, and, as a result, their suitability for certain surgical procedures. See, for example, U.S. Pat. No. 5,273,056.... Cataracts are opacities of the ocular lens which generally arise in the elderly. In order to improve eyesight, the cataractous lens is surgically removed and an artificial intraocular lens is inserted in its place. During these surgical procedures, viscoelastic materials are typically injected in the anterior chamber and capsular bag to prevent collapse of the anterior chamber and to protect tissue from damage resulting from physical manipulation.

Web site: http://appft1.uspto.gov/netahtml/PTO/search-bool.html

- **Treatment of posterior capsule opacification**

Inventor(s): Allan, Bruce Duncan Samuel; (London, GB)

Correspondence: Dickstein Shapiro Morin & Oshinsky; 41st Floor; 1177 Avenue of the Americas; New York; NY; 10036-2714; US

Patent Application Number: 20040047900

Date filed: September 23, 2003

Abstract: Posterior capsular opacification is inhibited by administration of polymer, having immobilised on the surface, a ligand for a death receptor, preferably joined by a spacer into the lens capsule following **cataract surgery.** The ligand is preferably Fas ligand. A spacer is preferably polyethyiene glycol. The polymer preferably constitutes an intraocular lens.

Excerpt(s): The present invention relates to the treatment of posterior lens opacification, a complication arising after **cataract surgery.** In particular the invention relates to the prevention of the proliferation and migration of lens epithelial cells after such surgery by the attachment to surface of the intraocular lens (IOL) implanted during **cataract surgery** of a death receptor ligand. Preferably the ligand binds to Fas receptor.... Opacification of the natural lens of the eye--cataract--is the leading cause of visual impairment. Globally, 20 million people are bilaterally blind from cataract. With population aging, this is set to double by 2020.sup.1. **Cataract surgery** is the most common elective operation. Over 175,000 procedures are performed each year in the UK alone.... A 4-5 mm disc shaped piece of the anterior lens capsule is removed routinely during **cataract surgery** (anterior capsulotomy). Ultrasonic liquifaction and aspiration of the opacified natural lens is performed through this circular opening, leaving the remainder of the capsule (the capsular bag) intact. A synthetic intraocular lens (IOL) is implanted within the capsular bag. A scarring reaction to the procedure, posterior capsule opacification (PCO), is the commonest complication of contemporary **cataract surgery.**

Web site: http://appft1.uspto.gov/netahtml/PTO/search-bool.html

- **Treatment solution and method for preventing posterior capsular opacification by selectively inducing detachment and/or death of lens epithelial cells**

Inventor(s): Zhang, Jin Jun; (Shanghai, CN)

Correspondence: Mcandrews, Held & Malloy, Ltd.; 34th Floor; 500 W. Madison Street; Chicago; IL; 60661; US

Patent Application Number: 20040052823

Date filed: September 17, 2002

Abstract: A treatment solution used to prevent posterior capsular opacification is applied or introduced into the lens capsular bag before, during, or after **cataract surgery.** The treatment solution comprises an ion transport mechanism interference agent, which either alone or in combination with other treatment agents such as an osmotic stress agent and an agent to establish a suitable pH, selectively induces detachment and/or death of lens epithelial cells such that posterior capsular opacification is prevented. While the ion transport mechanism interference agent is capable of interfering with the cellular mechanisms and cell ion distribution of a broad range of cells, a concentration of agent is selected such that the treatment solution interferes selectively with the cellular mechanisms of lens epithelial cells while leaving other ocular cells substantially unharmed. The treatment solution selectively induces cellular death and/or detachment of lens epithelial cells while other ocular cells and tissue remain substantially unharmed and without lengthy preoperative pre-treatment.

Excerpt(s): The present invention relates to novel treatment solutions and methods comprising an ion transport mechanism interference agent, alone or in combination with other agents, used to prevent posterior capsular opacification by selectively inducing detachment and/or cell death of lens epithelial cells without damaging other ocular cells and tissue and without lengthy preoperative treatment.... The predominant role of the lens of the human eye is to focus light rays that have passed through the cornea and aqueous humour onto the retina. The structure and metabolism of the lens contributes directly toward maintaining its integrity and transparency. The lens is composed entirely of epithelial cells in different stages of maturation and is relatively unusual in that tissue is never discarded during the maturation process. As new lens cells are formed, older cells are displaced toward the interior of the lens. The lens soon becomes isolated from a direct blood supply and depends on the aqueous and vitreous humors for both nutrition and elimination pathways. The optical characteristics of the lens are much dependent on lens cells maintaining a constant cell volume and dense packing of the fibers to reduce the volume of intercellular space. Maintaining its delicate structure therefore becomes an essential characteristic of the lens. The lens has evolved its unique capabilities to maintain constant cell volume by regulating its ion, sugar, amino acid, and water balances.... A cataract of the human eye is the interruption of the transmission of light by loss of lens transparency. Cataracts, which cause blurring and clouding of vision, are by far the most common cause of low visual acuity. The clouded lens can be removed by surgical procedure, i.e. extra-capsular **cataract extraction** (ECCE). ECCE comprises the removal of the clinical nucleus with cortical cleanup using either manual or automated vacuuming techniques. The posterior and equatorial capsule is left intact as an envelope or bag into which a posterior chamber intraocular lens can be inserted. If the posterior capsule and zonules are intact, this lens will ordinarily remain in place throughout the patient's life without any complications. During the operation, the anterior portion of the lens capsule is carefully opened and the cataract is removed. The intraocular lens is inserted into the remaining (posterior) portion of the capsule. This results in a loss of natural lens accommodation.

Web site: http://appft1.uspto.gov/netahtml/PTO/search-bool.html

- **Use of hydroxyeicosatetraenoic acid derivatives in intraocular surgery**

Inventor(s): Chan, Kwan; (Fort Worth, TX), Karakelle, Mutlu; (Fort Worth, TX)

Correspondence: Alcon Research, Ltd.; Patrick M. Ryan(q-148); R&d Counsel; 6201 So. Freeway; Fort Worth; TX; 76134-2099; US

Patent Application Number: 20020103257

Date filed: September 27, 2001

Abstract: The use of HETE derivatives in intraocular surgery (e.g., cataract surgery) is disclosed. The HETE derivatives protect and maintain the corneal endothelium.

Excerpt(s): This application claims priority to U.S. Provisional Application, U.S. Ser. No. 60/242,501 filed Oct. 23, 2000.... The present invention is directed to the use of hydroxyeicosatetraenoic acid derivatives during intraocular surgery. In particular, the invention relates to the use of such derivatives for the protection of the corneal endothelium during intraocular surgery.... Mucins are proteins which are heavily glycosylated with glucosamine-based moieties. Mucins provide protective and lubricating effects to epithelial cells, especially those of mucosal membranes. Mucins have been shown to be secreted by vesicles and discharged on the surface of the conjunctival epithelium of human eyes (Greiner et al., Mucous Secretory Vesicles in Conjunctival Epithelial Cells of Wearers of Contact Lenses, Archives of Ophthalmology, volume 98, pages 1843-1846 (1980); and Dilly et al., Surface Changes in the Anaesthetic Conjunctiva in Man, with Special Reference to the Production of Mucous from a Non-Goblet-Cell Source, British Journal of Ophthalmology, volume 65, pages 833-842 (1981)). A number of human-derived mucins which reside in the apical and subapical corneal epithelium have been discovered and cloned (Watanabe et al., Human Corneal and Conjunctival Epithelia Produce a Mucin-Like Glycoprotein for the Apical Surface, Investigative Ophthalmology and Visual Science, volume 36, number 2, pages 337-344 (1995)). Recently, Watanabe discovered a new mucin which is secreted via the cornea apical and subapical cells as well as the conjunctival epithelium of the human eye (Watanabe et al., IOVS, volume 36, number 2, pages 337-344 (1995)). These mucins provide lubrication, and additionally attract and hold moisture and sebaceous material for lubrication and the corneal refraction of light.

Web site: http://appft1.uspto.gov/netahtml/PTO/search-bool.html

Keeping Current

In order to stay informed about patents and patent applications dealing with cataract surgery, you can access the U.S. Patent Office archive via the Internet at **http://www.uspto.gov/patft/index.html**. You will see two broad options: (1) Issued Patent, and (2) Published Applications. To see a list of issued patents, perform the following steps: Under "Issued Patents," click "Quick Search." Then, type "cataract surgery" (or synonyms) into the "Term 1" box. After clicking on the search button, scroll down to see the various patents which have been granted to date on cataract surgery.

You can also use this procedure to view pending patent applications concerning cataract surgery. Simply go back to the following Web address: **http://www.uspto.gov/patft/index.html**. Select "Quick Search" under "Published Applications." Then proceed with the steps listed above.

Vocabulary Builder

Ablation: The removal of an organ by surgery. [NIH]

Angulation: Deviation from the normal long axis, as in a fractured bone healed out of line. [NIH]

Aperture: A natural hole of perforation, especially one in a bone. [NIH]

Biconvex: A double-convex lens has two convex surfaces. It is used in various magnifying glasses. [NIH]

Ciliary: Inflammation or infection of the glands of the margins of the eyelids. [NIH]

Cleave: A double-stranded cut in DNA with a restriction endonuclease. [NIH]

Glycosidic: Formed by elimination of water between the anomeric hydroxyl of one sugar and a hydroxyl of another sugar molecule. [NIH]

Hypopyon: An accumulation of pus in the anterior chamber of the eye associated with infectious diseases of the cornea, the iris, and the ciliary body. [NIH]

Loop: A wire usually of platinum bent at one end into a small loop (usually 4 mm inside diameter) and used in transferring microorganisms. [NIH]

Nucleus: A body of specialized protoplasm found in nearly all cells and containing the chromosomes. [NIH]

Pole: The point at either end of the spindle, from which the spindle fibers radiate to the equator. [NIH]

Proenzyme: Inactive form of an enzyme which can then be converted to the active form, usually by excision of a polypeptide, e. g. trypsinogen is the zymogen of trypsin. [NIH]

Racemic: Optically inactive but resolvable in the way of all racemic compounds. [NIH]

Sebaceous: Gland that secretes sebum. [NIH]

Secretory: Secreting; relating to or influencing secretion or the secretions. [NIH]

Stromal: Large, veil-like cell in the bone marrow. [NIH]

Suspensory: Supporting a part. [NIH]

CHAPTER 5. BOOKS ON CATARACT SURGERY

Overview

This chapter provides bibliographic book references relating to cataract surgery. You have many options to locate books on cataract surgery. The simplest method is to go to your local bookseller and inquire about titles that they have in stock or can special order for you. Some patients, however, feel uncomfortable approaching their local booksellers and prefer online sources (e.g. **www.amazon.com** and **www.bn.com**). In addition to online booksellers, excellent sources for book titles on cataract surgery include the Combined Health Information Database and the National Library of Medicine. Once you have found a title that interests you, visit your local public or medical library to see if it is available for loan.

Book Summaries: Online Booksellers

Commercial Internet-based booksellers, such as Amazon.com and Barnes & Noble.com, offer summaries which have been supplied by each title's publisher. Some summaries also include customer reviews. Your local bookseller may have access to in-house and commercial databases that index all published books (e.g. Books in Print®). The following have been recently listed with online booksellers as relating to cataract surgery (sorted alphabetically by title; follow the hyperlink to view more details at Amazon.com):

- **32nd Report [session 1997-98]: Cataract Surgery in Scotland: [HC]: [1997-98]: House of Commons Papers: [1997-98]** by David Davis; ISBN: 0102481989;

http://www.amazon.com/exec/obidos/ASIN/0102481989/icongroupin
terna

- **Advances in Cataract Surgery** by Glen C. Cangelosi (Editor), Glenn Cangelosi (Editor); ISBN: 1556421648;
  http://www.amazon.com/exec/obidos/ASIN/1556421648/icongroupin
  terna

- **Atlas of Cataract Surgery** by William H. Havener; ISBN: 0801621003;
  http://www.amazon.com/exec/obidos/ASIN/0801621003/icongroupin
  terna

- **Cataract Surgery** by Andrew Coombes (Editor), et al; ISBN: 0727912011;
  http://www.amazon.com/exec/obidos/ASIN/0727912011/icongroupin
  terna

- **Cataract Surgery** by Ira A. Abrahamson (Editor); ISBN: 0070001731;
  http://www.amazon.com/exec/obidos/ASIN/0070001731/icongroupin
  terna

- **Cataract Surgery** by Jack M. Dodick; ISBN: 0316188298;
  http://www.amazon.com/exec/obidos/ASIN/0316188298/icongroupin
  terna

- **Cataract Surgery** by Robert C. Drews (Editor), Arthur D. Steele (Editor); ISBN: 0407023410;
  http://www.amazon.com/exec/obidos/ASIN/0407023410/icongroupin
  terna

- **Cataract Surgery**; ISBN: 0727911872;
  http://www.amazon.com/exec/obidos/ASIN/0727911872/icongroupin
  terna

- **Cataract Surgery - A Medical Dictionary, Bibliography, and Annotated Research Guide to Internet Refe** by Icon Health Publications; ISBN: 0597843694;
  http://www.amazon.com/exec/obidos/ASIN/0597843694/icongroupin
  terna

- **Cataract Surgery & Lens Implantation (Current Opinion in Ophthalmology 1994 Series)** by Richard L. Lindstrom; ISBN: 1859226248;
  http://www.amazon.com/exec/obidos/ASIN/1859226248/icongroupin
  terna

- **Cataract Surgery in Axial Myopia** by Buratto L. (Editor); ISBN: 8877802529;
  http://www.amazon.com/exec/obidos/ASIN/8877802529/icongroupin
  terna

- **Cataract Surgery in Complicated Cases** by Lucio Buratto (Editor), et al; ISBN: 1556424671;
  http://www.amazon.com/exec/obidos/ASIN/1556424671/icongroupin terna

- **Cataract Surgery in Scotland: Minutes of Evidence, Monday 9 February 1998: [HC]: [1997-98]: House of Commons Papers: [1997-98]** by David Davis; ISBN: 0102480982;
  http://www.amazon.com/exec/obidos/ASIN/0102480982/icongroupin terna

- **Cataract surgery patient-reported data on appropriateness and outcomes : report to congressional requesters (SuDoc GA 1.13:PEMD-93-14)** by U.S. General Accounting Office; ISBN: B00010LVSE;
  http://www.amazon.com/exec/obidos/ASIN/B00010LVSE/icongroupi nterna

- **Cataract Surgery: A Literature Review and Ratings of Appropriateness and Cruciality/Jra-06** by Paul P. Lee, et al; ISBN: 0833014056;
  http://www.amazon.com/exec/obidos/ASIN/0833014056/icongroupin terna

- **Cataract Surgery: Before and After** by Robert I. Johnson, Thomas J. Pusateri (Designer); ISBN: 1556421257;
  http://www.amazon.com/exec/obidos/ASIN/1556421257/icongroupin terna

- **Cataract Surgery: Current Options and Problems** by Joel M. Engelstein (Editor); ISBN: 0808916173;
  http://www.amazon.com/exec/obidos/ASIN/0808916173/icongroupin terna

- **Cataract Surgery: Perspectives from Ophthalmic Surgery** by George W. Weinstein, George L. Spaeth; ISBN: 1556420161;
  http://www.amazon.com/exec/obidos/ASIN/1556420161/icongroupin terna

- **Cataract Surgery: Technique, Complications, & Management** by Roger F. Steinert (Editor), I. Howard Fine (Editor); ISBN: 0721650449;
  http://www.amazon.com/exec/obidos/ASIN/0721650449/icongroupin terna

- **Cataract Surgery: The State of the Art** by H. Fine, et al; ISBN: 1556425481;
  http://www.amazon.com/exec/obidos/ASIN/1556425481/icongroupin terna

- **Cataract Surgery: The State of the Art** by James P. Gills (Editor), et al; ISBN: 1556423624;

http://www.amazon.com/exec/obidos/ASIN/1556423624/icongroupin
terna

- **Clear-Corneal Cataract Surgery and Topical Anesthesia** by I. Howard
  Fine, et al; ISBN: 1556422261;
  http://www.amazon.com/exec/obidos/ASIN/1556422261/icongroupin
  terna

- **Complications of Cataract Surgery: A Manual** by Bruce Noble, et al;
  ISBN: 075064799X;
  http://www.amazon.com/exec/obidos/ASIN/075064799X/icongroupin
  terna

- **Current Concepts in Cataract Surgery** by Jared M. Emery, Adrienne C.
  Jacobson; ISBN: 0838514057;
  http://www.amazon.com/exec/obidos/ASIN/0838514057/icongroupin
  terna

- **Current concepts in cataract surgery : selected proceedings of the Sixth
  Biennial Cataract Surgical Congress**; ISBN: 0801615275;
  http://www.amazon.com/exec/obidos/ASIN/0801615275/icongroupin
  terna

- **Current Concepts in Cataract Surgery: Selected Proceedings of the
  Eighth Biennial Cataract Surgical Congress** by Tex.)/ Jacobson,
  Adrienne C. Cataract Surgical Congress 1982 Houston (Editor), et al;
  ISBN: 0838514049;
  http://www.amazon.com/exec/obidos/ASIN/0838514049/icongroupin
  terna

- **Extracapsular Cataract Surgery** by Jared M. Emery; ISBN: 0801615526;
  http://www.amazon.com/exec/obidos/ASIN/0801615526/icongroupin
  terna

- **First International Congress on Cataract Surgery, Florence, 1978**; ISBN:
  9061931622;
  http://www.amazon.com/exec/obidos/ASIN/9061931622/icongroupin
  terna

- **Intercapsular cataract extraction : current developments in IOL
  implantation & design : proceedings of part of the seventh
  International Symposium on Anterior Segment Microsurgery, Hong
  Kong, February 1987**; ISBN: 0080359078;
  http://www.amazon.com/exec/obidos/ASIN/0080359078/icongroupin
  terna

- **Intercapsular Cataract Extraction: Current Developments in Iol
  Implantation & Design** by I. Kalb (Editor), Emanuel S. Rosen; ISBN:
  008035906X;

http://www.amazon.com/exec/obidos/ASIN/008035906X/icongroupin
terna

- **Manual of Cataract Surgery** by Gavin G. Bahadur (Editor), Robert M. Sinskey (Editor); ISBN: 0750670827;
http://www.amazon.com/exec/obidos/ASIN/0750670827/icongroupin
terna

- **Master Techniques in Cataract Surgery** by H. Roy, C. Arzabe; ISBN: 1556426186;
http://www.amazon.com/exec/obidos/ASIN/1556426186/icongroupin
terna

- **Medicare : withdrawing eyeglass coverage recommended following cataract surgery : report to congressional requesters (SuDoc GA 1.13:HRD-90-31)** by U.S. General Accounting Office; ISBN: B0001050EU;
http://www.amazon.com/exec/obidos/ASIN/B0001050EU/icongroupi
nterna

- **Modern Cataract Surgery** by Thomas Kohnen (Author); ISBN: 3805573642;
http://www.amazon.com/exec/obidos/ASIN/3805573642/icongroupin
terna

- **Modern cataract surgery and artificial lens implants** by Joe W. Morgan; ISBN: 0918464560;
http://www.amazon.com/exec/obidos/ASIN/0918464560/icongroupin
terna

- **Pediatric Cataract Surgery: Technique, Complications, and Management** by Edward M. Wilson, et al; ISBN: 0781743079;
http://www.amazon.com/exec/obidos/ASIN/0781743079/icongroupin
terna

- **Phacoemulsification and aspiration : the Kelman technique of cataract removal** by Charles D. Kelman; ISBN: 0912684089;
http://www.amazon.com/exec/obidos/ASIN/0912684089/icongroupin
terna

- **Preoperative and Postoperative Issues in Cataract Surgery** by Tyree Carr; ISBN: 0727913298;
http://www.amazon.com/exec/obidos/ASIN/0727913298/icongroupin
terna

- **Refractive Keratotomy for Cataract Surgery and Astigmatism** by Robert M. Kershner; ISBN: 1556422377;
http://www.amazon.com/exec/obidos/ASIN/1556422377/icongroupin
terna

- **Small Incision Cataract Surgery** by Donald R. Sanders (Editor), et al; ISBN: 1556421842; http://www.amazon.com/exec/obidos/ASIN/1556421842/icongroupin terna

- **Small Incision Manual Cataract Surgery** by Michael Blumenthal, Peter Kansas; ISBN: 9962613248; http://www.amazon.com/exec/obidos/ASIN/9962613248/icongroupin terna

- **Soft Implant Lenses in Cataract Surgery** by Thomas R. Mazzocco, et al; ISBN: 0943432782; http://www.amazon.com/exec/obidos/ASIN/0943432782/icongroupin terna

- **Sutureless Cataract Surgery: An Evolution Toward Minimally Invasive Technique** by James P. Gills (Editor), et al; ISBN: 1556421982; http://www.amazon.com/exec/obidos/ASIN/1556421982/icongroupin terna

- **Symposium on Cataract Surgery: Transactions of the New Orleans Academy of Ophthalmology** by H. Dwight Cavanagh; ISBN: 0801638216; http://www.amazon.com/exec/obidos/ASIN/0801638216/icongroupin terna

Chapters on Cataract Surgery

Frequently, cataract surgery will be discussed within a book, perhaps within a specific chapter. In order to find chapters that are specifically dealing with cataract surgery, an excellent source of abstracts is the Combined Health Information Database. You will need to limit your search to book chapters and cataract surgery using the "Detailed Search" option. Go directly to the following hyperlink: **http://chid.nih.gov/detail/detail.html**. To find book chapters, use the drop boxes at the bottom of the search page where "You may refine your search by." Select the dates and language you prefer, and the format option "Book Chapter." By making these selections and typing in "cataract surgery" (or synonyms) into the "For these words:" box, you will only receive results on chapters in books.

General Home References

In addition to references for cataract surgery, you may want a general home medical guide that spans all aspects of home healthcare. The following list is a recent sample of such guides (sorted alphabetically by title; hyperlinks provide rankings, information, and reviews at Amazon.com):

- **American College of Physicians Complete Home Medical Guide (with Interactive Human Anatomy CD-ROM)** by David R. Goldmann (Editor), American College of Physicians; Hardcover - 1104 pages, Book & CD-Rom edition (1999), DK Publishing; ISBN: 0789444127; http://www.amazon.com/exec/obidos/ASIN/0789444127/icongroupinterna

- **The American Medical Association Guide to Home Caregiving** by the American Medical Association (Editor); Paperback - 256 pages 1 edition (2001), John Wiley & Sons; ISBN: 0471414093; http://www.amazon.com/exec/obidos/ASIN/0471414093/icongroupinterna

- **Anatomica : The Complete Home Medical Reference** by Peter Forrestal (Editor); Hardcover (2000), Book Sales; ISBN: 1740480309; http://www.amazon.com/exec/obidos/ASIN/1740480309/icongroupinterna

- **The HarperCollins Illustrated Medical Dictionary : The Complete Home Medical Dictionary** by Ida G. Dox, et al; Paperback - 656 pages 4th edition (2001), Harper Resource; ISBN: 0062736469; http://www.amazon.com/exec/obidos/ASIN/0062736469/icongroupinterna

- **Mayo Clinic Guide to Self-Care: Answers for Everyday Health Problems** by Philip Hagen, M.D. (Editor), et al; Paperback - 279 pages, 2nd edition (December 15, 1999), Kensington Publishing Corp.; ISBN: 0962786578; http://www.amazon.com/exec/obidos/ASIN/0962786578/icongroupinterna

- **The Merck Manual of Medical Information : Home Edition (Merck Manual of Medical Information Home Edition (Trade Paper)** by Robert Berkow (Editor), Mark H. Beers, M.D. (Editor); Paperback - 1536 pages (2000), Pocket Books; ISBN: 0671027263; http://www.amazon.com/exec/obidos/ASIN/0671027263/icongroupinterna

CHAPTER 6. PERIODICALS AND NEWS ON CATARACT SURGERY

Overview

Keeping up on the news relating to cataract surgery can be challenging. Subscribing to targeted periodicals can be an effective way to stay abreast of recent developments on cataract surgery. Periodicals include newsletters, magazines, and academic journals.

In this chapter, we suggest a number of news sources and present various periodicals that cover cataract surgery beyond and including those which are published by patient associations mentioned earlier. We will first focus on news services, and then on periodicals. News services, press releases, and newsletters generally use more accessible language, so if you do chose to subscribe to one of the more technical periodicals, make sure that it uses language you can easily follow.

News Services and Press Releases

Well before articles show up in newsletters or the popular press, they may appear in the form of a press release or a public relations announcement. One of the simplest ways of tracking press releases on cataract surgery is to search the news wires. News wires are used by professional journalists, and have existed since the invention of the telegraph. Today, there are several major "wires" that are used by companies, universities, and other organizations to announce new medical breakthroughs. In the following sample of sources, we will briefly describe how to access each service. These services only post recent news intended for public viewing.

PR Newswire

Perhaps the broadest of the wires is PR Newswire Association, Inc. To access this archive, simply go to **http://www.prnewswire.com**. Below the search box, select the option "The last 30 days." In the search box, type "cataract surgery" or synonyms. The search results are shown by order of relevance. When reading these press releases, do not forget that the sponsor of the release may be a company or organization that is trying to sell a particular product or therapy. Their views, therefore, may be biased. The following is typical of press releases that can be found on PR Newswire:

- **AcrySof(R) ReSTOR(R) Intraocular Lens Demonstrates Ability to Provide Excellent Near and Distance Vision After Cataract Removal**

Reuters Health

The Reuters' Medical News and Health eLine databases can be very useful in exploring news archives relating to cataract surgery. While some of the listed articles are free to view, others can be purchased for a nominal fee. To access this archive, go to **http://www.reutershealth.com/en/index.html** and search by "cataract surgery" (or synonyms). The following was recently listed in this archive for cataract surgery:

- **Cataract surgery device earns conditional backing from FDA advisors**
  Source: Reuters Industry Breifing
  Date: January 17, 2002

- **Anterior capsular opening is smaller in diabetics after cataract surgery**
  Source: Reuters Medical News
  Date: January 26, 2001

- **Age strongly affects visual outcome after cataract surgery**
  Source: Reuters Medical News
  Date: December 25, 2000

- **Cataract surgery beneficial for patients with macular degeneration**
  Source: Reuters Medical News
  Date: December 01, 2000

- **Laser receives first FDA approval for cataract removal**
  Source: Reuters Industry Breifing
  Date: July 05, 2000

- **FDA approves first laser for cataract removal**
  Source: Reuters Health eLine
  Date: July 04, 2000

- **FDA approves Staar's Collamer intraocular lens for cataract surgery**
  Source: Reuters Industry Breifing
  Date: April 07, 2000

- **Medical testing before cataract surgery does not improve safety**
  Source: Reuters Medical News
  Date: January 20, 2000

- **Tests before cataract surgery not always needed**
  Source: Reuters Health eLine
  Date: January 19, 2000

- **Cataract surgery on a second eye has clinical benefits**
  Source: Reuters Medical News
  Date: September 18, 1998

- **"Clear benefit" from cataract surgery on 2nd eye**
  Source: Reuters Health eLine
  Date: September 18, 1998

- **Cataract surgery benefits patients with age-related maculopathy**
  Source: Reuters Medical News
  Date: July 08, 1998

- **Cataract Surgery Linked To Vision Loss**
  Source: Reuters Health eLine
  Date: April 16, 1998

- **Cataract Surgery Linked To Risk Of Age-Related Maculopathy**
  Source: Reuters Medical News
  Date: April 16, 1998

- **Rate of cataract surgery in 50+ age group assessed at about 6% in Australia**
  Source: Reuters Medical News
  Date: February 05, 2003

- **Cataract surgery reduces car accident rate in older drivers**
  Source: Reuters Medical News
  Date: August 20, 2002

- **Retinopathy progression not worsened after cataract surgery**
  Source: Reuters Medical News
  Date: May 31, 2002

- **Cataract Extraction Rates May Have Plateaued Or Declined Slightly**
  Source: Reuters Medical News
  Date: November 26, 1997

- **HMOs: Less Access to Cataract Surgery?**
  Source: Reuters Health eLine
  Date: June 10, 1997

The NIH

Within MEDLINEplus, the NIH has made an agreement with the New York Times Syndicate, the AP News Service, and Reuters to deliver news that can be browsed by the public. Search news releases at **http://www.nlm.nih.gov/medlineplus/alphanews_a.html.** MEDLINEplus allows you to browse across an alphabetical index. Or you can search by date at **http://www.nlm.nih.gov/medlineplus/newsbydate.html**. Often, news items are indexed by MEDLINEplus within their search engine.

Business Wire

Business Wire is similar to PR Newswire. To access this archive, simply go to **http://www.businesswire.com**. You can scan the news by industry category or company name.

Market Wire

Market Wire is more focused on technology than the other wires. To browse the latest press releases by topic, such as alternative medicine, biotechnology, fitness, healthcare, legal, nutrition, and pharmaceuticals, log on to Market Wire's Medical/Health channel at the following hyperlink **http://www.marketwire.com/mw/release_index?channel=MedicalHealth**. Market Wire's home page is **http://www.marketwire.com/mw/home**. From here, type "cataract surgery" (or synonyms) into the search box, and click on "Search News." As this service is technology oriented, you may wish to use it when searching for press releases covering diagnostic procedures or tests.

Search Engines

Free-to-view news can also be found in the news section of your favorite search engines (see the health news page at Yahoo: **http://dir.yahoo.com/Health/News_and_Media/,** or use this Web site's general news search page **http://news.yahoo.com/.** Type in "cataract surgery" (or synonyms). If you know the name of a company that has business interests related to cataract surgery, you can go to any stock trading Web site (such as **www.etrade.com**) and search for the company name there. News items across various news sources are reported on indicated hyperlinks.

BBC

Covering news from a more European perspective, the British Broadcasting Corporation (BBC) allows the public free access to their news archive located at **http://www.bbc.co.uk/**. Search by "cataract surgery" (or synonyms).

CHAPTER 7. PHYSICIAN GUIDELINES AND DATABASES

Overview

Doctors and medical researchers rely on a number of information sources to learn about procedures and treatments. Many will subscribe to journals or newsletters published by their professional associations or refer to specialized textbooks or clinical guides published for the medical profession. In this chapter, we focus on databases and Internet-based guidelines created or written for this professional audience.

NIH Guidelines

For the more common medical procedures and treatments, the National Institutes of Health publish guidelines that are frequently consulted by physicians. Publications are typically written by one or more of the various NIH Institutes. For physician guidelines, commonly referred to as "clinical" or "professional" guidelines, you can visit the following Institutes:

- Office of the Director (OD); guidelines consolidated across agencies available at **http://www.nih.gov/health/consumer/conkey.htm**

- National Institute of General Medical Sciences (NIGMS); fact sheets available at **http://www.nigms.nih.gov/news/facts/**

- National Library of Medicine (NLM); extensive encyclopedia (A.D.A.M., Inc.) with guidelines:
  http://www.nlm.nih.gov/medlineplus/healthtopics.html

- National Eye Institute (NEI); guidelines available at
  http://www.nei.nih.gov/order/index.htm

NIH Databases

In addition to the various Institutes of Health that publish professional guidelines, the NIH has designed a number of databases for professionals.[20] Physician-oriented resources provide a wide variety of information related to the biomedical and health sciences, both past and present. The format of these resources varies. Searchable databases, bibliographic citations, full text articles (when available), archival collections, and images are all available. The following are referenced by the National Library of Medicine:[21]

- **Bioethics:** Access to published literature on the ethical, legal and public policy issues surrounding healthcare and biomedical research. This information is provided in conjunction with the Kennedy Institute of Ethics located at Georgetown University, Washington, D.C.: **http://www.nlm.nih.gov/databases/databases_bioethics.html**

- **HIV/AIDS Resources:** Describes various links and databases dedicated to HIV/AIDS research: **http://www.nlm.nih.gov/pubs/factsheets/aidsinfs.html**

- **NLM Online Exhibitions:** Describes "Exhibitions in the History of Medicine": **http://www.nlm.nih.gov/exhibition/exhibition.html**. Additional resources for historical scholarship in medicine: **http://www.nlm.nih.gov/hmd/hmd.html**

- **Biotechnology Information:** Access to public databases. The National Center for Biotechnology Information conducts research in computational biology, develops software tools for analyzing genome data, and disseminates biomedical information for the better understanding of molecular processes affecting human health and disease: **http://www.ncbi.nlm.nih.gov/**

- **Population Information:** The National Library of Medicine provides access to worldwide coverage of population, family planning, and related health issues, including family planning technology and programs, fertility, and population law and policy: **http://www.nlm.nih.gov/databases/databases_population.html**

- **Cancer Information:** Access to caner-oriented databases: **http://www.nlm.nih.gov/databases/databases_cancer.html**

---

[20] Remember, for the general public, the National Library of Medicine recommends the databases referenced in MEDLINE*plus* (**http://medlineplus.gov/** or **http://www.nlm.nih.gov/medlineplus/databases.html**).

[21] See **http://www.nlm.nih.gov/databases/databases.html**.

- **Profiles in Science:** Offering the archival collections of prominent twentieth-century biomedical scientists to the public through modern digital technology: **http://www.profiles.nlm.nih.gov/**

- **Chemical Information:** Provides links to various chemical databases and references: **http://sis.nlm.nih.gov/Chem/ChemMain.html**

- **Clinical Alerts:** Reports the release of findings from the NIH-funded clinical trials where such release could significantly affect morbidity and mortality: **http://www.nlm.nih.gov/databases/alerts/clinical_alerts.html**

- **Space Life Sciences:** Provides links and information to space-based research (including NASA): **http://www.nlm.nih.gov/databases/databases_space.html**

- **MEDLINE:** Bibliographic database covering the fields of medicine, nursing, dentistry, veterinary medicine, the healthcare system, and the pre-clinical sciences: **http://www.nlm.nih.gov/databases/databases_medline.html**

- **Toxicology and Environmental Health Information (TOXNET):** Databases covering toxicology and environmental health: **http://sis.nlm.nih.gov/Tox/ToxMain.html**

- **Visible Human Interface:** Anatomically detailed, three-dimensional representations of normal male and female human bodies: **http://www.nlm.nih.gov/research/visible/visible_human.html**

While all of the above references may be of interest to physicians who conduct research on cataract surgery, the following are particularly noteworthy.

The NLM Gateway[22]

The NLM (National Library of Medicine) Gateway is a Web-based system that lets users search simultaneously in multiple retrieval systems at the U.S. National Library of Medicine (NLM). It allows users of NLM services to initiate searches from one Web interface, providing "one-stop searching" for many of NLM's information resources or databases.[23] One target audience for the Gateway is the Internet user who is new to NLM's online resources and does not know what information is available or how best to search for it. This

---

[22] Adapted from NLM: **http://gateway.nlm.nih.gov/gw/Cmd?Overview.x.**
[23] The NLM Gateway is currently being developed by the Lister Hill National Center for Biomedical Communications (LHNCBC) at the National Library of Medicine (NLM) of the National Institutes of Health (NIH).

audience may include physicians and other healthcare providers, researchers, librarians, students, and, increasingly, patients, their families, and the public.[24] To use the NLM Gateway, simply go to the search site at **http://gateway.nlm.nih.gov/gw/Cmd**. Type "cataract surgery" (or synonyms) into the search box and click "Search." The results will be presented in a tabular form, indicating the number of references in each database category.

Results Summary

Category	Items Found
Journal Articles	18259
Books / Periodicals / Audio Visual	301
Consumer Health	755
Meeting Abstracts	42
Other Collections	40
Total	19397

HSTAT[25]

HSTAT is a free, Web-based resource that provides access to full-text documents used in healthcare decision-making.[26] HSTAT's audience includes healthcare providers, health service researchers, policy makers, insurance companies, consumers, and the information professionals who serve these groups. HSTAT provides access to a wide variety of publications, including clinical practice guidelines, quick-reference guides for clinicians, consumer health brochures, evidence reports and technology assessments from the Agency for Healthcare Research and Quality (AHRQ), as well as AHRQ's Put Prevention Into Practice.[27] Simply search by "cataract surgery" (or synonyms) at the following Web site: **http://text.nlm.nih.gov**.

---

[24] Other users may find the Gateway useful for an overall search of NLM's information resources. Some searchers may locate what they need immediately, while others will utilize the Gateway as an adjunct tool to other NLM search services such as PubMed® and MEDLINEplus®. The Gateway connects users with multiple NLM retrieval systems while also providing a search interface for its own collections. These collections include various types of information that do not logically belong in PubMed, LOCATORplus, or other established NLM retrieval systems (e.g., meeting announcements and pre-1966 journal citations). The Gateway will provide access to the information found in an increasing number of NLM retrieval systems in several phases.

[25] Adapted from HSTAT: **http://www.nlm.nih.gov/pubs/factsheets/hstat.html**.

[26] The HSTAT URL is **http://hstat.nlm.nih.gov/**.

[27] Other important documents in HSTAT include: the National Institutes of Health (NIH) Consensus Conference Reports and Technology Assessment Reports; the HIV/AIDS

Coffee Break: Tutorials for Biologists[28]

Some patients may wish to have access to a general healthcare site that takes a scientific view of the news and covers recent breakthroughs in biology that may one day assist physicians in developing treatments. To this end, we recommend "Coffee Break," a collection of short reports on recent biological discoveries. Each report incorporates interactive tutorials that demonstrate how bioinformatics tools are used as a part of the research process. Currently, all Coffee Breaks are written by NCBI staff.[29] Each report is about 400 words and is usually based on a discovery reported in one or more articles from recently published, peer-reviewed literature.[30] This site has new articles every few weeks, so it can be considered an online magazine of sorts, and intended for general background information. You can access Coffee Break at **http://www.ncbi.nlm.nih.gov/Coffeebreak/**.

Other Commercial Databases

In addition to resources maintained by official agencies, other databases exist that are commercial ventures addressing medical professionals. Here are some examples that may interest you:

- **CliniWeb International:** Index and table of contents to selected clinical information on the Internet; see **http://www.ohsu.edu/cliniweb/**.

- **Medical World Search:** Searches full text from thousands of selected medical sites on the Internet; see **http://www.mwsearch.com/**.

Treatment Information Service (ATIS) resource documents; the Substance Abuse and Mental Health Services Administration's Center for Substance Abuse Treatment (SAMHSA/CSAT) Treatment Improvement Protocols (TIP) and Center for Substance Abuse Prevention (SAMHSA/CSAP) Prevention Enhancement Protocols System (PEPS); the Public Health Service (PHS) Preventive Services Task Force's *Guide to Clinical Preventive Services*; the independent, nonfederal Task Force on Community Services *Guide to Community Preventive Services*; and the Health Technology Advisory Committee (HTAC) of the Minnesota Health Care Commission (MHCC) health technology evaluations.

[28] Adapted from **http://www.ncbi.nlm.nih.gov/Coffeebreak/Archive/FAQ.html**.

[29] The figure that accompanies each article is frequently supplied by an expert external to NCBI, in which case the source of the figure is cited. The result is an interactive tutorial that tells a biological story.

[30] After a brief introduction that sets the work described into a broader context, the report focuses on how a molecular understanding can provide explanations of observed biology and lead to therapies for diseases. Each vignette is accompanied by a figure and hypertext links that lead to a series of pages that interactively show how NCBI tools and resources are used in the research process.

Specialized References

The following books are specialized references written for professionals interested in cataract surgery (sorted alphabetically by title, hyperlinks provide rankings, information, and reviews at Amazon.com):

- **Clinical Ophthalmic Pathology: Test Yourself** by John Harry, Gary Misson; Paperback (January 2004); Butterworth-Heinemann; ISBN: 0750622644;
  http://www.amazon.com/exec/obidos/ASIN/007137325X/icongroupinter na

- **Dictionary of Ophthalmology** by Michel Millodot, Ph.D., Daniel Laby, MD; Paperback, 1st edition (January 15, 2002), Butterworth-Heinemann Medical; ISBN: 0750647973;
  http://www.amazon.com/exec/obidos/ASIN/0750647973/icongroupinter na

- **Emergency Ophthalmology** by Kenneth C. Chern (Editor); Hardcover (October 2002), McGraw Hill Text; ISBN: 007137325X;
  http://www.amazon.com/exec/obidos/ASIN/007137325X/icongroupinter na

- **The Epidemiology of Eye Disease** by Gordon Johnson, et al; Hardcover (January 1999), Lippincott Williams & Wilkins Publishers; ISBN: 0412643103;
  http://www.amazon.com/exec/obidos/ASIN/0412643103/icongroupinter na

- **The Epidemiology of Eye Disease** by Gordon Johnson, et al; Paperback - 436 pages, 1st edition (March 15, 1998), Lippincott, Williams & Wilkins Publishers; ISBN: 0412845008;
  http://www.amazon.com/exec/obidos/ASIN/0412845008/icongroupinter na

- **External Eye Disease : A Systematic Approach** by Ian A. MacKie; Hardcover, Illustrated edition (January 1999), Butterworth-Heinemann; ISBN: 0750617446;
  http://www.amazon.com/exec/obidos/ASIN/0750617446/icongroupinter na

- **External Eye Disease (Clinical Ophthalmology Slide Set , Vol 2)** by Jack J. Kanski; Hardcover, Vol 2 (September 1997), Butterworth-Heinemann Medical; ISBN: 0750626461;

http://www.amazon.com/exec/obidos/ASIN/0750626461/icongroupinter
na

- **External Eye Disease (Clinical Ophthalmology Photo CD Set , Vol 2)** by Jack J. Kanski; Unknown Binding (September 1997), Butterworth-Heinemann Medical; ISBN: 0750626941;
http://www.amazon.com/exec/obidos/ASIN/0750626941/icongroupinter
na

- **The Eye Book: A Complete Guide to Eye Disorders and Health (Large Print)** by Gary H. Cassel, M.D., et al; Paperback - 528 pages, 1st edition (February 15, 2001), Johns Hopkins University Press; ISBN: 0801865204;
http://www.amazon.com/exec/obidos/ASIN/0801865204/icongroupinter
na

- **The Eye: Basic Sciences in Practice** by John V. Forrester (Editor), et al; Hardcover - 447 pages, 2nd edition (January 15, 2002), W B Saunders Co; ISBN: 0702025410;
http://www.amazon.com/exec/obidos/ASIN/0702025410/icongroupinter
na

- **Functional Anatomy and Histology of the Eye** by Gordon Ruskell; Hardcover, Illustrate edition (April 2002), Butterworth-Heinemann; ISBN: 0750637749;
http://www.amazon.com/exec/obidos/ASIN/0750637749/icongroupinter
na

- **The Little Eye Book: A Pupil's Guide to Understanding Ophthalmology** by Janice K. Comt Ledford, Roberto Pineda, MD; Paperback - 149 pages, 1st edition (January 15, 2002) Slack, Inc.; ISBN: 1556425600;
http://www.amazon.com/exec/obidos/ASIN/1556425600/icongroupinter
na

- **Ophthalmic Pocket Companion** by Dean Dornic; Paperback, 6th edition (March 15, 2002); Butterworth-Heinemann; ISBN: 0750673818;
http://www.amazon.com/exec/obidos/ASIN/0750673818/icongroupinter
na

- **Ophthalmology Review Manual** by Kenneth C. Chern, Michael E. Zegans (Editors); Paperback (550 pages), 1st edition (2000); Lippincott, Williams & Wilkins; ISBN: 0683303643;
http://www.amazon.com/exec/obidos/ASIN/0683303643/icongroupinter
na

- **Ophthalmic Research and Epidemiology: Evaluation and Application** by Stanley W. Hatch (Editor), Paperback - 298 pages, 1st edition (1998), Butterworth-Heinemann Medical; ISBN: 0750699140;

http://www.amazon.com/exec/obidos/ASIN/0750699140/icongroupinterna

- **Ophthalmic Surgery: Principles & Practice** by George L. Spaeth; Hardcover (January 2002), W B Saunders Co; ISBN: 0721669727; http://www.amazon.com/exec/obidos/ASIN/0721669727/icongroupinterna

- **Review Questions for Treatment and Management of Ocular Disease (Review Questions)** by Gurwood; Paperback (2001), Parthenon Pub Group; ISBN: 1850707502; http://www.amazon.com/exec/obidos/ASIN/1850707502/icongroupinterna

- **The Wills Eye Manual: Office and Emergency Room Diagnosis and Treatment of Eye Disease** by Douglas J. Rhee (Editor), et al; Paperback - 563 pages, 3rd edition (March 15, 1999), Lippincott, Williams & Wilkins Publishers; ISBN: 0781716020; http://www.amazon.com/exec/obidos/ASIN/0781716020/icongroupinterna

PART III. APPENDICES

ABOUT PART III

Part III is a collection of appendices on general medical topics which may be of interest to patients undergoing cataract surgery.

APPENDIX A. RESEARCHING YOUR MEDICATIONS

Overview

There are a number of sources available on new or existing medications which could be prescribed to patients undergoing cataract surgery. Often these medications can be taken in preparation for cataract surgery, or immediately following it. While a number of hard copy or CD-Rom resources are available to patients and physicians for research purposes, a more flexible method is to use Internet-based databases. In this chapter, we will begin with a general overview of medications. We will then proceed to outline official recommendations on how you should view your medications. You may also want to research medications that you are currently taking for other conditions as they may interact with medications prescribed specifically for cataract surgery. Research can give you information on the side effects, interactions, and limitations of prescription drugs used in conjunction with cataract surgery. Broadly speaking, there are two sources of information on approved medications: public sources and private sources. We will emphasize free-to-use public sources.

Your Medications: The Basics[31]

Taking medicines is not always as simple as swallowing a pill. It can involve many steps and decisions each day. The AHCRQ recommends that patients take part in treatment decisions. Do not be afraid to ask questions and talk about your concerns. By taking a moment to ask questions early, you may avoid problems later. Here are some points to cover each time a new medicine is prescribed:

---

[31] This section is adapted from AHCRQ: **http://www.ahcpr.gov/consumer/ncpiebro.htm**.

- Ask about all parts of your treatment, including diet changes, exercise, and medicines.

- Ask about the risks and benefits of each medicine or other treatment you might receive.

- Ask how often you or your doctor will check for side effects from a given medication.

Do not hesitate to ask what is important to you about your medicines. You may want a medicine with the fewest side effects, or the fewest doses to take each day. You may care most about cost, or how the medicine might affect your daily activities. Or, you may want the medicine your doctor believes will work the best. Telling your doctor will help him or her select the best medication for you.

Do not be afraid to "bother" your doctor with your concerns and questions about your medications. You can also talk to a nurse or a pharmacist. Feel free to bring a friend or family member with you when you visit your doctor. Talking over your options with someone you trust can help you make better choices, especially if you are not feeling well. Specifically, ask your doctor the following:

- The name of the medicine and what it is supposed to do.

- How and when to take the medicine, how much to take, and for how long.

- What food, drinks, other medicines, or activities you should avoid while taking the medicine.

- What side effects the medicine may have, and what to do if they occur.

- If you can get a refill, and how often.

- About any terms or directions you do not understand.

- What to do if you miss a dose.

- If there is written information you can take home (most pharmacies have information sheets on your prescription medicines; some even offer large-print or Spanish versions).

Do not forget to tell your doctor about all the medicines you are currently taking. This includes prescription medicines and the medicines that you buy over the counter. Then your doctor can avoid giving you a new medicine that may not work well with the medications you take now. When talking to your doctor, you may wish to prepare a list of medicines you currently take, the reason you take them, and how you take them. Be sure to include the following information for each:

- Name of medicine
- Reason taken
- Dosage
- Time(s) of day

Also include any over-the-counter medicines, such as:

- Laxatives
- Diet pills
- Vitamins
- Cold medicine
- Aspirin or other pain, headache, or fever medicine
- Cough medicine
- Allergy relief medicine
- Antacids
- Sleeping pills
- Others (include names)

Learning More about Your Medications

Because of historical investments by various organizations and the emergence of the Internet, it has become rather simple to learn about the medications your doctor has recommended. One such source is the United States Pharmacopeia. In 1820, eleven physicians met in Washington, D.C. to establish the first compendium of standard drugs for the United States. They called this compendium the "U.S. Pharmacopeia (USP)." Today, the USP is a non-profit organization consisting of 800 volunteer scientists, eleven elected officials, and 400 representatives of state associations and colleges of medicine and pharmacy. The USP is located in Rockville, Maryland, and its home page is located at **www.usp.org**. The USP currently provides standards for over 3,700 medications. The resulting USP DI® Advice for the Patient® can be accessed through the National Library of Medicine of the National Institutes of Health. The database is partially derived from lists of federally approved medications in the Food and Drug Administration's (FDA) Drug Approvals database.[32]

While the FDA database is rather large and difficult to navigate, the Phamacopeia is both user-friendly and free to use. It covers more than 9,000 prescription and over-the-counter medications. To access this database, simply type the following hyperlink into your Web browser: **http://www.nlm.nih.gov/medlineplus/druginformation.html**. To view examples of a given medication (brand names, category, description, preparation, proper use, precautions, side effects, etc.), simply follow the hyperlinks indicated within the United States Pharmacopeia (USP).

Of course, we as editors cannot be certain as to what medications you are taking. Therefore, we have compiled a list of medications associated with cataract surgery. Once again, due to space limitations, we only list a sample of medications and provide hyperlinks to ample documentation (e.g. typical dosage, side effects, drug-interaction risks, etc.). The following drugs have been mentioned in the Pharmacopeia and other sources as being potentially applicable to cataract surgery:

Anti-inflammatory Drugs, Nonsteroidal

- **Ophthalmic - U.S. Brands:** Ocufen; Profenal; Voltaren Ophthalmic
  http://www.nlm.nih.gov/medlineplus/druginfo/uspdi/202647.html

Hydroxypropyl Methylcellulose

- **Parenteral-Local - U.S. Brands:** Ocucoat
  http://www.nlm.nih.gov/medlineplus/druginfo/uspdi/203682.html

Ketorolac

- **Ophthalmic - U.S. Brands:** Acular
  http://www.nlm.nih.gov/medlineplus/druginfo/uspdi/202714.html

Commercial Databases

In addition to the medications listed in the USP above, a number of commercial sites are available by subscription to physicians and their

---

[32] Though cumbersome, the FDA database can be freely browsed at the following site: **www.fda.gov/cder/da/da.htm.**

institutions. You may be able to access these sources from your local medical library or your doctor's office.

Reuters Health Drug Database

The Reuters Health Drug Database can be searched by keyword at the hyperlink: **http://www.reutershealth.com/frame2/drug.html**.

Mosby's GenRx

Mosby's GenRx database (also available on CD-Rom and book format) covers 45,000 drug products including generics and international brands. It provides prescribing information, drug interactions, and patient information. Information can be obtained at the following hyperlink: **http://www.genrx.com/Mosby/PhyGenRx/group.html**.

PDR*health*

The PDR*health* database is a free-to-use, drug information search engine that has been written for the public in layman's terms. It contains FDA-approved drug information adapted from the Physicians' Desk Reference (PDR) database. PDR*health* can be searched by brand name, generic name, or indication. It features multiple drug interactions reports. Search PDR*health* at **http://www.pdrhealth.com/drug_info/index.html**.

Other Web Sites

A number of additional Web sites discuss drug information. As an example, you may like to look at **www.drugs.com** which reproduces the information in the Pharmacopeia as well as commercial information. You may also want to consider the Web site of the Medical Letter, Inc. which allows users to download articles on various drugs and therapeutics for a nominal fee: **http://www.medletter.com/**.

Contraindications and Interactions (Hidden Dangers)

Some of the medications mentioned in the previous discussions can be problematic for patients undergoing cataract surgery--not because they are used in the treatment process, but because of contraindications, or side effects. You should ask your physician about any contraindications, especially as these might apply to other medications that you may be taking for common ailments.

Drug-drug interactions occur when two or more drugs react with each other. This drug-drug interaction may cause you to experience an unexpected side effect. Drug interactions may make your medications less effective, cause unexpected side effects, or increase the action of a particular drug. Some drug interactions can even be harmful to you.

Be sure to read the label every time you use a nonprescription or prescription drug, and take the time to learn about drug interactions. These precautions may be critical to your health. You can reduce the risk of potentially harmful drug interactions and side effects with a little bit of knowledge and common sense.

Drug labels contain important information about ingredients, uses, warnings, and directions which you should take the time to read and understand. Labels also include warnings about possible drug interactions. Further, drug labels may change as new information becomes available. This is why it's especially important to read the label every time you use a medication. When your doctor prescribes a new drug, discuss all over-the-counter and prescription medications, dietary supplements, vitamins, botanicals, minerals and herbals you take as well as the foods you eat. Ask your pharmacist for the package insert for each prescription drug you take. The package insert provides more information about potential drug interactions.

A Final Warning

At some point, you may hear of alternative medications from friends, relatives, or in the news media. Advertisements may suggest that certain alternative drugs can produce positive results for patients. Exercise caution-- some of these drugs may have fraudulent claims, and others may actually hurt you. The Food and Drug Administration (FDA) is the official U.S. agency charged with discovering which medications are likely to benefit patients having cataract surgery. The FDA warns patients to watch out for[33]:

- Secret formulas (real scientists share what they know)

---

[33] This section has been adapted from **http://www.fda.gov/opacom/lowlit/medfraud.html**.

- Amazing breakthroughs or miracle cures (real breakthroughs don't happen very often; when they do, real scientists do not call them amazing or miracles)

- Quick, painless, or guaranteed cures

- If it sounds too good to be true, it probably isn't true.

If you have any questions about any kind of medical treatment, the FDA may have an office near you. Look for their number in the blue pages of the phone book. You can also contact the FDA through its toll-free number, 1-888-INFO-FDA (1-888-463-6332), or on the World Wide Web at **www.fda.gov**.

General References

In addition to the resources provided earlier in this chapter, the following general references describe medications (sorted alphabetically by title; hyperlinks provide rankings, information and reviews at Amazon.com):

- **Handbook of Drugs In Primary Eyecare** by D. Reid Woodard, R. Blair Woodard; Paperback - 477 pages, 2nd edition (March 13, 1997), McGraw-Hill Professional Publishing; ISBN: 0838536034;
  http://www.amazon.com/exec/obidos/ASIN/0838536034/icongroupinterna

- **O'Connor Davies's Ophthalmic Drugs: Diagnostic and Therapeutic Uses** by P. H. O'Connor Davies, et al; Paperback, 4th edition (June 1998), Butterworth-Heinemann Medical; ISBN: 0750629665;
  http://www.amazon.com/exec/obidos/ASIN/0750629665/icongroupinterna

- **Ophthalmic Drug Facts, 2002** by Jimmie D. Bartlett (Editor), et al; Paperback - 427 pages, 1st edition (January 15, 2002); Facts & Comparisons; ISBN: 1574391135;
  http://www.amazon.com/exec/obidos/ASIN/1574391135/icongroupinterna

- **Ophthalmic Medications and Pharmacology** by Brian Duvall, O.D., Robert M. Kershner, MD; Paperback - 118 pages, 1st edition (January 15, 1998), Slack, Inc.; ISBN: 1556423284;
  http://www.amazon.com/exec/obidos/ASIN/1556423284/icongroupinterna

- **Pocket Companion Clinical Ocular Pharmacology** by Bartlett, et al; Paperback, 4th edition (March 15, 2002), Butterworth-Heinemann; ISBN: 0750673443;

http://www.amazon.com/exec/obidos/ASIN/0750673443/icongroupinter
na

- **Textbook of Ocular Pharmacology** by Thom J. Zimmerman, Ph.D. (Editor), et al; Hardcover (September 1997), Lippincott, Williams & Wilkins Publishers; ISBN: 0781703069;
  http://www.amazon.com/exec/obidos/ASIN/0781703069/icongroupinter
  na

- **The Wills Eye Drug Guide** by Douglas J. Rhee, Vincent A. Deramo; Paperback, 2nd edition (May 15, 2001), Lippincott, Williams & Wilkins Publishers; ISBN: 0781732778;
  http://www.amazon.com/exec/obidos/ASIN/0781732778/icongroupinter
  na

Vocabulary Builder

The following vocabulary builder gives definitions of words used in this chapter that have not been defined in previous chapters:

Contraindications: Any factor or sign that it is unwise to pursue a certain kind of action or treatment, e. g. giving a general anesthetic to a person with pneumonia. [NIH]

Therapeutics: The branch of medicine which is concerned with the treatment of diseases, palliative or curative. [NIH]

Voltaren: Anti-inflammatory drug. [NIH]

APPENDIX B. RESEARCHING NUTRITION

Overview

Since the time of Hippocrates, doctors have understood the importance of diet and nutrition to patients' health and well-being. Since then, they have accumulated an impressive archive of studies and knowledge dedicated to this subject. Based on their experience, doctors and healthcare providers may recommend particular dietary supplements to patients having cataract surgery. Any dietary recommendation is based on a patient's age, body mass, gender, lifestyle, eating habits, food preferences, and health condition. It is therefore likely that different patients having cataract surgery may be given different recommendations. Some recommendations may be directly related to cataract surgery, while others may be more related to the patient's general health. These recommendations, themselves, may differ from what official sources recommend for the average person.

In this chapter we will begin by briefly reviewing the essentials of diet and nutrition that will broadly frame more detailed discussions of cataract surgery. We will then show you how to find studies dedicated specifically to nutrition and cataract surgery.

Food and Nutrition: General Principles

What Are Essential Foods?

Food is generally viewed by official sources as consisting of six basic elements: (1) fluids, (2) carbohydrates, (3) protein, (4) fats, (5) vitamins, and (6) minerals. Consuming a combination of these elements is considered to be a healthy diet:

- **Fluids** are essential to human life as 80-percent of the body is composed of water. Water is lost via urination, sweating, diarrhea, vomiting, diuretics (drugs that increase urination), caffeine, and physical exertion.

- **Carbohydrates** are the main source for human energy (thermoregulation) and the bulk of typical diets. They are mostly classified as being either simple or complex. Simple carbohydrates include sugars which are often consumed in the form of cookies, candies, or cakes. Complex carbohydrates consist of starches and dietary fibers. Starches are consumed in the form of pastas, breads, potatoes, rice, and other foods. Soluble fibers can be eaten in the form of certain vegetables, fruits, oats, and legumes. Insoluble fibers include brown rice, whole grains, certain fruits, wheat bran and legumes.

- **Proteins** are eaten to build and repair human tissues. Some foods that are high in protein are also high in fat and calories. Food sources for protein include nuts, meat, fish, cheese, and other dairy products.

- **Fats** are consumed for both energy and the absorption of certain vitamins. There are many types of fats, with many general publications recommending the intake of unsaturated fats or those low in cholesterol.

Vitamins and minerals are fundamental to human health, growth, and, in some cases, disease prevention. Most are consumed in your diet (exceptions being vitamins K and D which are produced by intestinal bacteria and sunlight on the skin, respectively). Each vitamin and mineral plays a different role in health. The following outlines essential vitamins:

- **Vitamin A** is important to the health of your eyes, hair, bones, and skin; sources of vitamin A include foods such as eggs, carrots, and cantaloupe.

- **Vitamin B[1]**, also known as thiamine, is important for your nervous system and energy production; food sources for thiamine include meat, peas, fortified cereals, bread, and whole grains.

- **Vitamin B[2]**, also known as riboflavin, is important for your nervous system and muscles, but is also involved in the release of proteins from nutrients; food sources for riboflavin include dairy products, leafy vegetables, meat, and eggs.

- **Vitamin B[3]**, also known as niacin, is important for healthy skin and helps the body use energy; food sources for niacin include peas, peanuts, fish, and whole grains

- **Vitamin B[6]**, also known as pyridoxine, is important for the regulation of cells in the nervous system and is vital for blood formation; food sources for pyridoxine include bananas, whole grains, meat, and fish.

- **Vitamin B^{12}** is vital for a healthy nervous system and for the growth of red blood cells in bone marrow; food sources for vitamin B^{12} include yeast, milk, fish, eggs, and meat.

- **Vitamin C** allows the body's immune system to fight various diseases, strengthens body tissue, and improves the body's use of iron; food sources for vitamin C include a wide variety of fruits and vegetables.

- **Vitamin D** helps the body absorb calcium which strengthens bones and teeth; food sources for vitamin D include oily fish and dairy products.

- **Vitamin E** can help protect certain organs and tissues from various degenerative diseases; food sources for vitamin E include margarine, vegetables, eggs, and fish.

- **Vitamin K** is essential for bone formation and blood clotting; common food sources for vitamin K include leafy green vegetables.

- **Folic Acid** maintains healthy cells and blood and, when taken by a pregnant woman, can prevent her fetus from developing neural tube defects; food sources for folic acid include nuts, fortified breads, leafy green vegetables, and whole grains.

It should be noted that it is possible to overdose on certain vitamins which become toxic if consumed in excess (e.g. vitamin A, D, E and K).

Like vitamins, minerals are chemicals that are required by the body to remain in good health. Because the human body does not manufacture these chemicals internally, we obtain them from food and other dietary sources. The more important minerals include:

- **Calcium** is needed for healthy bones, teeth, and muscles, but also helps the nervous system function; food sources for calcium include dry beans, peas, eggs, and dairy products.

- **Chromium** is helpful in regulating sugar levels in blood; food sources for chromium include egg yolks, raw sugar, cheese, nuts, beets, whole grains, and meat.

- **Fluoride** is used by the body to help prevent tooth decay and to reinforce bone strength; sources of fluoride include drinking water and certain brands of toothpaste.

- **Iodine** helps regulate the body's use of energy by synthesizing into the hormone thyroxine; food sources include leafy green vegetables, nuts, egg yolks, and red meat.

- **Iron** helps maintain muscles and the formation of red blood cells and certain proteins; food sources for iron include meat, dairy products, eggs, and leafy green vegetables.

- **Magnesium** is important for the production of DNA, as well as for healthy teeth, bones, muscles, and nerves; food sources for magnesium include dried fruit, dark green vegetables, nuts, and seafood.

- **Phosphorous** is used by the body to work with calcium to form bones and teeth; food sources for phosphorous include eggs, meat, cereals, and dairy products.

- **Selenium** primarily helps maintain normal heart and liver functions; food sources for selenium include wholegrain cereals, fish, meat, and dairy products.

- **Zinc** helps wounds heal, the formation of sperm, and encourage rapid growth and energy; food sources include dried beans, shellfish, eggs, and nuts.

The United States government periodically publishes recommended diets and consumption levels of the various elements of food. Again, your doctor may encourage deviations from the average official recommendation. To learn more about basic dietary guidelines, visit the Web site: **http://www.health.gov/dietaryguidelines/**. Based on these guidelines, many foods are required to list the nutrition levels on the food's packaging. Labeling Requirements are listed at the following site maintained by the Food and Drug Administration: **http://www.cfsan.fda.gov/~dms/lab-cons.html**. When interpreting these requirements, the government recommends that consumers become familiar with the following abbreviations before reading FDA literature:[34]

- **DVs (Daily Values):** A new dietary reference term that will appear on the food label. It is made up of two sets of references, DRVs and RDIs.

- **DRVs (Daily Reference Values):** A set of dietary references that applies to fat, saturated fat, cholesterol, carbohydrate, protein, fiber, sodium, and potassium.

- **RDIs (Reference Daily Intakes):** A set of dietary references based on the Recommended Dietary Allowances for essential vitamins and minerals and, in selected groups, protein. The name "RDI" replaces the term "U.S. RDA."

---

[34] Adapted from the FDA: **http://www.fda.gov/fdac/special/foodlabel/dvs.html**.

- **RDAs (Recommended Dietary Allowances):** A set of estimated nutrient allowances established by the National Academy of Sciences. It is updated periodically to reflect current scientific knowledge.

What Are Dietary Supplements?[35]

Dietary supplements are widely available through many commercial sources, including health food stores, grocery stores, pharmacies, and by mail. Dietary supplements are provided in many forms including tablets, capsules, powders, gel-tabs, extracts, and liquids. Historically in the United States, the most prevalent type of dietary supplement was a multivitamin/mineral tablet or capsule that was available in pharmacies, either by prescription or "over the counter." Supplements containing strictly herbal preparations were less widely available. Currently in the United States, a wide array of supplement products are available, including vitamin, mineral, other nutrients, and botanical supplements as well as ingredients and extracts of animal and plant origin.

According to the Office of Dietary Supplements (ODS), dietary supplements can have an important impact on the prevention and management of disease and on the maintenance of health.[36] The ODS notes that considerable research on the effects of dietary supplements has been conducted in Asia and Europe where the use of plant products, in particular, has a long tradition. However, the overwhelming majority of supplements have not been studied scientifically. To explore the role of dietary supplements in the improvement of health care, the ODS plans, organizes, and supports conferences, workshops, and symposia on scientific topics related to dietary supplements. The ODS often works in conjunction with other NIH Institutes and Centers, other government agencies, professional organizations, and public advocacy groups.

---

[35] This discussion has been adapted from the NIH:
http://ods.od.nih.gov/showpage.aspx?pageid=46.

[36] Adapted from **http://ods.od.nih.gov/showpage.aspx?pageid=2**. The Dietary Supplement Health and Education Act defines dietary supplements as "a product (other than tobacco) intended to supplement the diet that bears or contains one or more of the following dietary ingredients: a vitamin, mineral, amino acid, herb or other botanical; or a dietary substance for use to supplement the diet by increasing the total dietary intake; or a concentrate, metabolite, constituent, extract, or combination of any ingredient described above; and intended for ingestion in the form of a capsule, powder, softgel, or gelcap, and not represented as a conventional food or as a sole item of a meal or the diet."

To learn more about official information on dietary supplements, visit the ODS site at **http://dietary-supplements.info.nih.gov/**. Or contact:

> **The Office of Dietary Supplements**
> National Institutes of Health
> Building 31, Room 1B29
> 31 Center Drive, MSC 2086
> Bethesda, Maryland 20892-2086
> Tel: (301) 435-2920
> Fax: (301) 480-1845
> E-mail: ods@nih.gov

Finding Studies on Cataract Surgery

The NIH maintains an office dedicated to patient nutrition and diet. The National Institutes of Health's Office of Dietary Supplements (ODS) offers a searchable bibliographic database called the IBIDS (International Bibliographic Information on Dietary Supplements). The IBIDS contains over 460,000 scientific citations and summaries about dietary supplements and nutrition as well as references to published international, scientific literature on dietary supplements such as vitamins, minerals, and botanicals.[37] IBIDS is available to the public free of charge through the ODS Internet page: **http://ods.od.nih.gov/databases/ibids.html**.

After entering the search area, you have three choices: (1) IBIDS Consumer Database, (2) Full IBIDS Database, or (3) Peer Reviewed Citations Only. We recommend that you start with the Consumer Database. While you may not find references for the topics that are of most interest to you, check back periodically as this database is frequently updated. More studies can be found by searching the Full IBIDS Database. Healthcare professionals and researchers generally use the third option, which lists peer-reviewed citations. In all cases, we suggest that you take advantage of the "Advanced Search" option that allows you to retrieve up to 100 fully explained references in a comprehensive format. Type "cataract surgery" (or synonyms) into the search box. To narrow the search, you can also select the "Title" field.

---

[37] Adapted from **http://ods.od.nih.gov**. IBIDS is produced by the Office of Dietary Supplements (ODS) at the National Institutes of Health to assist the public, healthcare providers, educators, and researchers in locating credible, scientific information on dietary supplements. IBIDS was developed and will be maintained through an interagency partnership with the Food and Nutrition Information Center of the National Agricultural Library, U.S. Department of Agriculture.

The following information is typical of that found when using the "Full IBIDS Database" when searching using "cataract surgery" (or a synonym):

- **Anticoagulants and cataract surgery.**
  Source: Hall, D L Steen, W H Drummond, J W Byrd, W A Ophthalmic-Surg. 1988 March; 19(3): 221-2 0022-023X

- **Aspergillus niger endophthalmitis after cataract surgery.**
  Author(s): Department of Ophthalmology, Postgraduate Institute of Medical Education and Research, Chandigarh, India.
  Source: Brar, G S Ram, J Kaushik, S Chakraborti, A Dogra, M R Gupta, A J-Cataract-Refract-Surg. 2002 October; 28(10): 1882-3 0886-3350

- **Comparison of four viscoelastic substances for cataract surgery in eyes with cornea guttata.**
  Author(s): Department of Ophthalmology, Bundesknappschaft's Hospital Sulzbach, Germany. augen@kk-sulzbach.de
  Source: Mester, U Hauck, C Anterist, N Low, M Dev-Ophthalmol. 2002; 34: 25-31 0250-3751

- **Consultation section. Attitudes regarding the concomitant use of anti-coagulants with elective cataract surgery.**
  Source: Anonymous J-Cataract-Refract-Surg. 1992 September; 18(5): 531-5 0886-3350

- **Do inhaled corticosteroids significantly increase cataract surgery in elderly patients?**
  Source: Franfelder, F T Arch-Ophthalmol. 1998 October; 116(10): 1369 0003-9950

- **Effect of cataract extraction and posterior chamber lens implantation on outflow facility and its response to pilocarpine in Korean subjects.**
  Author(s): Department of Ophthalmology, Samsung Medical Center College of Medicine, Sungkyunkwan University, Seoul 135-710, Korea. cwkee@ophthalmology.org
  Source: Kee, C Moon, S H Br-J-Ophthalmol. 2000 September; 84(9): 987-9 0007-1161

- **Effect of dorzolamide and latanoprost on intraocular pressure after small incision cataract surgery.**
  Author(s): Department of Ophthalmology, University of Vienna, Austria.
  Source: Rainer, G Menapace, R Schmetterer, K Findl, O Georgopoulos, M Vass, C J-Cataract-Refract-Surg. 1999 December; 25(12): 1624-9 0886-3350

- **Effect of Healon5 and 4 other viscoelastic substances on intraocular pressure and endothelium after cataract surgery.**
  Author(s): Department of Ophthalmology, Humboldt University Berlin, Campus Virchow Klinikum, Germany.

Source: Holzer, M P Tetz, M R Auffarth, G U Welt, R Volcker, H E J-Cataract-Refract-Surg. 2001 February; 27(2): 213-8 0886-3350

- **Effects of flurbiprofen and indomethacin on acute cystoid macular edema after cataract surgery: functional vision and contrast sensitivity.**
  Author(s): Vision Psychophysics Lab, Allergan, Inc., San Ramon, California 94583, USA.
  Source: Ginsburg, A P Cheetham, J K DeGryse, R E Abelson, M J-Cataract-Refract-Surg. 1995 January; 21(1): 82-92 0886-3350

- **Effects of NG-nitro L-arginine and corticosteroids on aqueous humor levels of nitric oxide and cytokines after cataract surgery.**
  Author(s): University of Inonu School of Medicine, Turgut Ozal Medical Center, Department of Ophthalmology, Malatya, Turkey.
  Source: Er, H Gunduz, A Turkoz, Y Cigli, A Isci, N J-Cataract-Refract-Surg. 1999 June; 25(6): 795-9 0886-3350

- **Efficacy of preoperative versus postoperative ketorolac tromethamine 0.5% in reducing inflammation after cataract surgery.**
  Author(s): Department of Ophthalmology and Visual Science, University of Texas Health Science Center-Houston, Houston, Texas, USA.
  Source: El Harazi, S M Ruiz, R S Feldman, R M Villanueva, G Chuang, A Z J-Cataract-Refract-Surg. 2000 November; 26(11): 1626-30 0886-3350

- **Extracellular matrix of opacified anterior capsule after endocapsular cataract surgery.**
  Author(s): Department of Ophthalmology, National Children's Hospital, Tokyo, Japan. nazuma@nch.go.jp
  Source: Azuma, N Hara, T Hara, T Graefes-Arch-Clin-Exp-Ophthalmol. 1998 July; 236(7): 531-6 0721-832X

- **Influence of viscoelastic substances used in cataract surgery on corneal metabolism and endothelial morphology: comparison of Healon and Viscoat(1).**
  Author(s): Department of Opthalmology, University of Vienna, Vienna, Austria
  Source: Maar, N Graebe, A Schild, G Stur, M Amon, M J-Cataract-Refract-Surg. 2001 November; 27(11): 1756-61 0886-3350

- **Intraindividual comparison of the effects of a fixed dorzolamide-timolol combination and latanoprost on intraocular pressure after small incision cataract surgery.**
  Author(s): Department of Ophthalmology, University of Vienna, Vienna, Austria. georg.rainer@akh-wien.ac.at
  Source: Rainer, G Menapace, R Findl, O Petternel, V Kiss, B Georgopoulos, M J-Cataract-Refract-Surg. 2001 May; 27(5): 706-10 0886-3350

- **Intraocular pressure after small incision cataract surgery with Healon5 and Viscoat.**
Author(s): Department of Ophthalmology, University of Vienna, Austria.
Source: Rainer, G Menapace, R Findl, O Georgopoulos, M Kiss, B Petternel, V J-Cataract-Refract-Surg. 2000 February; 26(2): 271-6 0886-3350

- **Ketorolac-tobramycin combination vs fluorometholone-tobramycin combination in reducing inflammation following phacoemulsification cataract extraction with scleral tunnel incision.**
Author(s): Department of Ophthalmology, Harran University School of Medicine and Faculty of Agriculture, Sanliurfa, Turkey. guzey@turk.net
Source: Guzey, M Karadede, S Dogan, Z Satici, A Ophthalmic-Surg-Lasers. 2000 Nov-December; 31(6): 451-6 1082-3069

- **Ocufen and pupillary dilation during cataract surgery.**
Author(s): Department of Ophthalmology, Washington University, St. Louis, Missouri.
Source: Drews, R C Katsev, D A J-Cataract-Refract-Surg. 1989 July; 15(4): 445-8 0886-3350

- **Presumed photic retinopathy after cataract surgery: an angiographic study.**
Author(s): Department of Ophthalmology, Sir Mortimer B. Davis-Jewish General Hospital, Montreal, PQ.
Source: Gomolin, J E Koenekoop, R K Can-J-Ophthalmol. 1993 August; 28(5): 221-4 0008-4182

- **Progression of diabetic retinopathy after cataract extraction.**
Author(s): Ophthalmology Department, Kaplan Hospital, Rehovot, Israel.
Source: Pollack, A Dotan, S Oliver, M Br-J-Ophthalmol. 1991 September; 75(9): 547-51 0007-1161

- **Pupillary dilatation during cataract surgery--relative efficacy of indomethacin and flurbiprofen.**
Author(s): Dr Rajendra Prasad Center for Ophthalmic Sciences, All India Institute of Medical Sciences, Ansari Nagar, New Delhi.
Source: Sachdev, M S Mehta, M R Dada, V K Jain, A K Garg, S P Gupta, S K Ophthalmic-Surg. 1990 August; 21(8): 557-9 0022-023X

- **Recurrent severe hypotony after cataract surgery in an eye with previous trabeculectomy.**
Author(s): Department of Ophthalmology, Turku University Hospital, Finland.
Source: Vuori, M L J-Cataract-Refract-Surg. 1998 January; 24(1): 136-8 0886-3350

- **Reduction of inflammation following cataract surgery by the nonsteroidal anti-inflammatory drug, flurbiprofen.**
  Author(s): University of Illinois at Chicago, College of Medicine.
  Source: Sabiston, D Tessler, H Sumers, K Osterle, C Cheetham, J K Duzman, E DeGryse, R Ophthalmic-Surg. 1987 December; 18(12): 873-7 0022-023X

- **Removal of viscoelastic materials after experimental cataract surgery in vitro.**
  Author(s): Department of Ophthalmology, Medical University of South Carolina, Charleston 29425.
  Source: Assia, E I Apple, D J Lim, E S Morgan, R C Tsai, J C J-Cataract-Refract-Surg. 1992 January; 18(1): 3-6 0886-3350

- **Tear lactoferrin concentration during postoperative ocular inflammation in cataract surgery.**
  Author(s): Department of Ophthalmology, Pt. B.D. Sharma Post Graduate Institute of Medical Sciences, Rohtak, India.
  Source: KuMarch, R Parmar, I P Chhillar, N Lal, H Acta-Ophthalmol-Scand. 1997 April; 75(2): 142-4 1395-3907

- **The association of cataract and cataract surgery with the long-term incidence of age-related maculopathy: the Beaver Dam eye study.**
  Author(s): Department of Ophthalmology and Visual Sciences, University of Wisconsin-Madison, 610 N Walnut St, 460 WARF, Madison, WI 53726-2397, USA. kleinr@epi.ophth.wisc.edu
  Source: Klein, R Klein, B E Wong, T Y Tomany, S C Cruickshanks, K J Arch-Ophthalmol. 2002 November; 120(11): 1551-8 0003-9950

- **The effect of indomethacin 1% ophthalmic suspension in preventing surgically induced miosis at extracapsular cataract surgery.**
  Author(s): Department of Ophthalmology, Odense University Hospital, Denmark.
  Source: Nielsen, P J Gregersen, P Mortensen, K K Kalstrup, N Acta-Ophthalmol-Suppl. 1987; 182115-8

- **The effect of treatment with topical nonsteroidal anti-inflammatory drugs with and without intraoperative epinephrine on the maintenance of mydriasis during cataract surgery.**
  Author(s): University of Calgary, Alberta, Canada.
  Source: Gimbel, H V Ophthalmology. 1989 May; 96(5): 585-8 0161-6420

- **Topical 0.1% indomethacin solution versus topical 0.1% dexamethasone solution in the prevention of inflammation after cataract surgery. The Study Group.**
  Author(s): Universitair Ziekenhuis, Leuven, Belgium.

Source: Missotten, L Richard, C Trinquand, C Ophthalmologica. 2001 Jan-February; 215(1): 43-50 0030-3755

- **Topical indomethacin in extracapsular cataract surgery. A photographic study.**
  Author(s): Department of Ophthalmology, Kuopio University Central Hospital, Finland.
  Source: Terasvirta, M Acta-Ophthalmol-(Copenh). 1989 June; 67(3): 339-41 0001-639X

- **Trends in cataract surgery.**
  Author(s): Department of Ophthalmology, Mount Sinai School of Medicine, New York, New York.
  Source: Eichenbaum, J W Bull-N-Y-Acad-Med. 1992 July; 68(3): 367-89 0028-7091

- **Use of collagen shields in cataract surgery.**
  Author(s): Rikshospitalet, Department of Ophthalmology, University of Oslo, Norway.
  Source: Haaskjold, E Ohrstrom, A Uusitalo, R J Krootila, K Sandvig, K U Sonne, H Mahlberg, K J-Cataract-Refract-Surg. 1994 March; 20(2): 150-3 0886-3350

Federal Resources on Nutrition

In addition to the IBIDS, the United States Department of Health and Human Services (HHS) and the United States Department of Agriculture (USDA) provide many sources of information on general nutrition and health. Recommended resources include:

- healthfinder®, HHS's gateway to health information, including diet and nutrition:
  http://www.healthfinder.gov/scripts/SearchContext.asp?topic=238&page=0

- The United States Department of Agriculture's Web site dedicated to nutrition information: **www.nutrition.gov**

- The Food and Drug Administration's Web site for federal food safety information: **www.foodsafety.gov**

- The National Action Plan on Overweight and Obesity sponsored by the United States Surgeon General:
  http://www.surgeongeneral.gov/topics/obesity/

- The Center for Food Safety and Applied Nutrition has an Internet site sponsored by the Food and Drug Administration and the Department of Health and Human Services: **http://vm.cfsan.fda.gov/**

- Center for Nutrition Policy and Promotion sponsored by the United States Department of Agriculture: **http://www.usda.gov/cnpp/**

- Food and Nutrition Information Center, National Agricultural Library sponsored by the United States Department of Agriculture: **http://www.nal.usda.gov/fnic/**

- Food and Nutrition Service sponsored by the United States Department of Agriculture: **http://www.fns.usda.gov/fns/**

Additional Web Resources

A number of additional Web sites offer encyclopedic information covering food and nutrition. The following is a representative sample:

- AOL: **http://search.aol.com/cat.adp?id=174&layer=&from=subcats**

- Family Village: **http://www.familyvillage.wisc.edu/med_nutrition.html**

- Google: **http://directory.google.com/Top/Health/Nutrition/**

- Open Directory Project: **http://dmoz.org/Health/Nutrition/**

- Yahoo.com: **http://dir.yahoo.com/Health/Nutrition/**

- WebMD®Health: **http://my.webmd.com/nutrition**

- WholeHealthMD.com: **http://www.wholehealthmd.com/reflib/0,1529,,00.html**

The following is a specific Web list relating to cataract surgery; please note that any particular subject below may indicate either a therapeutic use, or a contraindication (potential danger), and does not reflect an official recommendation:

- **Vitamins**

  Vitamin C
  Source: Prima Communications, Inc.www.personalhealthzone.com

Vocabulary Builder

The following vocabulary builder defines words used in the references in this chapter that have not been defined in previous chapters:

Potassium: It is essential to the ability of muscle cells to contract. [NIH]

Sperm: The fecundating fluid of the male. [NIH]

APPENDIX C. FINDING MEDICAL LIBRARIES

Overview

At a medical library you can find medical texts and reference books, consumer health publications, specialty newspapers and magazines, as well as medical journals. In this Appendix, we show you how to quickly find a medical library in your area.

Preparation

Before going to the library, highlight the references mentioned in this sourcebook that you find interesting. Focus on those items that are not available via the Internet, and ask the reference librarian for help with your search. He or she may know of additional resources that could be helpful to you. Most importantly, your local public library and medical libraries have Interlibrary Loan programs with the National Library of Medicine (NLM), one of the largest medical collections in the world. According to the NLM, most of the literature in the general and historical collections of the National Library of Medicine is available on interlibrary loan to any library. NLM's interlibrary loan services are only available to libraries. If you would like to access NLM medical literature, then visit a library in your area that can request the publications for you.[38]

---

[38] Adapted from the NLM: **http://www.nlm.nih.gov/psd/cas/interlibrary.html**.

Finding a Local Medical Library

The quickest method to locate medical libraries is to use the Internet-based directory published by the National Network of Libraries of Medicine (NN/LM). This network includes 4626 members and affiliates that provide many services to librarians, health professionals, and the public. To find a library in your area, simply visit **http://nnlm.gov/members/adv.html** or call 1-800-338-7657.

Medical Libraries in the U.S. and Canada

In addition to the NN/LM, the National Library of Medicine (NLM) lists a number of libraries with reference facilities that are open to the public. The following is the NLM's list and includes hyperlinks to each library's Web site. These Web pages can provide information on hours of operation and other restrictions. The list below is a small sample of libraries recommended by the National Library of Medicine (sorted alphabetically by name of the U.S. state or Canadian province where the library is located)[39]:

- **Alabama:** Health InfoNet of Jefferson County (Jefferson County Library Cooperative, Lister Hill Library of the Health Sciences), **http://www.uab.edu/infonet/**

- **Alabama:** Richard M. Scrushy Library (American Sports Medicine Institute)

- **Arizona:** Samaritan Regional Medical Center: The Learning Center (Samaritan Health System, Phoenix, Arizona), **http://www.samaritan.edu/library/bannerlibs.htm**

- **California:** Kris Kelly Health Information Center (St. Joseph Health System, Humboldt), **http://www.humboldt1.com/~kkhic/index.html**

- **California:** Community Health Library of Los Gatos, **http://www.healthlib.org/orgresources.html**

- **California:** Consumer Health Program and Services (CHIPS) (County of Los Angeles Public Library, Los Angeles County Harbor-UCLA Medical Center Library) - Carson, CA, **http://www.colapublib.org/services/chips.html**

- **California:** Gateway Health Library (Sutter Gould Medical Foundation)

- **California:** Health Library (Stanford University Medical Center), **http://www-med.stanford.edu/healthlibrary/**

---

[39] Abstracted from http://www.nlm.nih.gov/medlineplus/libraries.html.

- **California:** Patient Education Resource Center - Health Information and Resources (University of California, San Francisco), **http://sfghdean.ucsf.edu/barnett/PERC/default.asp**

- **California:** Redwood Health Library (Petaluma Health Care District), **http://www.phcd.org/rdwdlib.html**

- **California:** Los Gatos PlaneTree Health Library, **http://planetreesanjose.org/**

- **California:** Sutter Resource Library (Sutter Hospitals Foundation, Sacramento), **http://suttermedicalcenter.org/library/**

- **California:** Health Sciences Libraries (University of California, Davis), **http://www.lib.ucdavis.edu/healthsci/**

- **California:** ValleyCare Health Library & Ryan Comer Cancer Resource Center (ValleyCare Health System, Pleasanton), **http://gaelnet.stmarys-ca.edu/other.libs/gbal/east/vchl.html**

- **California:** Washington Community Health Resource Library (Fremont), **http://www.healthlibrary.org/**

- **Colorado:** William V. Gervasini Memorial Library (Exempla Healthcare), **http://www.saintjosephdenver.org/yourhealth/libraries/**

- **Connecticut:** Hartford Hospital Health Science Libraries (Hartford Hospital), **http://www.harthosp.org/library/**

- **Connecticut:** Healthnet: Connecticut Consumer Health Information Center (University of Connecticut Health Center, Lyman Maynard Stowe Library), **http://library.uchc.edu/departm/hnet/**

- **Connecticut:** Waterbury Hospital Health Center Library (Waterbury Hospital, Waterbury), **http://www.waterburyhospital.com/library/consumer.shtml**

- **Delaware:** Consumer Health Library (Christiana Care Health System, Eugene du Pont Preventive Medicine & Rehabilitation Institute, Wilmington), **http://www.christianacare.org/health_guide/health_guide_pmri_health_info.cfm**

- **Delaware:** Lewis B. Flinn Library (Delaware Academy of Medicine, Wilmington), **http://www.delamed.org/chls.html**

- **Georgia:** Family Resource Library (Medical College of Georgia, Augusta), **http://cmc.mcg.edu/kids_families/fam_resources/fam_res_lib/frl.htm**

- **Georgia:** Health Resource Center (Medical Center of Central Georgia, Macon), **http://www.mccg.org/hrc/hrchome.asp**

- **Hawaii:** Hawaii Medical Library: Consumer Health Information Service (Hawaii Medical Library, Honolulu), **http://hml.org/CHIS/**

- **Idaho:** DeArmond Consumer Health Library (Kootenai Medical Center, Coeur d'Alene), **http://www.nicon.org/DeArmond/index.htm**

- **Illinois:** Health Learning Center of Northwestern Memorial Hospital (Chicago), **http://www.nmh.org/health_info/hlc.html**

- **Illinois:** Medical Library (OSF Saint Francis Medical Center, Peoria), **http://www.osfsaintfrancis.org/general/library/**

- **Kentucky:** Medical Library - Services for Patients, Families, Students & the Public (Central Baptist Hospital, Lexington), **http://www.centralbap.com/education/community/library.cfm**

- **Kentucky:** University of Kentucky - Health Information Library (Chandler Medical Center, Lexington), **http://www.mc.uky.edu/PatientEd/**

- **Louisiana:** Alton Ochsner Medical Foundation Library (Alton Ochsner Medical Foundation, New Orleans), **http://www.ochsner.org/library/**

- **Louisiana:** Louisiana State University Health Sciences Center Medical Library-Shreveport, **http://lib-sh.lsuhsc.edu/**

- **Maine:** Franklin Memorial Hospital Medical Library (Franklin Memorial Hospital, Farmington), **http://www.fchn.org/fmh/lib.htm**

- **Maine:** Gerrish-True Health Sciences Library (Central Maine Medical Center, Lewiston), **http://www.cmmc.org/library/library.html**

- **Maine:** Hadley Parrot Health Science Library (Eastern Maine Healthcare, Bangor), **http://www.emh.org/hll/hpl/guide.htm**

- **Maine:** Maine Medical Center Library (Maine Medical Center, Portland), **http://www.mmc.org/library/**

- **Maine:** Parkview Hospital (Brunswick), **http://www.parkviewhospital.org/**

- **Maine:** Southern Maine Medical Center Health Sciences Library (Southern Maine Medical Center, Biddeford), **http://www.smmc.org/services/service.php3?choice=10**

- **Maine:** Stephens Memorial Hospital's Health Information Library (Western Maine Health, Norway), **http://www.wmhcc.org/Library/**

- **Manitoba, Canada:** Consumer & Patient Health Information Service (University of Manitoba Libraries), **http://www.umanitoba.ca/libraries/units/health/reference/chis.html**

- **Manitoba, Canada:** J.W. Crane Memorial Library (Deer Lodge Centre, Winnipeg), **http://www.deerlodge.mb.ca/crane_library/about.asp**

- **Maryland:** Health Information Center at the Wheaton Regional Library (Montgomery County, Dept. of Public Libraries, Wheaton Regional Library), **http://www.mont.lib.md.us/healthinfo/hic.asp**

- **Massachusetts:** Baystate Medical Center Library (Baystate Health System), **http://www.baystatehealth.com/1024/**

- **Massachusetts:** Boston University Medical Center Alumni Medical Library (Boston University Medical Center), **http://med-libwww.bu.edu/library/lib.html**

- **Massachusetts:** Lowell General Hospital Health Sciences Library (Lowell General Hospital, Lowell), **http://www.lowellgeneral.org/library/HomePageLinks/WWW.htm**

- **Massachusetts:** Paul E. Woodard Health Sciences Library (New England Baptist Hospital, Boston), **http://www.nebh.org/health_lib.asp**

- **Massachusetts:** St. Luke's Hospital Health Sciences Library (St. Luke's Hospital, Southcoast Health System, New Bedford), **http://www.southcoast.org/library/**

- **Massachusetts:** Treadwell Library Consumer Health Reference Center (Massachusetts General Hospital), **http://www.mgh.harvard.edu/library/chrcindex.html**

- **Massachusetts:** UMass HealthNet (University of Massachusetts Medical School, Worchester), **http://healthnet.umassmed.edu/**

- **Michigan:** Botsford General Hospital Library - Consumer Health (Botsford General Hospital, Library & Internet Services), **http://www.botsfordlibrary.org/consumer.htm**

- **Michigan:** Helen DeRoy Medical Library (Providence Hospital and Medical Centers), **http://www.providence-hospital.org/library/**

- **Michigan:** Marquette General Hospital - Consumer Health Library (Marquette General Hospital, Health Information Center), **http://www.mgh.org/center.html**

- **Michigan:** Patient Education Resouce Center - University of Michigan Cancer Center (University of Michigan Comprehensive Cancer Center, Ann Arbor), **http://www.cancer.med.umich.edu/learn/leares.htm**

- **Michigan:** Sladen Library & Center for Health Information Resources - Consumer Health Information (Detroit), **http://www.henryford.com/body.cfm?id=39330**

- **Montana:** Center for Health Information (St. Patrick Hospital and Health Sciences Center, Missoula)

- **National:** Consumer Health Library Directory (Medical Library Association, Consumer and Patient Health Information Section), **http://caphis.mlanet.org/directory/index.html**

- **National:** National Network of Libraries of Medicine (National Library of Medicine) - provides library services for health professionals in the United States who do not have access to a medical library, **http://nnlm.gov/**

- **National:** NN/LM List of Libraries Serving the Public (National Network of Libraries of Medicine), **http://nnlm.gov/members/**

- **Nevada:** Health Science Library, West Charleston Library (Las Vegas-Clark County Library District, Las Vegas), **http://www.lvccld.org/special_collections/medical/index.htm**

- **New Hampshire:** Dartmouth Biomedical Libraries (Dartmouth College Library, Hanover), **http://www.dartmouth.edu/~biomed/resources.htmld/conshealth.htmld**

- **New Jersey:** Consumer Health Library (Rahway Hospital, Rahway), **http://www.rahwayhospital.com/library.htm**

- **New Jersey:** Dr. Walter Phillips Health Sciences Library (Englewood Hospital and Medical Center, Englewood), **http://www.englewoodhospital.com/links/index.htm**

- **New Jersey:** Meland Foundation (Englewood Hospital and Medical Center, Englewood), **http://www.geocities.com/ResearchTriangle/9360/**

- **New York:** Choices in Health Information (New York Public Library) - NLM Consumer Pilot Project participant, **http://www.nypl.org/branch/health/links.html**

- **New York:** Health Information Center (Upstate Medical University, State University of New York, Syracuse), **http://www.upstate.edu/library/hic/**

- **New York:** Health Sciences Library (Long Island Jewish Medical Center, New Hyde Park), **http://www.lij.edu/library/library.html**

- **New York:** ViaHealth Medical Library (Rochester General Hospital), **http://www.nyam.org/library/**

- **Ohio:** Consumer Health Library (Akron General Medical Center, Medical & Consumer Health Library), **http://www.akrongeneral.org/hwlibrary.htm**

- **Oklahoma:** The Health Information Center at Saint Francis Hospital (Saint Francis Health System, Tulsa), **http://www.sfh-tulsa.com/services/healthinfo.asp**

- **Oregon:** Planetree Health Resource Center (Mid-Columbia Medical Center, The Dalles), **http://www.mcmc.net/phrc/**

- **Pennsylvania:** Community Health Information Library (Milton S. Hershey Medical Center, Hershey), **http://www.hmc.psu.edu/commhealth/**

- **Pennsylvania:** Community Health Resource Library (Geisinger Medical Center, Danville), **http://www.geisinger.edu/education/commlib.shtml**

- **Pennsylvania:** HealthInfo Library (Moses Taylor Hospital, Scranton), **http://www.mth.org/healthwellness.html**

- **Pennsylvania:** Hopwood Library (University of Pittsburgh, Health Sciences Library System, Pittsburgh), **http://www.hsls.pitt.edu/guides/chi/hopwood/index_html**

- **Pennsylvania:** Koop Community Health Information Center (College of Physicians of Philadelphia), **http://www.collphyphil.org/kooppg1.shtml**

- **Pennsylvania:** Learning Resources Center - Medical Library (Susquehanna Health System, Williamsport), **http://www.shscares.org/services/lrc/index.asp**

- **Pennsylvania:** Medical Library (UPMC Health System, Pittsburgh), **http://www.upmc.edu/passavant/library.htm**

- **Quebec, Canada:** Medical Library (Montreal General Hospital), **http://www.mghlib.mcgill.ca/**

- **South Dakota:** Rapid City Regional Hospital Medical Library (Rapid City Regional Hospital), **http://www.rcrh.org/Services/Library/Default.asp**

- **Texas:** Houston HealthWays (Houston Academy of Medicine-Texas Medical Center Library), **http://hhw.library.tmc.edu/**

- **Washington:** Community Health Library (Kittitas Valley Community Hospital), **http://www.kvch.com/**

- **Washington:** Southwest Washington Medical Center Library (Southwest Washington Medical Center, Vancouver), **http://www.swmedicalcenter.com/body.cfm?id=72**

APPENDIX D. YOUR RIGHTS AND INSURANCE

Overview

Any patient undergoing cataract surgery faces a series of issues related more to the healthcare industry than to the medical procedure itself. This appendix covers two important topics in this regard: your rights and responsibilities as a patient, and how to get the most out of your medical insurance plan.

Your Rights as a Patient

The President's Advisory Commission on Consumer Protection and Quality in the Healthcare Industry has created the following summary of your rights as a patient.[40]

Information Disclosure

Consumers have the right to receive accurate, easily understood information. Some consumers require assistance in making informed decisions about health plans, health professionals, and healthcare facilities. Such information includes:

- *Health plans.* Covered benefits, cost-sharing, and procedures for resolving complaints, licensure, certification, and accreditation status, comparable measures of quality and consumer satisfaction, provider network composition, the procedures that govern access to specialists and emergency services, and care management information.

---

[40]Adapted from Consumer Bill of Rights and Responsibilities: http://www.hcqualitycommission.gov/press/cbor.html#head1.

- *Health professionals.* Education, board certification, and recertification, years of practice, experience performing certain procedures, and comparable measures of quality and consumer satisfaction.

- *Healthcare facilities.* Experience in performing certain procedures and services, accreditation status, comparable measures of quality, worker, and consumer satisfaction, and procedures for resolving complaints.

- *Consumer assistance programs.* Programs must be carefully structured to promote consumer confidence and to work cooperatively with health plans, providers, payers, and regulators. Desirable characteristics of such programs are sponsorship that ensures accountability to the interests of consumers and stable, adequate funding.

Choice of Providers and Plans

Consumers have the right to a choice of healthcare providers that is sufficient to ensure access to appropriate high-quality healthcare. To ensure such choice, the Commission recommends the following:

- *Provider network adequacy.* All health plan networks should provide access to sufficient numbers and types of providers to assure that all covered services will be accessible without unreasonable delay -- including access to emergency services 24 hours a day and 7 days a week. If a health plan has an insufficient number or type of providers to provide a covered benefit with the appropriate degree of specialization, the plan should ensure that the consumer obtains the benefit outside the network at no greater cost than if the benefit were obtained from participating providers.

- *Women's health services.* Women should be able to choose a qualified provider offered by a plan -- such as gynecologists, certified nurse midwives, and other qualified healthcare providers -- for the provision of covered care necessary to provide routine and preventative women's healthcare services.

- *Access to specialists.* Consumers having complex or serious medical procedures who require frequent specialty care should have direct access to a qualified specialist of their choice within a plan's network of providers. Authorizations, when required, should be for an adequate number of direct access visits under an approved treatment plan.

- *Transitional care.* Consumers who are undergoing a course of treatment for a chronic or disabling condition (or who are in the second or third trimester of a pregnancy) at the time they involuntarily change health plans or at a time when a provider is terminated by a plan for other than cause should be able to continue seeing their current specialty providers for up to 90 days (or through completion of postpartum care) to allow for transition of care.

- *Choice of health plans.* Public and private group purchasers should, wherever feasible, offer consumers a choice of high-quality health insurance plans.

Access to Emergency Services

Consumers have the right to access emergency healthcare services when and where the need arises. Health plans should provide payment when a consumer presents to an emergency department with acute symptoms of sufficient severity--including severe pain--such that a "prudent layperson" could reasonably expect the absence of medical attention to result in placing that consumer's health in serious jeopardy, serious impairment to bodily functions, or serious dysfunction of any bodily organ or part.

Participation in Treatment Decisions

Consumers have the right and responsibility to fully participate in all decisions related to their healthcare. Consumers who are unable to fully participate in treatment decisions have the right to be represented by parents, guardians, family members, or other conservators. Physicians and other health professionals should:

- Provide patients with sufficient information and opportunity to decide among treatment options consistent with the informed consent process.

- Discuss all treatment options with a patient in a culturally competent manner, including the option of no treatment at all.

- Ensure that persons with disabilities have effective communications with members of the health system in making such decisions.

- Discuss all current treatments a consumer may be undergoing.

- Discuss all risks, benefits, and consequences to treatment or nontreatment.

- Give patients the opportunity to refuse treatment and to express preferences about future treatment decisions.

- Discuss the use of advance directives -- both living wills and durable powers of attorney for healthcare -- with patients and their designated family members.

- Abide by the decisions made by their patients and/or their designated representatives consistent with the informed consent process.

Health plans, health providers, and healthcare facilities should:

- Disclose to consumers factors -- such as methods of compensation, ownership of or interest in healthcare facilities, or matters of conscience -- that could influence advice or treatment decisions.

- Assure that provider contracts do not contain any so-called "gag clauses" or other contractual mechanisms that restrict healthcare providers' ability to communicate with and advise patients about medically necessary treatment options.

- Be prohibited from penalizing or seeking retribution against healthcare professionals or other health workers for advocating on behalf of their patients.

Respect and Nondiscrimination

Consumers have the right to considerate, respectful care from all members of the healthcare industry at all times and under all circumstances. An environment of mutual respect is essential to maintain a quality healthcare system. To assure that right, the Commission recommends the following:

- Consumers must not be discriminated against in the delivery of healthcare services consistent with the benefits covered in their policy, or as required by law, based on race, ethnicity, national origin, religion, sex, age, mental or physical disability, sexual orientation, genetic information, or source of payment.

- Consumers eligible for coverage under the terms and conditions of a health plan or program, or as required by law, must not be discriminated against in marketing and enrollment practices based on race, ethnicity, national origin, religion, sex, age, mental or physical disability, sexual orientation, genetic information, or source of payment.

Confidentiality of Health Information

Consumers have the right to communicate with healthcare providers in confidence and to have the confidentiality of their individually identifiable healthcare information protected. Consumers also have the right to review and copy their own medical records and request amendments to their records.

Complaints and Appeals

Consumers have the right to a fair and efficient process for resolving differences with their health plans, healthcare providers, and the institutions that serve them, including a rigorous system of internal review and an independent system of external review. A free copy of the Patient's Bill of Rights is available from the American Hospital Association.[41]

Patient Responsibilities

Treatment is a two-way street between you and your healthcare providers. To underscore the importance of finance in modern healthcare as well as your responsibility for the financial aspects of your care, the President's Advisory Commission on Consumer Protection and Quality in the Healthcare Industry has proposed that patients understand the following "Consumer Responsibilities."[42] In a healthcare system that protects consumers' rights, it is reasonable to expect and encourage consumers to assume certain responsibilities. Greater individual involvement by the consumer in his or her care increases the likelihood of achieving the best outcome and helps support a quality-oriented, cost-conscious environment. Such responsibilities include:

- Take responsibility for maximizing healthy habits such as exercising, not smoking, and eating a healthy diet.

- Work collaboratively with healthcare providers in developing and carrying out agreed-upon treatment plans.

- Disclose relevant information and clearly communicate wants and needs.

- Use your health insurance plan's internal complaint and appeal processes to address your concerns.

- Avoid knowingly spreading disease.

---

[41] To order your free copy of the Patient's Bill of Rights, telephone 312-422-3000 or visit the American Hospital Association's Web site: **http://www.aha.org**. Click on "Resource Center," go to "Search" at bottom of page, and then type in "Patient's Bill of Rights." The Patient's Bill of Rights is also available from Fax on Demand, at 312-422-2020, document number 471124.

[42] Adapted from **http://www.hcqualitycommission.gov/press/cbor.html#head1**.

- Recognize the reality of risks, the limits of the medical science, and the human fallibility of the healthcare professional.

- Be aware of a healthcare provider's obligation to be reasonably efficient and equitable in providing care to other patients and the community.

- Become knowledgeable about your health plan's coverage and options (when available) including all covered benefits, limitations, and exclusions, rules regarding use of network providers, coverage and referral rules, appropriate processes to secure additional information, and the process to appeal coverage decisions.

- Show respect for other patients and health workers.

- Make a good-faith effort to meet financial obligations.

- Abide by administrative and operational procedures of health plans, healthcare providers, and Government health benefit programs.

Choosing an Insurance Plan

There are a number of official government agencies that help consumers understand their healthcare insurance choices.[43] The U.S. Department of Labor, in particular, recommends ten ways to make your health benefits choices work best for you.[44]

1. Your options are important. There are many different types of health benefit plans. Find out which one your employer offers, then check out the plan, or plans, offered. Your employer's human resource office, the health plan administrator, or your union can provide information to help you match your needs and preferences with the available plans. The more information you have, the better your healthcare decisions will be.

2. Reviewing the benefits available. Do the plans offered cover preventive care, well-baby care, vision or dental care? Are there deductibles? Answers to these questions can help determine the out-of-pocket expenses you may face. Matching your needs and those of your family members will result in the best possible benefits. Cheapest may not always be best. Your goal is high quality health benefits.

---

[43] More information about quality across programs is provided at the following AHRQ Web site: **http://www.ahrq.gov/consumer/qntascii/qnthplan.htm**.
[44] Adapted from the Department of Labor:
http://www.dol.gov/dol/pwba/public/pubs/health/top10-text.html.

3. Look for quality. The quality of healthcare services varies, but quality can be measured. You should consider the quality of healthcare in deciding among the healthcare plans or options available to you. Not all health plans, doctors, hospitals and other providers give the highest quality care. Fortunately, there is quality information you can use right now to help you compare your healthcare choices. Find out how you can measure quality. Consult the U.S. Department of Health and Human Services publication "Your Guide to Choosing Quality Health Care" on the Internet at **www.ahcpr.gov/consumer**.

4. Your plan's summary plan description (SPD) provides a wealth of information. Your health plan administrator can provide you with a copy of your plan's SPD. It outlines your benefits and your legal rights under the Employee Retirement Income Security Act (ERISA), the federal law that protects your health benefits. It should contain information about the coverage of dependents, what services will require a co-pay, and the circumstances under which your employer can change or terminate a health benefits plan. Save the SPD and all other health plan brochures and documents, along with memos or correspondence from your employer relating to health benefits.

5. Assess your benefit coverage as your family status changes. Marriage, divorce, childbirth or adoption, and the death of a spouse are all life events that may signal a need to change your health benefits. You, your spouse and dependent children may be eligible for a special enrollment period under provisions of the Health Insurance Portability and Accountability Act (HIPAA). Even without life-changing events, the information provided by your employer should tell you how you can change benefits or switch plans, if more than one plan is offered. If your spouse's employer also offers a health benefits package, consider coordinating both plans for maximum coverage.

6. Changing jobs and other life events can affect your health benefits. Under the Consolidated Omnibus Budget Reconciliation Act (COBRA), you, your covered spouse, and your dependent children may be eligible to purchase extended health coverage under your employer's plan if you lose your job, change employers, get divorced, or upon occurrence of certain other events. Coverage can range from 18 to 36 months depending on your situation. COBRA applies to most employers with 20 or more workers and requires your plan to notify you of your rights. Most plans require eligible individuals to make their COBRA election within 60 days of the plan's notice. Be sure to follow up with your plan sponsor if you don't receive notice, and make sure you respond within the allotted time.

7. HIPAA can also help if you are changing jobs, particularly if you have a medical condition. HIPAA generally limits pre-existing condition exclusions to a maximum of 12 months (18 months for late enrollees). HIPAA also requires this maximum period to be reduced by the length of time you had prior "creditable coverage." You should receive a certificate documenting your prior creditable coverage from your old plan when coverage ends.

8. Plan for retirement. Before you retire, find out what health benefits, if any, extend to you and your spouse during your retirement years. Consult with your employer's human resources office, your union, the plan administrator, and check your SPD. Make sure there is no conflicting information among these sources about the benefits you will receive or the circumstances under which they can change or be eliminated. With this information in hand, you can make other important choices, like finding out if you are eligible for Medicare and Medigap insurance coverage.

9. Know how to file an appeal if your health benefits claim is denied. Understand how your plan handles grievances and where to make appeals of the plan's decisions. Keep records and copies of correspondence. Check your health benefits package and your SPD to determine who is responsible for handling problems with benefit claims. Contact PWBA for customer service assistance if you are unable to obtain a response to your complaint.

10. You can take steps to improve the quality of the healthcare and the health benefits you receive. Look for and use things like Quality Reports and Accreditation Reports whenever you can. Quality reports may contain consumer ratings -- how satisfied consumers are with the doctors in their plan, for instance-- and clinical performance measures -- how well a healthcare organization prevents and treats illness. Accreditation reports provide information on how accredited organizations meet national standards, and often include clinical performance measures. Look for these quality measures whenever possible. Consult "Your Guide to Choosing Quality Health Care" on the Internet at **www.ahcpr.gov/consumer**.

Medicare and Medicaid

Illness strikes both rich and poor families. For low-income families, Medicaid is available to defer the costs of treatment. The Health Care Financing Administration (HCFA) administers Medicare, the nation's largest health insurance program, which covers 39 million Americans. In the following pages, you will learn the basics about Medicare insurance as well as useful contact information on how to find more in-depth information about Medicaid.[45]

Who Is Eligible for Medicare?

Generally, you are eligible for Medicare if you or your spouse worked for at least 10 years in Medicare-covered employment and you are 65 years old and a citizen or permanent resident of the United States. You might also qualify for coverage if you are under age 65 but have a disability or End-Stage Renal disease (permanent kidney failure requiring dialysis or transplant). Here are some simple guidelines:

You can get Part A at age 65 without having to pay premiums if:

- You are already receiving retirement benefits from Social Security or the Railroad Retirement Board.

- You are eligible to receive Social Security or Railroad benefits but have not yet filed for them.

- You or your spouse had Medicare-covered government employment.

If you are under 65, you can get Part A without having to pay premiums if:

- You have received Social Security or Railroad Retirement Board disability benefit for 24 months.

- You are a kidney dialysis or kidney transplant patient.

Medicare has two parts:

- Part A (Hospital Insurance). Most people do not have to pay for Part A.

- Part B (Medical Insurance). Most people pay monthly for Part B.

Part A (Hospital Insurance)

Helps Pay For: Inpatient hospital care, care in critical access hospitals (small facilities that give limited outpatient and inpatient services to people in rural areas) and skilled nursing facilities, hospice care, and some home healthcare.

---

[45] This section has been adapted from the Official U.S. Site for Medicare Information: **http://www.medicare.gov/Basics/Overview.asp**.

Cost: Most people get Part A automatically when they turn age 65. You do not have to pay a monthly payment called a premium for Part A because you or a spouse paid Medicare taxes while you were working.

If you (or your spouse) did not pay Medicare taxes while you were working and you are age 65 or older, you still may be able to buy Part A. If you are not sure you have Part A, look on your red, white, and blue Medicare card. It will show "Hospital Part A" on the lower left corner of the card. You can also call the Social Security Administration toll free at 1-800-772-1213 or call your local Social Security office for more information about buying Part A. If you get benefits from the Railroad Retirement Board, call your local RRB office or 1-800-808-0772. For more information, call your Fiscal Intermediary about Part A bills and services. The phone number for the Fiscal Intermediary office in your area can be obtained from the following Web site: **http://www.medicare.gov/Contacts/home.asp**.

Part B (Medical Insurance)

Helps Pay For: Doctors, services, outpatient hospital care, and some other medical services that Part A does not cover, such as the services of physical and occupational therapists, and some home healthcare. Part B helps pay for covered services and supplies when they are medically necessary.

Cost: As of 2001, you pay the Medicare Part B premium of $50.00 per month. In some cases this amount may be higher if you did not choose Part B when you first became eligible at age 65. The cost of Part B may go up 10% for each 12-month period that you were eligible for Part B but declined coverage, except in special cases. You will have to pay the extra 10% cost for the rest of your life.

Enrolling in Part B is your choice. You can sign up for Part B anytime during a 7-month period that begins 3 months before you turn 65. Visit your local Social Security office, or call the Social Security Administration at 1-800-772-1213 to sign up. If you choose to enroll in Part B, the premium is usually taken out of your monthly Social Security, Railroad Retirement, or Civil Service Retirement payment. If you do not receive any of the above payments, Medicare sends you a bill for your part B premium every 3 months. You should receive your Medicare premium bill in the mail by the 10th of the month. If you do not, call the Social Security Administration at 1-800-772-1213, or your local Social Security office. If you get benefits from the Railroad Retirement Board, call your local RRB office or 1-800-808-0772. For more information, call your Medicare carrier about bills and services. The phone number for the Medicare carrier in your area can be found at the following Web site: **http://www.medicare.gov/Contacts/home.asp**. You may have choices in how you get your healthcare including the Original Medicare Plan, Medicare Managed Care Plans (like HMOs), and Medicare Private Fee-for-Service Plans.

Medicaid

Medicaid is a joint federal and state program that helps pay medical costs for some people with low incomes and limited resources. Medicaid programs vary from state to state. People on Medicaid may also get coverage for nursing home care and outpatient prescription drugs which are not covered by Medicare. You can find more information about Medicaid on the HCFA.gov Web site at **http://www.hcfa.gov/medicaid/medicaid.htm**.

States also have programs that pay some or all of Medicare's premiums and may also pay Medicare deductibles and coinsurance for certain people who have Medicare and a low income. To qualify, you must have:

- Part A (Hospital Insurance),

- Assets, such as bank accounts, stocks, and bonds that are not more than $4,000 for a single person, or $6,000 for a couple, and

- A monthly income that is below certain limits.

For more information, look at the Medicare Savings Programs brochure, **http://www.medicare.gov/Library/PDFNavigation/PDFInterim.asp?Language=English&Type=Pub&PubID=10126**. There are also Prescription Drug Assistance Programs available. Find information on these programs which offer discounts or free medications to individuals in need at **http://www.medicare.gov/Prescription/Home.asp**.

NORD's Medication Assistance Programs

Finally, the National Organization for Rare Disorders, Inc. (NORD) administers medication programs sponsored by humanitarian-minded pharmaceutical and biotechnology companies to help uninsured or under-insured individuals secure life-saving or life-sustaining drugs.[46] NORD programs ensure that certain vital drugs are available "to those individuals whose income is too high to qualify for Medicaid but too low to pay for their

---

[46] Adapted from NORD: **http://www.rarediseases.org/programs/medication**.

prescribed medications." The program has standards for fairness, equity, and unbiased eligibility. It currently covers some 14 programs for nine pharmaceutical companies. NORD also offers early access programs for investigational new drugs (IND) under the approved "Treatment INDs" programs of the Food and Drug Administration (FDA). In these programs, a limited number of individuals can receive investigational drugs that have yet to be approved by the FDA. These programs are generally designed for rare treatments. For more information, visit **www.rarediseases.org**.

Additional Resources

In addition to the references already listed in this chapter, you may need more information on health insurance, hospitals, or the healthcare system in general. The NIH has set up an excellent guidance Web site that addresses these and other issues. Topics include:[47]

- Health Insurance:
  http://www.nlm.nih.gov/medlineplus/healthinsurance.html

- Health Statistics:
  http://www.nlm.nih.gov/medlineplus/healthstatistics.html

- HMO and Managed Care:
  http://www.nlm.nih.gov/medlineplus/managedcare.html

- Hospice Care: **http://www.nlm.nih.gov/medlineplus/hospicecare.html**

- Medicaid: **http://www.nlm.nih.gov/medlineplus/medicaid.html**

- Medicare: **http://www.nlm.nih.gov/medlineplus/medicare.html**

- Nursing Homes and Long-Term Care:
  http://www.nlm.nih.gov/medlineplus/nursinghomes.html

- Patient's Rights, Confidentiality, Informed Consent, Ombudsman Programs, Privacy and Patient Issues:
  http://www.nlm.nih.gov/medlineplus/patientissues.html

- Veteran's Health, Persian Gulf War, Gulf War Syndrome, Agent Orange:
  http://www.nlm.nih.gov/medlineplus/veteranshealth.html

---

[47] You can access this information at
http://www.nlm.nih.gov/medlineplus/healthsystem.html.

ONLINE GLOSSARIES

The Internet provides access to a number of free-to-use medical dictionaries and glossaries. The National Library of Medicine has compiled the following list of online dictionaries:

- ADAM Medical Encyclopedia (A.D.A.M., Inc.), comprehensive medical reference: **http://www.nlm.nih.gov/medlineplus/encyclopedia.html**

- MedicineNet.com Medical Dictionary (MedicineNet, Inc.): **http://www.medterms.com/Script/Main/hp.asp**

- Merriam-Webster Medical Dictionary (Inteli-Health, Inc.): **http://www.intelihealth.com/IH/**

- Multilingual Glossary of Technical and Popular Medical Terms in Eight European Languages (European Commission) - Danish, Dutch, English, French, German, Italian, Portuguese, and Spanish: **http://allserv.rug.ac.be/~rvdstich/eugloss/welcome.html**

- On-line Medical Dictionary (CancerWEB): **http://www.graylab.ac.uk/omd/**

- Technology Glossary (National Library of Medicine) - Health Care Technology: **http://www.nlm.nih.gov/nichsr/ta101/ta10108.htm**

- Terms and Definitions (Office of Rare Diseases): **http://rarediseases.info.nih.gov/ord/glossary_a-e.html**

Beyond these, MEDLINEplus contains a very user-friendly encyclopedia covering every aspect of medicine (licensed from A.D.A.M., Inc.). The ADAM Medical Encyclopedia can be accessed via the following Web site address: **http://www.nlm.nih.gov/medlineplus/encyclopedia.html**. ADAM is also available on commercial Web sites such as Web MD (**http://my.webmd.com/adam/asset/adam_disease_articles/a_to_z/a**) and drkoop.com (**http://www.drkoop.com/**). Topics of interest can be researched by using keywords before continuing elsewhere, as these basic definitions and concepts will be useful in more advanced areas of research. You may choose to print various pages specifically relating to cataract surgery and keep them on file. The NIH, in particular, suggests that patients with cataract surgery visit the following Web sites in the ADAM Medical Encyclopedia:

- **Basic Guidelines for Cataract Surgery**

   Cataract removal
   Web site:
   http://www.nlm.nih.gov/medlineplus/ency/article/002957.htm

- **Signs & Symptoms for Cataract Surgery**

  Loss of vision
  Web site:
  http://www.nlm.nih.gov/medlineplus/ency/article/003040.htm

  Vision abnormalities
  Web site:
  http://www.nlm.nih.gov/medlineplus/ency/article/003029.htm

  Visual abnormalities
  Web site:
  http://www.nlm.nih.gov/medlineplus/ency/article/003029.htm

- **Background Topics for Cataract Surgery**

  Retina
  Web site:
  http://www.nlm.nih.gov/medlineplus/ency/article/002291.htm

Online Dictionary Directories

The following are additional online directories compiled by the National Library of Medicine, including a number of specialized medical dictionaries and glossaries:

- Medical Dictionaries: Medical & Biological (World Health Organization):
  http://www.who.int/hlt/virtuallibrary/English/diction.htm#Medical

- MEL-Michigan Electronic Library List of Online Health and Medical Dictionaries (Michigan Electronic Library):
  http://mel.lib.mi.us/health/health-dictionaries.html

- Patient Education: Glossaries (DMOZ Open Directory Project):
  http://dmoz.org/Health/Education/Patient_Education/Glossaries/

- Web of Online Dictionaries (Bucknell University):
  http://www.yourdictionary.com/diction5.html#medicine

CATARACT SURGERY GLOSSARY

The following is a complete glossary of terms used in this sourcebook. The definitions are derived from official public sources including the National Institutes of Health [NIH] and the European Union [EU]. After this glossary, we list a number of additional hardbound and electronic glossaries and dictionaries that you may wish to consult.

Ablation: The removal of an organ by surgery. [NIH]

Abscess: A localized, circumscribed collection of pus. [NIH]

Adjustment: The dynamic process wherein the thoughts, feelings, behavior, and biophysiological mechanisms of the individual continually change to adjust to the environment. [NIH]

Angulation: Deviation from the normal long axis, as in a fractured bone healed out of line. [NIH]

Antibiotic: A substance usually produced by vegetal micro-organisms capable of inhibiting the growth of or killing bacteria. [NIH]

Aperture: A natural hole of perforation, especially one in a bone. [NIH]

Applicability: A list of the commodities to which the candidate method can be applied as presented or with minor modifications. [NIH]

Biconvex: A double-convex lens has two convex surfaces. It is used in various magnifying glasses. [NIH]

Branch: Most commonly used for branches of nerves, but applied also to other structures. [NIH]

Breakdown: A physical, metal, or nervous collapse. [NIH]

Cataracts: In medicine, an opacity of the crystalline lens of the eye obstructing partially or totally its transmission of light. [NIH]

Catheters: A small, flexible tube that may be inserted into various parts of the body to inject or remove liquids. [NIH]

Ciliary: Inflammation or infection of the glands of the margins of the eyelids. [NIH]

Cleave: A double-stranded cut in DNA with a restriction endonuclease. [NIH]

Consultation: A deliberation between two or more physicians concerning the diagnosis and the proper method of treatment in a case. [NIH]

Consumption: Pulmonary tuberculosis. [NIH]

Contraindications: Any factor or sign that it is unwise to pursue a certain kind of action or treatment, e. g. giving a general anesthetic to a person with pneumonia. [NIH]

Cornea: The transparent anterior portion of the fibrous coat of the eye consisting of five layers. [NIH]

Cystoid: Like a bladder or a cyst. [NIH]

Cytokine: Small but highly potent protein that modulates the activity of many cell types, including T and B cells. [NIH]

Density: The logarithm to the base 10 of the opacity of an exposed and processed film. [NIH]

Diaphragm: Contraceptive intra-uterine device. [NIH]

Dissection: Cutting up of an organism for study. [NIH]

Duke: A lamp which produces ultraviolet radiations for certain ophthalmologic therapy. [NIH]

Effector: It is often an enzyme that converts an inactive precursor molecule into an active second messenger. [NIH]

Enhancer: Transcriptional element in the virus genome. [NIH]

Epstein: Failure of the upper eyelid to move downward on downward movement of the eye, occurring in premature and nervous infants. [NIH]

Glycosidic: Formed by elimination of water between the anomeric hydroxyl of one sugar and a hydroxyl of another sugar molecule. [NIH]

Gould: Turning of the head downward in walking to bring the image of the ground on the functioning position of the retina, in destructive disease of the peripheral retina. [NIH]

Grafting: The operation of transfer of tissue from one site to another. [NIH]

Growth: The progressive development of a living being or part of an organism from its earliest stage to maturity. [NIH]

Hospice: Institution dedicated to caring for the terminally ill. [NIH]

Host: Any animal that receives a transplanted graft. [NIH]

Hyaluronidase: An enzyme that splits hyaluronic acid and thus lowers the viscosity of the acid and facilitates the spreading of fluids through tissues either advantageously or disadvantageously. [NIH]

Hypopyon: An accumulation of pus in the anterior chamber of the eye associated with infectious diseases of the cornea, the iris, and the ciliary body. [NIH]

Impairment: In the context of health experience, an impairment is any loss or abnormality of psychological, physiological, or anatomical structure or function. [NIH]

Infections: The illnesses caused by an organism that usually does not cause disease in a person with a normal immune system. [NIH]

Insight: The capacity to understand one's own motives, to be aware of one's own psychodynamics, to appreciate the meaning of symbolic behavior. [NIH]

Jefferson: A fracture produced by a compressive downward force that is transmitted evenly through occipital condyles to superior articular surfaces of the lateral masses of C1. [NIH]

Koch: It was an early form of tuberculin of low specificity, devised by Robert Koch and made by heat concentration of a broth culture of Mycobacterium tuberculosis. [NIH]

Linkage: The tendency of two or more genes in the same chromosome to remain together from one generation to the next more frequently than expected according to the law of independent assortment. [NIH]

Loop: A wire usually of platinum bent at one end into a small loop (usually 4 mm inside diameter) and used in transferring microorganisms. [NIH]

Microsurgery: Surgical procedures on the cellular level; a light microscope and miniaturized instruments are used. [NIH]

Migration: The systematic movement of genes between populations of the same species, geographic race, or variety. [NIH]

Morphological: Relating to the configuration or the structure of live organs. [NIH]

Myopia: Astigmatism in which one principal meridian is myopic and the other enmetropic, or in which both meridians are myopic. [NIH]

Need: A state of tension or dissatisfaction felt by an individual that impels him to action toward a goal he believes will satisfy the impulse. [NIH]

Nerve: A cordlike structure of nervous tissue that connects parts of the nervous system with other tissues of the body and conveys nervous impulses to, or away from, these tissues. [NIH]

Networks: Pertaining to a nerve or to the nerves, a meshlike structure of interlocking fibers or strands. [NIH]

Neutrophil: A motile, short-lived polymorphonuclear leucocyte with a multilobed nucleus and a cytoplasm filled with numerous minute granules, which is primarily responsible for maintaining normal host defenses against invading microorganisms. [NIH]

Nucleus: A body of specialized protoplasm found in nearly all cells and containing the chromosomes. [NIH]

Nystagmus: Rhythmical oscillation of the eyeballs, either pendular or jerky. [NIH]

Opacity: Degree of density (area most dense taken for reading). [NIH]

Outpatient: A patient who is not an inmate of a hospital but receives diagnosis or treatment in a clinic or dispensary connected with the hospital. [NIH]

Patch: A piece of material used to cover or protect a wound, an injured part, etc.: a patch over the eye. [NIH]

Pathologies: The study of abnormality, especially the study of diseases. [NIH]

Pharmacokinetic: The mathematical analysis of the time courses of absorption, distribution, and elimination of drugs. [NIH]

Phosphorylated: Attached to a phosphate group. [NIH]

Pole: The point at either end of the spindle, from which the spindle fibers radiate to the equator. [NIH]

Potassium: It is essential to the ability of muscle cells to contract. [NIH]

Probe: An instrument used in exploring cavities, or in the detection and dilatation of strictures, or in demonstrating the potency of channels; an elongated instrument for exploring or sounding body cavities. [NIH]

Proenzyme: Inactive form of an enzyme which can then be converted to the active form, usually by excision of a polypeptide, e. g. trypsinogen is the zymogen of trypsin. [NIH]

Protocol: The detailed plan for a clinical trial that states the trial's rationale, purpose, drug or vaccine dosages, length of study, routes of administration, who may participate, and other aspects of trial design. [NIH]

Psychoactive: Those drugs which alter sensation, mood, consciousness or other psychological or behavioral functions. [NIH]

Racemic: Optically inactive but resolvable in the way of all racemic compounds. [NIH]

Reassurance: A procedure in psychotherapy that seeks to give the client confidence in a favorable outcome. It makes use of suggestion, of the prestige of the therapist. [NIH]

Refer: To send or direct for treatment, aid, information, de decision. [NIH]

Reliability: Used technically, in a statistical sense, of consistency of a test with itself, i. e. the extent to which we can assume that it will yield the same result if repeated a second time. [NIH]

Resolving: The ability of the eye or of a lens to make small objects that are close together, separately visible; thus revealing the structure of an object. [NIH]

Restoration: Broad term applied to any inlay, crown, bridge or complete denture which restores or replaces loss of teeth or oral tissues. [NIH]

Retractor: An instrument designed for pulling aside tissues to improve exposure at operation; an instrument for drawing back the edge of a wound. [NIH]

Sebaceous: Gland that secretes sebum. [NIH]

Secretory: Secreting; relating to or influencing secretion or the secretions.

[NIH]

Sensor: A device designed to respond to physical stimuli such as temperature, light, magnetism or movement and transmit resulting impulses for interpretation, recording, movement, or operating control. [NIH]

Sharpness: The apparent blurring of the border between two adjacent areas of a radiograph having different optical densities. [NIH]

Sinclair: A special glue for applying extension in fractures. [NIH]

Snellen: Congestion of the ear from stimulating of the cut end of the great auricular nerve. [NIH]

Specialist: In medicine, one who concentrates on 1 special branch of medical science. [NIH]

Sperm: The fecundating fluid of the male. [NIH]

Spike: The activation of synapses causes changes in the permeability of the dendritic membrane leading to changes in the membrane potential. This difference of the potential travels along the axon of the neuron and is called spike. [NIH]

Streptococci: A genus of spherical Gram-positive bacteria occurring in chains or pairs. They are widely distributed in nature, being important pathogens but often found as normal commensals in the mouth, skin, and intestine of humans and other animals. [NIH]

Stromal: Large, veil-like cell in the bone marrow. [NIH]

Suspensory: Supporting a part. [NIH]

Temporal: One of the two irregular bones forming part of the lateral surfaces and base of the skull, and containing the organs of hearing. [NIH]

Therapeutics: The branch of medicine which is concerned with the treatment of diseases, palliative or curative. [NIH]

Threshold: For a specified sensory modality (e. g. light, sound, vibration), the lowest level (absolute threshold) or smallest difference (difference threshold, difference limen) or intensity of the stimulus discernible in prescribed conditions of stimulation. [NIH]

Thrush: A disease due to infection with species of fungi of the genus Candida. [NIH]

Ubiquitin: A highly conserved 76 amino acid-protein found in all eukaryotic cells. [NIH]

Vitreoretinal: A rare familial condition characterized by a clear vitreous, except for preretinal filaments and veils which have been loosened from the retina, a dense hyaloid membrane which is perforated and detached, and masses of peripheral retinal pigmentation inters. [NIH]

Vitro: Descriptive of an event or enzyme reaction under experimental investigation occurring outside a living organism. Parts of an organism or microorganism are used together with artificial substrates and/or conditions. [NIH]

Vivo: Outside of or removed from the body of a living organism. [NIH]

Voltaren: Anti-inflammatory drug. [NIH]

Wound: Any interruption, by violence or by surgery, in the continuity of the external surface of the body or of the surface of any internal organ. [NIH]

General Dictionaries and Glossaries

While the above glossary is essentially complete, the dictionaries listed here cover virtually all aspects of medicine, from basic words and phrases to more advanced terms (sorted alphabetically by title; hyperlinks provide rankings, information and reviews at Amazon.com):

- **Dictionary of Medical Acronymns & Abbreviations** by Stanley Jablonski (Editor), Paperback, 4th edition (2001), Lippincott Williams & Wilkins Publishers, ISBN: 1560534605, http://www.amazon.com/exec/obidos/ASIN/1560534605/icongroupinterna

- **Dictionary of Medical Terms : For the Nonmedical Person (Dictionary of Medical Terms for the Nonmedical Person, Ed 4)** by Mikel A. Rothenberg, M.D, et al, Paperback - 544 pages, 4th edition (2000), Barrons Educational Series, ISBN: 0764112015, http://www.amazon.com/exec/obidos/ASIN/0764112015/icongroupinterna

- **A Dictionary of the History of Medicine** by A. Sebastian, CD-Rom edition (2001), CRC Press-Parthenon Publishers, ISBN: 185070368X, http://www.amazon.com/exec/obidos/ASIN/185070368X/icongroupinterna

- **Dorland's Illustrated Medical Dictionary (Standard Version)** by Dorland, et al, Hardcover - 2088 pages, 29th edition (2000), W B Saunders Co, ISBN: 0721662544, http://www.amazon.com/exec/obidos/ASIN/0721662544/icongroupinterna

- **Dorland's Electronic Medical Dictionary** by Dorland, et al, Software, 29th Book & CD-Rom edition (2000), Harcourt Health Sciences, ISBN: 0721694934, http://www.amazon.com/exec/obidos/ASIN/0721694934/icongroupinterna

- **Dorland's Pocket Medical Dictionary (Dorland's Pocket Medical Dictionary, 26th Ed)** Hardcover - 912 pages, 26th edition (2001), W B Saunders Co, ISBN: 0721682812, http://www.amazon.com/exec/obidos/ASIN/0721682812/icongroupinterna/103-4193558-7304618

- **Melloni's Illustrated Medical Dictionary (Melloni's Illustrated Medical Dictionary, 4th Ed)** by Melloni, Hardcover, 4th edition (2001), CRC Press-Parthenon Publishers, ISBN: 85070094X, http://www.amazon.com/exec/obidos/ASIN/85070094X/icongroupinterna

- **Stedman's Electronic Medical Dictionary Version 5.0 (CD-ROM for Windows and Macintosh, Individual)** by Stedmans, CD-ROM edition (2000), Lippincott Williams & Wilkins Publishers, ISBN: 0781726328, http://www.amazon.com/exec/obidos/ASIN/0781726328/icongroupinterna

- **Stedman's Medical Dictionary** by Thomas Lathrop Stedman, Hardcover - 2098 pages, 27th edition (2000), Lippincott, Williams & Wilkins, ISBN: 068340007X, http://www.amazon.com/exec/obidos/ASIN/068340007X/icongroupinterna

- **Tabers Cyclopedic Medical Dictionary (Thumb Index)** by Donald Venes (Editor), et al, Hardcover - 2439 pages, 19th edition (2001), F A Davis Co, ISBN: 0803606540, http://www.amazon.com/exec/obidos/ASIN/0803606540/icongroupinterna

INDEX

A

Ablation 130
Abscess...99
Adjustment...120
Angulation 151
Antibiotic......................................40, 161
Aperture 129, 142
Applicability 128

B

Biconvex...160, 164
Branch 26, 206, 226, 247
Breakdown 46, 83

C

Cataracts 11, 12, 14, 15, 21, 24, 38, 40, 41,
    49, 54, 102, 126, 128, 139, 144, 157, 159,
    161, 162, 163
Catheters...40
Ciliary 120, 134, 136, 137, 150, 151, 164,
    167, 173, 244
Consultation............................ii, iii, 3, 35
Consumption 38, 210
Contraindications............................ii, 204
Cystoid.............................94, 125, 214

D

Density.............................67, 116, 245
Diaphragm..62
Dissection 45

E

Enhancer...42

G

Glycosidic..166
Grafting..111, 143
Growth...42, 46, 93, 114, 144, 157, 208, 209,
    210, 243

H

Hospice...237
Host...................................45, 64, 116, 245
Hyaluronidase 68, 166
Hypopyon 161

I

Impairment....10, 25, 38, 39, 40, 48, 49, 130,
    158, 169, 231, 244
Infections 39

L

Linkage 48
Loop 133, 135, 138, 173, 245

M

Migration.............................46, 52, 125, 169
Morphological.................................44, 148

N

Myopia 16, 66, 91, 154, 167, 168

Nerve.................11, 110, 116, 166, 245, 247
Networks..230
Neutrophil 80
Nystagmus...93

O

Opacity ...25, 57, 74, 115, 120, 125, 126, 150,
    161, 162, 164, 243, 244
Outpatient........................18, 237, 238, 239

P

Patch 17, 26, 246
Pathologies..40
Phosphorylated 46
Pole 148, 164
Potassium..210
Probe.................................16, 131, 140
Proenzyme 148
Protocol 53
Psychoactive 49

R

Racemic 122, 173, 246
Reassurance 76
Refer.....................3, 4, 15, 24, 130, 151, 189
Reliability...46
Resolving 229, 230, 233
Restoration.....................................55, 157

S

Sebaceous...172
Sensor 44
Sharpness 12, 13
Specialist 15, 19, 28, 29, 33, 230
Sperm...210
Spike 117, 168, 247
Streptococci..73
Stromal 154
Suspensory..148

T

Temporal..61
Therapeutics 203
Threshold 46, 117, 247
Thrush 39

V

Vitreoretinal...45
Vitro..46, 216
Vivo..50

W

Wound......26, 51, 53, 77, 116, 121, 122, 124,
    136, 144, 149, 154, 156, 246

Printed in the United States
28781LVS00001B/228

best
sports
stories
1976

best sports stories 1976

A PANORAMA OF THE 1975 SPORTS WORLD
INCLUDING THE 1975 CHAMPIONS OF ALL SPORTS
WITH THE YEAR'S TOP PHOTOGRAPHS

Edited by Irving T. Marsh and Edward Ehre

E. P. DUTTON & CO., INC. / NEW YORK

Published simultaneously in Canada by Clarke, Irwin & Company
Limited, Toronto and Vancouver

ISBN: 0-525-06622-5
Library of Congress Catalog Card Number: 45-35124

76=08307

Contents

Preface   13

THE PRIZE-WINNING STORIES

BEST MAGAZINE STORY
(Unanimous Choice of Judges)
Boxing: *Pride of the Tiger* by Robert M. Lipsyte
The Atlantic Monthly   23

BEST NEWS-COVERAGE STORY
(With a Six-Point Score)
World Series: *"An Event for the Ages"* by Maury Allen
New York Post   33

BEST NEWS-FEATURE STORY
(With a Six-Point Score)
Baseball: *There Was Only One Casey* by Wells Twombly
San Francisco Examiner   37

OTHER POINT-SCORERS
Football: *A Hard Man to Find* by Jim Murray
Los Angeles Times   41
Tennis: *Ashe's Lucky Saturday* by Bud Collins
The Boston Globe   44
Boxing: *That Thrilla in Manila* by Dick Schaap
Washington Star   48
World Series: *Rose Sticks It to the Red Sox* by Bill Conlin
Philadelphia Daily News   52
Hockey: *Bernie Parent Misses the Boat* by Stan Hochman
Philadelphia Daily News   55
Tennis: *Virginia Wade, Whatever Became of Her "Brilliant
Future"?* by Catherine Bell
Tennis Magazine   58

Baseball: *A Rookie League* by Dave Kindred
The Louisville Courier-Journal   66
Tennis: *Orantes's Triumph: Portrait of Ecstasy* by Barry Lorge
The Washington Post   71
Baseball: *All New England Feels Feverish* by Thomas Boswell
The Washington Post   76
Football: *Trying Out for the Jets* by Mark Jacobson
New York   79
General: *Play-by-Play Before Its Heyday* by Hubert Mizell
The Floridian   86
Football: *Swarthmore Finally Has Champagne* by Frank Dolson
Philadelphia Inquirer   95
Fishing: *Fishing with My Father—and Other Outlandish Partners*
by Nord Riley, Outdoor Life   98
Football: *Defense, the Old Equalizer* by Blackie Sherrod
Dallas Times Herald   106
General: *He's Not as Simple as ABC* by Paul Hendrickson
The National Observer   110
Golf: *"The Only-Ness"* by Nick Seitz
Golf Digest   115

THE OTHER STORIES OF THE YEAR
World Series: *It Was Tiant's Show* by Allen Lewis
Philadelphia Inquirer   121
World Series: *The Old Cat-and-Mouse Game* by Si Burick
Dayton Daily News   124
World Series: *Play That Again, Sam* by Art Spander
The Sporting News   127
Golf: *A Landslide It Wasn't* by Furman Bisher
The Atlanta Journal   130
Horse Racing: *The Lady in Red* by Hal Lebovitz
Cleveland Plain Dealer   133
Horse Racing: *The Great Dictator of the Thoroughbred World*
by Neil Milbert, Chicago Tribune   136
General: *Muhammad Ali Takes on Harvard* by Larry Eldridge
The Christian Science Monitor   139
Basketball: *Wayne Estes's Final Game* by Harvey Kirkpatrick
Sport   142
Golf: *The Quiet Golfer from Nashville* by Bob Addie
The Washington Post   145
General: *China Through Different Eyes* by Will Grimsley
The Associated Press   148

Basketball: *Little Looie* by Tony Kornheiser
 Street & Smith Basketball Annual   152
Auto Racing: *The Indy "Float"* by John S. Radosta
 The New York Times   156
Football: *Football Trophies: Their Stories* by Ron Martz
 The St. Petersburg Times   160
Horse Racing: *Ruffian's Last Race* by Pete Axthelm
 Newsweek   164
Basketball: *The Ultimate Pol* by Murray Olderman
 Newspaper Enterprise Association   167
General: *Can Sports Survive Money?* by Roger Kahn
 Esquire   170
Basketball: *A Grand Finale* by Joe Gergen
 Newsday   180
General: *Namath's Mother Also Scores* by Gerald Eskenazi
 The New York Times   184
General: *Name the U.S. Congressman Who Holds the NFL Record
for the Most Fumbles Recovered, Lifetime* by Stanley Frank
 TV Guide   186
Basketball: *The Cardiac Kids End an Incredible Season*
by John Simmonds
 The Oakland Tribune   190
General: *How Ivan Does It* by Wally Provost
 Omaha World-Herald   194
Football: *A Throwback to Football's Stone Age* by Glenn Dickey
 San Francisco Chronicle   197
General: *Cure for the Blues* by Regis McAuley
 Tucson Daily Citizen   201
Golf: *Women's Golf: The Rewards Are Elusive* by Joan Libman
 The Wall Street Journal   203
General: *They Do It to Hear Bubbles* by Phil Hersh
 Baltimore Evening Sun   208
Basketball: *Million-Dollar Question: Bucks or Books?*
by Dave Hirshey, New York Daily News   210
Boxing: *Shelby's Moment of Glory* by Royal Brougham
 The Seattle Post-Intelligencer   213
Basketball: *The Mystery Man of the Blazers* by John Schulian
 The Washington Post   217
General: *Mama Clears the Smoke* by John Soucheray
 Minneapolis Tribune   220

FOR THE RECORD
Champions of 1975   223

WHO'S WHO IN BEST SPORTS STORIES—1976

Writers in Best Sports Stories—1976   244
Photographers in Best Sports Stories—1976   254

THE YEAR'S BEST SPORTS PHOTOS   259

Illustrations

THE PRIZE-WINNING PHOTOS

BEST ACTION PHOTO
Head in Groin, Shoe in Belly, Cleats in Face & Other Items by George
D. Waldman, Colorado Springs Sun   261

BEST FEATURE PHOTO
"Now the Way to Prevent a Slice. . . ." by Cletus M. (Pete) Hohn,
Minneapolis Tribune   262

OTHER PHOTOS
The Mighty Luis at Bat by Mike Anderson, Boston Herald
    American   263
Aaron Doesn't Break Only Home-Run Records by John E. Biever,
    The Milwaukee Journal   264
Saving Face by Ron Burda, San Jose Mercury-News   265
Two to Tangle by Karen Engstrom, The Portland Oregonian   266
Almost Measured by a Foot by Marvin M. Greene, Cleveland Plain
    Dealer   267
"Hang On, I'm Coming" by Charles Kirman, Chicago Sun
    Times   268
Bitter End in End Zone by Rich McCarthy, San Diego Evening
    Tribune   270
"Gotcha!" by James Roark, Los Angeles Herald-Examiner   271
"What Team You Playin' With?" by Robert Johnson, The Nash-
    ville Tennessean   272
The Feminine Touch by Ron Jett, Sarasota Journal   273
The Moose Shuffle by Elwood P. Smith, Philadelphia Daily
    News   274
A Winning Story by Sports Editor by John Pineda, Miami
    Herald   275
Man Left at Starting Gate by John H. White, Chicago Daily
    News   276

A Mother's Kiss by Harrison A. Howard, The Indianapolis
Star   278
No Last Hurrah by William Meyer, The Milwaukee Journal   279
Bored Blazers in a Laugher by Dave Weintraub,
The Oregon Journal   280
Ref Makes Like the Statue of Liberty by W. F. (Bill) Thompson,
The Houston Post   281
"First and Ten, Let's Do It Again" by Richard Mackson,
Santa Monica Outlook   282
Golden State Played 12 Feet Tall by Richard Darcey,
The Washington Post   283
Polarity by Tom Merryman, Cedar Rapids Gazette   284
A Nightmare Start by Fred Matthes, San Jose Mercury-News   285
A Family Affair by John P. Foster, The Seattle Times   286

best
sports
stories
1976

Preface

The late chief justice of the United States Supreme Court, Earl Warren, once said, "I always turn to the sports page first. The sports page records people's accomplishments; the front page has nothing but man's failures."

So, in this, the thirty-second annual compendium of the *Best Sports Stories* annuals, the editors are happy to list on the first reading page of the anthology the accomplishments of at least some of the men who help turn out some of those sports pages, newspaper and magazine, of America.

According to our distinguished panel of judges—John Chamberlain, John Hutchens, and Jerry Nason, sports aficionados all—perhaps the outstanding accomplishment in this regard has been turned in by Robert M. Lipsyte, former sports columnist for *The New York Times* and currently a novelist and free-lancer. His magazine boxing story, "Pride of the Tiger," which appeared in *The Atlantic Monthly,* gained the unanimous vote of the Messrs. Chamberlain (a national news columnist and former book reviewer for King Features Syndicate), Hutchens (former book reviewer and now a member of the Selection Board of The Book-of-the-Month Club), and Nason (retired sports editor of *The Boston Globe*), a feat that hasn't happened too often in the history of (your editors hope) this long and distinguished series.

This is the fourth top prize for Lipsyte. In previous efforts he won the news-coverage award once and the news-feature award twice, so the magazine prize he took this year completes the gamut. He has now taken the No. 1 prize in all three classifications.

Not, we hasten to interpose, that the story winners in the other two classifications are far behind. We and the judges salute Maury Allen, of the *New York Post,* for his magnificent story on the sixth World Series game, "An Event for the Ages," and Wells Twombly, sports columnist of the *San Francisco Examiner,* for his warm story on Casey Stengel, "There Was Only One Casey." Twombly is a repeater. He won the news-coverage story in 1970 with his account of the Super Bowl game between the New York Jets and the Baltimore Colts, high spot of his 12 or 15 stories that have appeared during the years of the competition. Allen, whose latest book effort is the story of Joe DiMaggio, also has appeared 12 to 15 times during the years but this is his first victory.

Each of these writers garnered the first-place vote of two of the three judges. The other first places were captured by Jim Murray, syndicated columnist of the *Los Angeles Times,* for his column on Fran Tarkenton, and Dick Schaap, for his account of the Ali-Frazier fight, which appeared in the *Washington Star.* The closest competition came in the news-feature category, where Jim Murray was second to his Pacific Coast confrere, Wells Twombly. Altogether, 19 of the stories submitted to the judges earned points.

Through the years, there has been no dimunition of story entries. This year there were well over 1,100 of them—the high-water mark in the series thus far—read by the editors.

As in the past, the stories that were sent to the judges went to them "blind." That is, they were identified only by a word or two (known in newspaperese as a "slug") with no indication as to the writer or his publication. You may note that's how the stories are identified by the judges in the box score and in their comments, which follow.

THE BOX SCORE

News-Coverage Stories	Chamber-lain	Hutchens	Nason	Total Points*
Sixth Series ["An Event for the Ages" by Maury Allen]	—	3	3	6
Wimbledon [Ashe's Lucky Saturday by Bud Collins]	2	—	2	4
Ali [That Thrilla in Manila by Dick Schaap]	3	—	—	3
Seventh Series [Rose Sticks It to the Red Sox by Bill Conlin]	1	—	1	2
Forest [Orantes's Triumph: Portrait of Ecstasy by Barry Lorge]	—	2	—	2
Oklahoma [Defense, the Old Equalizer by Blackie Sherrod]	—	1	—	1
News-Feature Stories				
Casey [There Was Only One Casey by Wells Twombly]	—	3	3	6
Fran [A Hard Man to Find by Jim Murray]	3	2	—	5
Sox [All New England Feels Feverish by Thomas Boswell]	2	—	—	2
Parent [Bernie Parent Misses the Boat by Stan Hochman]	—	—	2	2
Rookie [A Rookie League by Dave Kindred]	1	1	—	2
Swarthmore [Swarthmore Finally Has Champagne by Frank Dolson]	—	—	1	1
Magazine Stories				
Tiger [Pride of the Tiger by Robert M. Lipsyte]	3	3	3	9
Virginia [Virginia Wade: Whatever Became of Her "Brilliant Future"? by Catherine Bell]	2	—	—	2

*Based on 3 points for a first-place vote, 2 for a second, 1 for a third.

Radio [Play-by-Play Before Its Heyday by Hubert Mizell]	—	2	—	2
Jets [Trying Out for the Jets by Mark Jacobson]	—	—	2	2
Irwin ["The Only-Ness" by Nick Seitz]	1	—	—	1
Fishing [Fishing with My Father by Nord Riley]	—	1	—	1
Karras [He's Not as Simple as ABC by Paul Hendrickson]	—	—	1	1

JUDGES' COMMENTS

John Chamberlain
News-Coverage Stories

1. Ali [That Thrilla in Manila by Dick Schaap]
2. Wimbledon [Ashe's Lucky Saturday by Bud Collins]
3. Seventh Series [Rose Sticks It to the Red Sox by Bill Conlin]

1. "Ali," of course, is the greatest. But his character has unexpected facets and it is good to read a news story about the "greatest" that lets a little unexpected humility come through. This is Joe Frazier's story as much as it is Ali's. "He is greater than I thought he was," said Ali—and the respect in that confession gives the tonal quality to my choice for No. 1.

2. "Wimbledon" was always Arthur Ashe's nemesis. But he didn't choke when he had his chance to cut Jimmy Connors down. A good come-uppance flavor to this one.

3. "Seventh Series" was anti-climactic to "Sixth Series," but the author gets plenty of climax out of a single hard slide by Pete Rose, the world's greatest journeyman ball player. The little move that won the big one.

News-Feature Stores

1. Fran [A Hard Man to Find by Jim Murray]
2. Sox [All New England Feels Feverish by Thomas Boswell]
3. Rookie [A Rookie League by Dave Kindred]

1. As a spectator who thinks quarterback-in-the-pocket strategy can make for consummate dullness, I'm glad to see someone do a real appreciation of Fran Tarkenton. The pro game needed something that Tarkenton and Roger Staubach have given it. This is an

inspiriting feature. Hope the style that it celebrates becomes contagious.

2. Who said that Bostonians were proper? They know how to let their emotions run whenever a good team—such as the Sox of 1975 —gives them a chance. A good story of midsummer madness.

3. They have lots of towels in the bigs. But they pass the single towel around in the bus leagues. This is a good story of how a pitcher has to scramble for a three-figure bonus in his scramble to make the majors.

Magazine Stories

1. Tiger [Pride of the Tiger by Robert M. Lipsyte]
2. Virginia [Virginia Wade: Whatever Became of Her "Brilliant Future"? by Catherine Bell]
3. Irwin ["The Only-Ness" by Nick Seitz]

1. The story of Dick Tiger, the Ibo fighter from Biafra in Nigeria who had to contend with everything from third-rate Manhattan hotels to the British Empire, is one of the most affecting I have ever read. It's not only about a boxer, it is about all the forces that have made the twentieth century the most frightful ever.

2. A good psychograph of an interesting woman who happens to have been cast as a tennis player.

3. Golf is played against yourself, which makes Hale Irwin's description of the state of "only-ness" something special. The individual gets no real emotional outlet in golf—control of the emotions is everything. The tension builds and builds. A good story of men under a most peculiar stress.

John Hutchens
News-Coverage Stories

1. Sixth Series ["An Event for the Ages" by Maury Allen]
2. Forest [Orantes's Triumph: Portrait of Ecstasy by Barry Lorge]
3. Oklahoma [Defense, the Old Equalizer by Blackie Sherrod]

1. Just about the most exciting World Series game anyone can remember is all here, as nearly as the printed word can bring it— the tension, the color, the finely described technical detail. It's a story that rose splendidly to the occasion.

2. The courteous, controlled Manuel Orantes over the brash Jimmy Connors—surely one of the most popular tennis triumphs on record, and one of the most startling upsets, pictured with exemplary skill and verve.

3. A stirring report, even for a reader with no loyalty for either team, of a battle between two old foes. And, along with the drama, writing marked by dash and style.

News-Feature Stories

1. Casey [There Was Only One Casey by Wells Twombly]
2. Fran [A Hard Man to Find by Jim Murray]
3. Rookie [A Rookie League by Dave Kindred]

1. Of all the countless words written since his death about the ineffable Casey, these carry a special tone of authenticity. Admiration without hero-worship, humor with dignity, above all the real, astute, straight Casey behind the clowning façade.

2. The Vikings' stylish quarterback, a one-man revolution in that position, sits for a first-rate portrait by an analyst clearly acquainted with all the Tarkenton techniques and performances from the very beginning of a dazzling career. Painful reading, I suspect, for certain coaches and owners who traded him away, but a pleasure for the rest of us.

3. It's edifying to get away from the lofty majors now and then and have a look at the far-down minors from which a future major leaguer now and then fights his way upward. In this case, it's the Appalachian League—dismal bus rides from one town to another, four towels in the dressing room for a whole team, etc. For glory and romance, substitute pathos and truth in this convincing account.

Magazine Stories

1. Tiger [Pride of the Tiger by Robert M. Lipsyte]
2. Radio [Play-by-Play Before Its Heyday by Hubert Mizell]
3. Fishing [Fishing with My Father by Nord Riley]

1. A deeply moving, quietly written portrait of a champion who may not have been among the all-time greatest but was a champion outside the ring as he was inside those ropes. Anyone who saw the old Tiger, almost always fighting against the odds but usually winning just the same, will file it away among cherished memories of him.

2. So a lot of us were taken in, and happily so, in the long ago, innocent days by those radio pioneers who "recreated" baseball games they presumably were seeing but actually were broadcasting from telegraph reports. Excellent anecdotal sports history, hilarious and informative.

Jerry Nason
News-Coverage Stories

1. Sixth Series ["An Event for the Ages" by Maury Allen]
2. Wimbledon [Ashe's Lucky Saturday by Bud Collins]
3. Seventh Series [Rose Sticks It to the Red Sox by Bill Conlin]

1. It was predictable that the boys would come up with some of the year's best sports-reporting at the scenes of the '75 World Series. In my experience, superb competition invariably inspires that extra touch that transmutes a good story into an outstanding one. And the confrontation of the Reds and Red Sox marked a pinnacle of Series competition. Of all the zesty reports of this epic baseball struggle none seemed to me to have equaled the clarity, the economy of verbiage, the controlled excitement of "Sixth Game"— which game may have been the most thrilling ever played in a World Series. This report was obviously the work of a top professional working "under the gun," so to speak, with a rare subject on the one hand and the words, and skill, to meet a press deadline in telling it. It won both my vote and my admiration.

2. "Wimbledon," too, is a fine example of a real pro's response to a memorable assignment. This writer was on familiar turf and took his reader along to stroll it.

3. The seventh and concluding game of the Series provided an excellent report in story selected. This writer felt that while this was a conclusive game, as a subject it lacked the drama of the sixth game.

News-Feature Stories

1. Casey [There Was Only One Casey by Wells Twombly]
2. Parent [Bernie Parent Misses the Boat by Stan Hochman]
3. Swarthmore [Swarthmore Finally Has Champagne by Frank Dolson]

1. This category, in today's fast-paced news scene, in many cases involves sports columns—and often today's sports column, like the news account on the same page—is written to appease an early deadline. "Casey," my choice, seemed to me to have been written right from the heart and from the news service wire just announcing the death of Casey Stengel. If, 50 years from now, somebody were to research Casey as man or myth the researcher would not have to probe beyond this one piece. It tells IT ALL—because there were two Casey Stengels and, with a knowing, delicate touch, the writer of this one paints portraits of both.

2. "Parent" was another piece that searched for and found its

mark. Reading it, you can understand why Ted Williams may be wrong—that stopping a rubber puck at 100 mph may be sport's toughest single act, not hitting a baseball pitched at 80 mph.

3. The story of the small college football team unexpectedly concluding its losing streak provided a rare opportunity for writing at a college football level and attaining stature in a contest such as this.

Magazine Stories

1. Tiger [Pride of the Tiger by Robert M. Lipsyte]
2. Jets [Trying Out for the Jets by Mark Jacobson]
3. Karras [He's Not as Simple as ABC by Paul Hendrickson]

1. Normally my preference in magazine reading is for articles themed to the meaningful present. Obviously "Tiger" is written, and beautifully written, of the past. Yet I suspect it is one of those timeless gems that leap effortlessly from one sporting era to another, gaining story momentum as it goes. The writer of this one unconsciously bared the bones of a marvelous Hollywood or TV script. Boxing will not forget Dick Tiger, and it will not be easy to forget this story of him once you've read it. I frankly felt that no magazine piece submitted, and there were some top-drawer efforts, seriously challenged "Tiger" in either story impact or in the technical quality of its presentation.

2. "Jets" was particularly well done on the more routine topic of pro football rookie tryouts.

3. "Karras" takes you to an enjoyable, informative off-day visit with a growing television personality.

As for the photos, the editors were struck by the tense action in the entry that won this award: the shot by George D. Waldman of the *Colorado Springs Sun* on a soccer game between the Air Force Academy and Colorado College. Note the expressions on the faces of the athletes. This is Waldman's first appearance in *Best Sports Stories*.

And the feature photo, showing Patty Berg giving a golf lesson, by Cletus M. (Pete) Hohn, of the *Minneapolis Tribune*, is, we think, a hilarious picture.

So, for your nostalgic enjoyment, here is *Best Sports Stories—1976*. Enjoy, enjoy.

IRVING T. MARSH
EDWARD EHRE

THE PRIZE-WINNING STORIES

Best Magazine Story

(Unanimous Choice of the Judges)

BOXING

PRIDE OF THE TIGER

By Robert M. Lipsyte

From The Atlantic Monthly
Copyright, ©, 1975, by Robert M. Lipsyte

The first time I saw Dick Tiger he was waiting for me in front of the old Madison Square Garden, a homburg perched on top of his head. The homburg was much too small, and I thought he looked comical. It was years before I learned that he always bought his hats a size too small, so he could share them with his brothers back home in Nigeria.

I introduced myself to Tiger and he shook my hand gravely. Then he turned and began moving down Eighth Avenue on the balls of his feet, like a big black cat. His manager and I followed.

"Nigerian fighters are very good, very tough," said his manager. "They're closer to the jungle."

Over his shoulder, Tiger said, "There is no jungle in Nigeria."

"It's just an expression, Dick, just a figure of speech," said the manager. "I mean they're hungry fighters."

Tiger stopped. "Hungry fighters." He winked at me. "We eat hoo-mon bee-inks. Medium rare."

We walked a mile and a half to the gym where he was training because Tiger would not consider a cab, even if I paid. It was said around that Tiger had the terminal cheaps. I followed him into a dressing room and watched him shed the comedy of his clothes. As the homburg, the brown sports jacket, the blue tie, and white shirt disappeared into a rusty metal locker, Tiger seemed to grow larger. The blue tribal tattoos across his chest and back rippled over knotty muscle. He seemed suddenly savage, dangerous.

But there was only gentleness in his eyes, and humor twitched at the corners of his wide mouth. I watched him tape his hands slowly and with great care, first winding the dirty gray bandages around and around, then placing the sponge across the knuckles, then wrapping on the adhesive. I asked him why he didn't have his manager or trainer perform this daily chore, now that he was middleweight champion of the world.

"I am a travelin' man, and I got to do things myself, a fighter should know these things," he said. "This is my business. I don't want to spoil myself for someday when there is no one around to help me."

He was thirty-four years old at the time and had been champion for less than a year. He was training in New York, where facilities and sparring partners were the best, for the second defense of that championship, to be held in Ibadan, Nigeria. Tiger was taking this fight very seriously. It would be Nigeria's first world title fight, and his own real homecoming. "It is very important I win," he said. "For pride. They receive me different, people, when I am champion."

This was June 1963 and I had interviewed few fighters. I watched Tiger work out for two hours, methodically, intensely, oblivious of sound and movement around him. Great silver globules of sweat formed, swelled, exploded on his forehead, and he never wiped them away. He weighed about 160 pounds then, and his 5-foot-8 body was unusually hard and fit. His calisthenics were so violent that they seemed beyond human tolerance; I was sure his eyes would pop out of his head as he twisted his neck, that his muscles and veins would burst through his skin.

We talked again after he was finished. His voice was softer now, his body more relaxed. He had been born in Amaigbo, a remote eastern Nigerian town in the rain forests of the Binin River delta, a town that appeared on few maps. He was raised on a farm and educated in English and Ibo at an Anglican mission school. At nineteen he went to the city of Aba to work in his brother's grocery store. At a local boys' club he learned to box.

He had been christened Richard Ihetu, Ibo for "what I want," but assumed the ring name Dick Tiger for his early pro fights against the likes of Easy Dynamite and Super Human Power. He kept the name when a British promoter brought him to England to fight on the Blackpool-Liverpool circuit. He was lonely and chilled in the dank foreign gyms, and he lost his first four fights. Letters from his family in Nigeria were beseeching him to give up the foolishness and return to his father's farm or his brother's grocery store. Tiger gave himself one more chance. In his fifth fight, he knocked out a Liverpool boy in 90 seconds, and Richard Ihetu, farmer and clerk, disappeared forever.

He first came to America in 1959 and lived with his pregnant wife in third-rate Manhattan hotels, cooking meals on a hot plate and running in Central Park. He slowly gained a reputation among boxing promoters as an honest workman. He was always in top condition, he always gave his best. He would never be spectacular, he did not have a great deal of boxing finesse or personal "color," but he was dependable and tough. His wife gave birth to twins, then to a third child in 1960. Tiger sent her back to Nigeria and began commuting between New York and Aba. Now he lived in fourth-rate hotels, walked whenever possible, window-shopped for entertainment, sent every penny home. After he won the title in 1962, he was able to send more money home, but he did not improve the quality of his living conditions or his clothing. I asked him if he was saving his money for something special.

"This will not always be my business. I want money," he said, rubbing his fingers together. "Six hundred thousand to start a big business. Now all I have is a house and a Peugeot, that is all."

We left the gym together and took the subway uptown. We made small talk on the ride, and he told me the only tiger he had ever seen was in a cage in the Liverpool zoo. My stop came first. I got off the train and looked back at him through the window. In his clothes again, he was just a chunky man in a too-small homburg, hanging from an overhead strap, jostled by a rush-hour crowd.

I went back to the office and wrote a tidy Sunday feature story, my specialty. A month later, I read that he had won his bout in Ibadan. I was glad of that; something about Tiger had touched me.

In December of that year, 1963, he defended his title against Joey Giardello in Atlantic City. It was my first championship fight, and my notes were unusually voluminous, including the first stanza of the Nigerian anthem, which was played before the fight began.

> Nigeria, we hail thee,
> Our own dear native land.
> Though tribe and tongue may differ
> In brotherhood we stand.

Tiger lost the 15-round fight by a decision. I knew he would be very upset. He had become a national hero in Nigeria: he had been awarded a medal, Member of the British Empire, in Lagos, and he was amassing property in Aba. In a few days he would be returning home a loser.

But the next morning he smiled at me and said amiably, "Look at my face. I don't look like I was in a fight last night. I did a bit of dancing last night with Giardello, and I am a fighter, not a dancer. I thought I did enough to win, as he kept running away."

He shrugged and sighed. "These days you get a title by running away."

We shook hands gravely and said good-bye. I would have liked to tell him that I was sorry he had lost, but the words stuck in my throat. It seemed somehow unprofessional, and Tiger was a professional.

Giardello promised Tiger a rematch within six months, but it was two years before they met again. Giardello enjoyed his championship hugely and did nothing to endanger it, like fighting someone who might take it away. Tiger, meanwhile waited patiently and rarely fought: his reputation as a head-down, hands-up, straight-ahead slugger who plodded into his opponent and beat away scared off anyone who didn't need to fight him for a payday or a shot at the title.

By the time they met again I was a regular boxing writer, veteran of the Clay-Liston spectacles, a seasoned observer who almost knew A. J. Liebling's *The Sweet Science* by heart. I even kept my own scorecard, which usually conflicted with the judges'. I was also a great deal more appreciative of Dick Tiger, now that I had interviewed many other boxers and watched them train and fight. Of all athletes, boxers are generally the friendliest and the most dedicated, and Tiger had the most heart and soul of them all.

I liked Joey Giardello, but I was secretly rooting for Tiger to win back his title the night of the rematch in Madison Square Garden. Tiger was shorter and lighter and older than Giardello, but from the opening bell, when a Nigerian *etulago* set a thumping drumbeat, Tiger doggedly followed Giardello around the ring, pressing and battering and slugging. Giardello stayed on his feet as a point of pride. At the start of the fifteenth and last round, with the decision certain for Tiger, Giardello leaned forward and whispered, "Nice fight."

Tiger did not hold the title very long this time, either. He was over thirty-six years old, and the strain of keeping his weight below the 160-pound middleweight limit sapped his strength. Emile Griffith, the welterweight champion, who could no longer keep his weight below 147 pounds, moved up in class and beat him. So, logically, Tiger decided to move up in class, too. In the winter of 1966 he beat the brilliant but erratic José Torres and became light heavyweight champion. The morning after that fight I visited his shabby hotel room. He greeted me with the same amiable, win-or-lose smile.

"The people all said that Tiger is finished, that he looks a hundred years old, and now they come around to pat my head and tell me I'm a good boy." He shrugged. "That's life."

His investments in Nigeria were doing well, he told me, although he was concerned by the mounting violence and political instability. Many thousands of his fellow Ibo tribesmen had been slaughtered in pogroms in northern Nigeria. The Ibo, who were Christians, were civil servants and small businessmen in the Moslem north. Ibo were fleeing back to their native lands in eastern Nigeria. Tiger's holdings were in Aba, in the eastern region, where he lived in a large, air-conditioned home, owned several buildings, operated several businesses and shops, and had a chauffeur for his Mercedes-Benz limousine. He was still optimistic about the future of his six children and the many nieces and nephews that he took pride and joy in supporting.

Tiger fought Torres again the following spring, as usual giving away height and weight and age, and he beat him again. This time, when the decision was announced, fights broke out in the balcony and bottles of wine and rum smashed on the Garden floor and sprayed the crowd with shards of glass. There was blood and there were a number of injuries. I wrote most of my story crouched under the Garden ring, with my typewriter on my knees. The incident was discussed and written about for several days, and then dismissed as one of those cultural-ethnic-economic-sporting inevitabilities. Garden officials blamed "a few nuts or hoodlums" who wanted to read about themselves in the papers. Torres said he was proud of his fellow Puerto Ricans for showing their "support" of him, and Lipsyte analyzed the random violence as an expression of the class struggle. The boxing commissioner declared: "A hundred years ago Charles Dickens went to a fight with William Makepeace Thackeray and wrote about a riot in London."

It was an ironic send-off for Tiger, who flew back home into the Nigerian civil war.

The next time I saw him, in March of 1968, the smile was gone. His mouth was twisted, his voice high and tense. His square hands plucked at his baggy gray suit pants.

"I used to be a happy man, but now I have seen something I have never seen before. I read about killing and war, but I had never seen such things. Now, I have seen massacres."

He bounded from the straight-backed hotel chair and began fishing in his bureau drawers, through pamphlets and books and newspaper clippings. "Ah, here," he said, almost reverentially opening tissue paper. "This is Aba." He spread the photographs on the bed.

"The hospital. There were eight patients and a doctor when the planes came and threw bombs around. Hired pilots. The Nigerians can't fly planes. They are a thousand years behind civilization, that is why they are doing everything wrong.

"The open market, look at that. In that corner, that is a hand. A little girl's hand. What does she know of war? This woman burned. These men dead, not even soldiers. This is a woman, too. No, it is not rags, it was a woman."

He carefully repacked the photographs and sat down again. "The Nigerian radio says Dick Tiger of Nigeria will defend his light heavy-weight championship against Bob Foster in Madison Square Garden on May 24. Dick Tiger of Nigeria. They still claim me and they would kill me, they want to kill us all. I am a Biafran. And we just want to live."

I asked him about his family, which now included seven children. He said he had moved them back to Amaigbo while he tended his businesses in Aba. "I do not worry so much anymore. The children have learned to take cover quickly when they hear the planes. It is the fighter planes we worry about. The bombs fall slowly. If you see them you can run away. But you never see the bullets."

Foster knocked him cold in the fourth round of the fight. Tiger went straight down, his head smacked the canvas sickeningly. He twitched on his back like a turtle on its shell. He had to be helped up. In his dressing room he managed a smile at the crowd, which included various countrymen, boxing buffs, and Giardello. "Since I been winning I never had my fans stay in my dressing room so long. Now, I'm a loser and everybody's here. I guess I am a good man."

He left the United States without his light heavyweight title, but with enough currency to buy a planeload of tinned meat and pow-dered milk in Lisbon and fly it into Biafra.

In the summer of 1968 there were reports of 6,000 Ibos a day dying of malnutrition and disease and wounds. Occasionally we would hear that Tiger was dead, too. And sometimes we would hear that he was hiding out in Brooklyn.

He reappeared in September to fight an upcoming young light heavyweight, Frankie DePaula.

I visited him in training. I was completing my first year as a columnist, and I had tried to stay away from boxing, to break the identification and establish my credentials in other sports. But Tiger had become a touchstone for me; I think I derived some symbolic nourishment from watching him tape his own hands. The honest, independent workman, a man of dignity and courage.

"If I had been a flashy fellow," he told me, "with fancy clothes and many women and big cars and nightclubs every night, I would have trouble. But I have never been a flashy fellow; I eat what is there to eat, I just dress, you know . . ."

"And still you have nothing now."

"This is true. I saved all my money and brought it home. I had apartment buildings in Lagos and Port Harcourt and Aba, and a movie and factories and shops and now, with the shelling, I guess it is all gone. Everything I have saved. But I am not sorry. If I had been a flashy fellow when I had lots of money, what would I do with myself now?"

He was training in the evening because he could no longer afford professional sparring partners; he sparred against dockers coming off work. He spent his days at the Biafra Mission, reading cables and dispatches. He disputed reports in American newspapers that the Nigerians were in complete control of almost all the cities.

"In every city they are still fighting," he said. "The Biafran fights to the end; the Nigerian will kill him anyway. The plan is to kill every Biafran over two years old. Then all the children will pray to the sun and moon instead of God, and never know who their fathers were. That is why we fight to survive."

We walked out of the dressing room to the training ring. In the hallway, a schoolboy caught his own reflection in the mirror of a vending machine and jabbed at it.

Tiger smiled. "When I was young, if I ever saw my shadow I had to fight it, I always boxed at mirrors. No more. I am just one old man."

He was thirty-nine, and he looked even older in his fight with DePaula. Tiger won, but in the late rounds he seemed to be melting like a candle.

He took his money and disappeared again.

I didn't see him for more than a year: my second year as a columnist, and probably the most interesting. The Mexico City Olympics. The Jets Super Bowl. The Aqueduct Boycott. The Mets World Series. The start of the Knicks' first championship season.

The rehabilitation of Muhammad Ali began: liberals discovered that his antiwar stand was compatible with theirs, even if his racial views were not, and sprang to defend his constitutional rights. Together they would prove that the American legal system worked perfectly for anyone with the money and the power to go all the way.

I began to wish I had more time to think and read and talk to people, to stop writing so much and with such assurance. Columnists have to write with assurance because they are paid to raise The Truth. As that second year slipped into a third year, as the column became progressively easier to write, as my work brought me greater access to people I wanted to talk with, I found I was less and less sure of what I knew absolutely. Was I growing wiser, losing my nerve, taking myself too seriously, getting bored? Was I over the hill, choking in the clutch, hearing footsteps, getting fat?

In November of 1969, Tiger sluggishly won a dreary decision over a light heavyweight no one had heard of before, or would hear of again. A victory that had meaning only when translated into milk and salt and meat. On December 5 we sat down at a table in a publicity office of the Garden to discuss a matter that had suddenly become very urgent to Tiger. The medal he had received in Lagos in 1963 had grown too heavy in his mind to keep. When he read that John Lennon had returned his M.B.E. award for reasons that included Britain's involvement in the Nigerian civil war, Tiger decided to mail back his medal, too. But he needed help with the accompanying letter. Garden officials had not wanted to become involved in his protest and had called Dave Anderson, then covering boxing for *The New York Times*. Dave called me. I had misgivings. I had always been contemptuous of sports writers who acted as go-betweens for professional clubs and city governments, for high school athletes and college recruiters, for out-of-work coaches and potential employers. They were no longer honest journalists. I thought, they could no longer be trusted by their readers. They were supposed to cover stories, not make them happen.

But I had known and written about Tiger for more than six years; he had always been cooperative and friendly. I would be his amanuensis, no more: not a single idea or even word of mine would slip into the letter; it would make a good column for my readers, my kind of column, a famous athlete taking a principled stand on a headline issue that transcended sports. I didn't think, This is a very important cause, life, freedom, justice, I should be involved and make a worthwhile contribution as a human being. In those days I thought being an honest journalist was enough.

We wrote the letter and addressed it to the British ambassador, Washington, D.C.

"I am hereby returning the M.B.E. because every time I look at it I think of millions of men, women, and children who died and are still dying in Biafra because of the arms and ammunition the British government is sending to Nigeria and its continued moral support of this genocidal war against the people of Biafra."

He signed it "Dick Tiger Ihetu."

We walked across Eighth Avenue in the brilliant chilly afternoon and up the post-office steps. Tiger said, "If they ask me how much it's worth, what should I say?"

I shrugged. "We should try to pawn it and find out."

"I'll say a million dollars." Tiger laughed for the first time. "I'll say fifty or a hundred, just so it gets there."

The clerk behind the registry wicket hefted the package and shook his head. "No good, you got Scotch tape on it. Go around the corner, they'll give you some brown paper."

Another line. He stood very quietly, a small black hat perched on his head, his body muffled in a fur-lined coat. I would always remember him for being overdressed and patient. He was always cold, and he was always willing to wait, for a bout, for a return bout, for a shot at a title. He was forty then, picking up fights wherever he could, waiting for one more big payday. If there had been no war, he would be retired in Aba, a rich man. He had been financially wiped out, but he said he could not complain, many others had lost all their property, and many, many others had lost their families and their lives.

A clerk finally handed him a long strip of gummed brown paper and a wet sponge in a glass dish. Tiger took it to a writing desk and began to tear the brown paper into small strips, his thick fingers careful and precise, the fingers of a man who taped his own hands.

When he finished the package he proudly held it up for me. "Now I know there is something else I can do."

We waited for the registry clerk silently. "Okay," he said, nodding at the package, then flipping it. "What's in it?"

"A medal," said Tiger softly.

"What's it worth?"

"I don't know. Fifty, hundred dollars?"

"No value," said the clerk, to himself. He weighed it, registered it, asked Tiger if he wanted it to go airmail. Tiger said, "Yes."

"One sixty."

Tiger gave him two dollar bills and counted his change. He adjusted his scarf as he walked out into the bright street, and smiled, and shook my hand gravely and could only say, "Well . . ." and shrug, and start down the steps. I never saw him again.

In the summer of 1971, after working briefly as a guard in the Metropolitan Museum of Art, Dick Tiger returned to his native land. He was penniless and brought nothing except the cancer in his liver. He died that December, in Aba, at the age of forty-two.

Best News-Coverage Story
(With a Six-Point Score)

WORLD SERIES

"AN EVENT FOR THE AGES"
(World Series Game VI)

By Maury Allen

From the New York Post
Copyright, ©, 1975, New York Post Corporation
Reprinted by permission of the New York Post

In the cosmic scale of things it was only a baseball game.

In the way human beings measure human drama, in the way 35,205 Fenway Park fans measure the beats of their hearts, in the way 50 million people stayed up until early morning to watch on television, in the way cold, professional athletes warmed to the excitement, it was an event for the ages.

World Series games have been played for 72 years. Only a dozen have survived the passage of time and been etched into history. At 12:34 this morning, as Carlton Fisk's two feet plopped on home plate with the 7–6 Boston win on his twelfth-inning homer, the number was raised to a baker's dozen.

The Red Sox had incredibly tied the 1975 World Series at three games each and the matter will be settled tonight with left-handers Don Gullett and Bill Lee in game seven of the Series and game 172 of the season.

"I'll give it all I've got," said the Cincinnati left hander who thinks like a right hander.

"I don't know if I'll be ready," said the Boston left hander who thinks like a guru. "I've had only 10 days of rest. Last time I pitched I had 23."

Sparky Anderson sat back last night with the comforting knowledge that he still had his best pitcher ready for his biggest game. He pitched Gary Nolan, said he never regretted it, followed him with seven more, lost, and still has his ace.

Darrell Johnson pitched his best man, Luis Tiant, saw him have a tough night, came out with a win, and now rests his case with his flaky lefty.

No matter what happens tonight, no matter which team wins, no matter how long it takes, the seventh game of this World Series almost has to be considered an anticlimax.

The sixth game was simply the most wonderful example of sustained baseball drama most veteran observers had ever seen. If four days without a game was the cause, the good people of Boston might rise as one tonight and sing an old refrain, "Spahn and Sain and Pray for Rain."

The drama began early as Tiant, the old warhorse from Havana, walked across the field from the bullpen on his way to the dugout before the game. He had won twice, and only four pitchers in modern times—Harry Brecheen, Lew Burdette, Bob Gibson, and Mickey Lolich—had ever won three games.

"I'm not nervous," Tiant said before the game. "Either you get the batters out or you go home."

He got Pete Rose out to start the game as Carl Yastrzemski, returned home to left field, made a slipping, sliding catch of a line drive. The motif was set. It wouldn't change for four hours.

Yastrzemski and Fisk singled off Nolan and Fred Lynn slugged a high fastball into the center-field seats for three quick runs. The Big Red Machine looked like a lemon and Red Sox were rolling.

Tiant looked impressive for four innings. With each out the noise grew louder, the banners waved in the stands, the Boston fans smelled a seventh game. The shouts of "Looie, Looie, Looie," filled the air. The dark-skinned, moustachioed, pot-bellied, elegant artist could be the mayor of Boston or Havana if only he would give the word.

Ed Armbrister, who seems to be in the midst of so much with so little time on the field, walked with one out in the fifth. Rose singled, then Ken Griffey lined a huge drive to the intersection of the left-field and center-field walls.

Fred Lynn raced back, leaped high against the concrete, couldn't reach the ball, and crashed hard into the wall. He lay still for several frightening moments as teammates raced to his aid. Griffey had a two-run triple.

"When I saw it," Fisk was to say later, "I thought he was hurt bad. He was an All-Star, all-world, the guy who carried us, I didn't want to lose him."

Lynn finally made it to his feet. He had smashed his lower back against the wall and suffered severe pain at the base of his spine. He was worked on between innings after recovering.

"I don't know about tonight," said manager Johnson. "We'll have to decide that after our trainer sees him."

"Don't worry," said Lynn, "I'll be there."

Johnny Bench became the first player to hit the left-field wall in the Series and the game was tied on his single.

"It isn't that easy," Bench said.

With the game tied 3–3 Tiant was beginning to weaken. His thirty-four-year-old body was entitled to a winter of rest. He made it through the sixth. In the seventh two singles and a double off the center-field wall by George Foster put the Reds ahead 5–3.

"I don't know if he was tired," said Johnson. "He just got some pitches where he didn't want them."

One of the places where he didn't want his pitches to be was the center-field wall. That is where Cesar Geronimo hit a lead-off homer in the eighth for an "invincible" 6–3 lead.

Johnson walked slowly to the mound. The crowd rose. Tiant faced center field. Johnson gently took the baseball from him. The applause was warm and kind. Tiant's season was over.

"Tonight," he said, "I'll be sitting in the corner of the dugout cheering very hard."

The game had barely begun. Lynn lined a ball off the leg of relief pitcher Pete Borbon for a hit. The count went to a 2–0 on Rico Petrocelli as Rawley Eastwick warmed up quickly in the bullpen.

"I couldn't bring him in to face Petrocelli," said Sparky. "I hadn't gotten the sign yet from the bullpen that he was ready."

Borbon finished walking Rico. Then Eastwick, who had two wins and a save, came in to strike out Dwight Evans, get Rick Burleson on a pop-up, and face pinch-hitter Bernie Carbo.

"I was trying to make contact," Carbo said. "I was trying not to strike out. It was a funny swing, like a Japanese swing."

The funny swing put the baseball into a funny place, the center-field seats, and Carbo had two World Series pinch-hit homers—the last man to do that was Chuck Essegian for the Dodgers in 1959—and the score was tied.

"When I came home, dancing all the way," Carbo said, "I guess it was the happiest moment of my life."

Carbo, who had complained about not playing, suddenly was in left-field in a lineup switch.

"I guess I was surprised about that," he said. "I do whatever the man (Johnson) wants." Not without some bitterness and lots of noise.

Now it was Boston's turn. A walk, a single by Yastrzemski on an 0–2 pitch after failing to bunt and an intentional walk to Fisk loaded the bases for Boston with nobody out in the ninth.

"It looked," said Anderson, "like we were in trouble."

Lynn hit a soft flyball toward short left, just inside the foul line, as Foster raced for the ball. Denny Doyle, on third, tagged as coach Don Zimmer, aware of the situation, screamed, "No, no, no."

Doyle decided "no, no, no," was "go, go, go" and he was gone. And soon forgotten as Foster's short but tough-angled throw got him at home. Bench put the tag on him and one out later the game was in extra innings.

In the eleventh Rose, so caught up in the drama that he had said to Fisk, "This is some kind of game," was hit by a pitch. He was forced at second on a bad bunt by Ken Griffey.

Now came the play of the night, of the Series, maybe of any Series. Joe Morgan, struggling to prove his MVP worth to American League fans, caught one of Dick Drago's fastballs on the signature. The ball zoomed off the bat, raced for the stands, and was headed for the seats.

"I saw it off the bat and went back as hard as I could," said Evans.

The young right fielder had earlier been called the most surprising player in the Series by Sparky Anderson. He now surprised himself, Griffey, the Reds, and the world by catching the ball with a headlong leap at the base of the low stands, similar to the catches often made at the low right-field seats at Yankee Stadium.

"It was the greatest catch I have ever seen," said Anderson. "The way I hurt all over I know it's as good as any I'll ever see."

The Red Sox would not be denied this night and maybe no night any longer in the year of 1975.

Fisk led off the twelfth against Pat Darcy. He took a ball. Then he smashed the next pitch on a high drive to the left-field screen. It was high enough and far enough. Fair or foul was the only question.

"I watched it and gave it the body English," Fisk said.

Then it crashed against the foul pole screen for a game-winning homer. The crowd went wild and Fisk ran his home run home.

"I made sure I touched every one of those sweet white bases," he said. "The fans jumped on the field but I would score even if I had to stiff-arm them."

The game was over. The Reds and Red Sox will settle it tonight. The pitching was shaky after the starters.

"I'll pitch tomorrow," Fisk said.

The way things are going he would probably do a hell of a job.

Best News-Feature Story

(With a Six-Point Score)

BASEBALL

THERE WAS ONLY ONE CASEY

By Wells Twombly

From the San Francisco Examiner
Copyright, ©, 1975, San Francisco Examiner

On casual inspection, the old man looked like a woodcarver's first attempt at a gargoyle. The face was crude and drooping, even when it was new. The eyes were watery and mournful, like a human basset hound. The ears were large and foolish. The hands were hopelessly gnarled. The legs looked like two Christmas stockings stuffed with oranges.

Luckily, greatness doesn't necessarily come in attractive wrappings. Up close, the old man was genuinely beautiful, not exactly in the category of Robert Redford, but beautiful just the same. It was the beauty of a rare antique, tenderly rendered and gracefully aged. It was the beauty of a three hundred-year-old handcrafted pipe, rubbed by a thousand hands and redolent of a thousand aromatic tobaccos. This was a precious original and, of the millions of words that will be written about Charles Dillon Stengel in the next few days, none of them will quite do him justice.

He was one of a handful of baseball characters whose reputations did not exceed their true personalities. The fact is that Yogi Berra was never anything but a quiet, humorless, somewhat grumpy New Jersey businessman, whose humor was largely created by Joe Garagiola anyway. Bo Belinsky was just another charming scoundrel who liked girls, which made him about as kooky as five-sixths of America's male population. Dizzy Dean was a big depression-era redneck who loved beer. As a young man he was bumptious. As a senior citizen, he was a bore.

But the Casey Stengel of real life was better than the Casey Stengel of the printed page. The problem was a mechanical one, which was never solved. He could not be properly transmitted. However, the best literary men of his time worked on it. Oh, how they worked. Still, it never came out quite right, especially the rambling, shattered syntax of his speech, which was a flagrant put-on. Only a very few people understood what Stengel was doing. He led them through a merry maze built entirely of semantic disgraces. He did it on purpose.

Early one morning when he was between jobs, he sat in the tower at Wrigley Field in Los Angeles trying to make Gene Autry a pauper by sucking up so much free booze that the singing cowboy would have to get his guitar and make a comeback. The more he tucked away, the more lucid he became. A twenty-five-year-old baseball writer who covered the Los Angeles Angels and delivered a column nobody read out in the San Fernando Valley was utterly amazed. "That jargon of yours is just a joke," he gasped.

"Son," said Casey in that gravel-driveway voice of his. "This is gonna be our little secret, isn't it?"

The man was a clever and articulate comic who spoke two languages. When he was unguarded he would talk in this straightforward, highly lucid English, which nobody paid any attention to. When there were reporters and other assorted individuals present he spoke in tongues. It was a tangled rat's nest of verbiage that bore only a scanty resemblance to the Mother Tongue so heartily endorsed by the queen of England. Even the mightiest of journalists cowed when he turned on the juice.

When he was managing the wretched New York Mets of the early 1960s he attempted to describe what the fans were like. It was a fine, feathered piece of literature. "These fans are very rabid like they were very collegiate or something because it takes four hours for us to leave our dressing room after a game, which is good because the concession people sell a lot of hot dogs, which is good for our business and I like that. I expect that very soon they will carry one of my players out on their shoulders like he just caught a touchdown for Yale. They are very patient and that's good. These fellows of ours are going to keep right on improving because they are better than most folks think and not as bad as they used to be, because it would be hard to be as bad as that."

There were people who thought Charles Dillon Stengel was a bad manager, just because he had wretched teams in Boston, Brooklyn, and New York. They said that Harpo Marx could have won ten pennants in 12 years with the Yankee clubs that Casey had. That was a mistake. Oh, occasionally he would fall asleep on the bench during night games when he was fronting for the Mets, but that was strictly an epilogue to his years with the Yankees. Even that most cynical of athletes-turned-author, Jim Bouton, said that Stengel knew exactly what he was doing when he had Mickey Mantle and Whitey Ford working for him.

There was this pitcher named Hal Stowe who thought that all he had to do to make the major-league roster was to act like he belonged. He did none of the things other rookies were asked to do. He drank and went to dinner with Mantle and Ford. He did not run in the outfield and he made no overt attempt to impress Stengel. There was one place open on the roster, but Stowe failed to qualify.

"It's true that Hal Stowe pitched pretty good this spring," said Stengel in straight language. "But I noticed that he never ran in the outfield, that he never did all the things he was supposed to do. He never really hustled and he never really worked at it. That's why he didn't make the squad cut, he could bull-bleep everybody but the manager."

Just two years later, Stowe used the same act and managed to put a move on Ralph Houk, the hand-clapping, cigar-chewing militarist who replaced Stengel. The pitcher went north and opened the season with the Yankees because Houk thought he looked and acted like a big leaguer and that was very, very important. Stengel was not so easily confused. When he worked for the Mets the club came up with a nineteen-year-old first baseman named Greg Goossen, whom everybody gurgled about.

"In ten years, Greg Goossen has a great chance of being twenty-nine years old," he said. It wasn't cruel. It was accurate. Sure enough, just ten years later, Goossen did turn twenty-nine, but not with any major-league baseball club.

One afternoon before a World Series game, Stengel took a young Mickey Mantle out to right field at the old ball park in Brooklyn and started to explain how to play caroms off the concave wall. Mantle wanted to know how his manager knew so much about it.

"I used to play right field for the Dodgers!" growled Stengel. "Do you think I was born old?"

So there will be a World Series this year and Casey Stengel will not be present. He was always good for a story. One afternoon it was raining in Baltimore and there he stood with a foot on the rail. "Pardon me, Casey," said a columnist, "it's lousy outside and I need help." He went on for an hour.

Standing nearby was a slim, quivering journalist from a small-town paper. When he was through rescuing the veteran, he turned to the rookie, gave him about 15 minutes and ended up with: "Listen, I got a secret, exclusive story I don't want to give to nobody else. I go to bed late and get up early. You gotta meet me at 6 A.M., but bring some Scotch and we'll break things together."

The man was beautiful. If he's dead, it is only a rumor. Don't bother to print it.

Other Point-Scorers

FOOTBALL

A HARD MAN TO FIND

By Jim Murray

From the Los Angeles Times
Copyright, ©, 1975, Los Angeles Times
Reprinted by permission

Francis Asbury Tarkenton, position, starting upstart for the Minnesota Vikings, has always been a player who drove NFL purists into mouth-frothing rage. But this time he's gone too far.

Frantic Francis, who plays quarterback like a Keystone Kop or a guy fleeing a bank heist, has just joined an unenviable fraternity. He is now at one with the ages with Gene Tunney, Sandy Saddler, Roger Maris, Henry Aaron, and the guy who shot Jesse James. He will have a hard time living it down. He joins a company of people who have knocked over a legend and who come out in history like a guy who would attack a statue with a hammer or put his feet on a Chippendale.

You have to understand, in the little world of football, the name John Unitas is up for sainthood. If he were English, it would be "Sir John." He's on a pedestal. You talk of him in awed whispers. You take your hat off passing his house. You go to one knee in front of his picture. Laid end-to-end, his passing yardage would crisscross the country like Route 66. He once threw touchdown passes in 47 straight games. The only thing in sports that can touch that is DiMaggio's 56-game hitting streak.

But the thing that Johnny U did best was, He Stayed In The Pocket. He was a classic stand-up passer. He was like an English fighter. He played the game The Way It Should Be Played.

The first time Francis Tarkenton showed up in the pro-set T, The Establishment couldn't have been more shocked if someone showed up in the Vatican in shorts. The first time Francis took the ball, he looked as if he were going to run home with it. He looked like a guy stealing a loaf of bread. He not only ran out of the pocket, he damn near ran out of the stadium.

The pros had never seen this before and the gnashing of teeth was coast to coast. Pro quarterbacks are supposed to play the position as if it were set in concrete. A good pro quarterback looks like a statue of Beethoven with a football.

The fraternity had one comfort: funning around that way, Francis wouldn't last long. (Of course, neither would the fat old parties of the front four who had to chase him week-to-week.) Francis, went the theory, would be in traction or a wheelchair by the fourth game. That was 16 years and 7,000 scrambles ago. Francis Tarkenton has started every single NFL game since that time and still has all his legs and eyes and ears, fingers, toes, and teeth.

A typical diagram of a Tarkenton play would look like a drawing of a constellation in the southern skies or a Rube Goldberg How-to-Make-a-Touchdown invention. Francis pioneered the three-minute pass completion. Pocket quarterbacks estimate they have 3.5 seconds to get rid of the football. Francis figures he has 60 minutes. "Some day, he's going to take the ball on the first play of the game from scrimmage and run out the clock," darkly predicted his former coach, Dutch Van Brocklin, who felt a quarterback running was a crime against nature like a horse talking or a lion lisping.

You have to remember Francis was on an expansion team, the last such to win its first league game (37–13). It won three games and scored more points (285) than most expansion teams score in a decade. But the pocket they asked Francis to operate out of frequently was torn. It was not a safe place to keep your money—or the football.

Van Brocklin finally wearied of his Tom-and-Jerry cartoon quarterbacking and dealt Francis off to the New York Giants. The Giants didn't care if their quarterback left the state with the football so long as he occasionally found receivers. Tarkenton took a 1–12 team and turned it into a 7–7 and, ultimately, a 9–5 team. It should be noted the Giant running attack consisted of Fran Tarkenton but he was always breaking the Commandments—"Thou shalt not run out of the pocket," "Thou shalt not win by scrambling," and the Giants soon dealt their sinner back to Minnesota while they went back to 2-and-12 football.

Meanwhile a funny thing was happening over in that funny little other league—quarterbacks began to roll out and pockets began to move up and down the line of scrimmage. You couldn't play quarterback in high cuts anymore. The old set-plant-count-to-three-and-fire! quarterback was as obsolete as the double wing. The other league suddenly had 14 Tarkentons. And all the Super Bowl trophies they could carry.

Tarkenton took the Vikings to two Super Bowls in a row but, in the first one, the Miami Dolphins scored seven points before the Vikings ever got the football and 14 points before Tarkenton had it for three downs. When he got the football, it had been spiked twice.

Last year, Tarkenton tore his shoulder muscle loose in game three. "I couldn't throw the ball more than 10 yards on the fly without screaming. If it wasn't for Butazolidin, I couldn't have lifted the football." Nevertheless, only one quarterback in the league threw for more yards. "It proves," laughed Francis the other day, "that the arm is only a small percentage of quarterbacking. Even when it was 100 percent, nobody ever compared it to Roman Gabriel's."

A series of exercises given him by the Dodgers' Mike Marshall restored the arm. This year, Francis Tarkenton became The Quarterback. He has passed Unitas's record for total completions and soon will pass his record for touchdown completions. All of this is cause for great wailing and anguish from old-timers. A pro quarterback who has passed for 286 touchdowns and 37,779 yards is tolerable. But one who has RUSHED for 26 touchdowns and 3,600 yards (and that's only PAST the line of scrimmage) is no member of the club.

The man who said, "I never thought a quarterback should be a statue," is about to become one. If they put him in the Hall of Fame at Canton, at least the eyes ought to move. If they want authenticity they will put it on rollers. And, every night, they'll come in and find Deacon Jones or Merlin Olsen looking around to see where it went.

TENNIS

ASHE'S LUCKY SATURDAY

By Bud Collins

From The Boston Globe
Copyright, ©, 1975, Globe Newspaper Co.
Courtesy of The Boston Globe

The day that he would win Wimbledon against heavy odds (and over the heavyweight champion of tennis, Jimmy Connors) began for Arthur Ashe at a gaming table in a London casino. "It was about 12:20, and I wanted to get to bed by 1, so I decided to play one last hand, and threw down $175 and said 'deal.' Ace, king—blackjack," Ashe grinned. "I picked up about $300 and went home."

Later yesterday, Ashe blackjacked the reigning king, Connors, 6–1, 6–1, 5–7, 6–4, and picked up about $23,000.

It was lucky Saturday for a guy whose chances of winning the Big W seemed buried six years ago in the semi-finals. But there was nothing lucky about the way Arthur performed in picking apart the brash basher, who had been all but canonized in his rush to a second straight final and 13 straight Wimbledon match victories.

The Fourth of July was past, but Ashe was waving the flag as well as his surgical racket at the kid from Belleville, Ill., in this first All-American male final at Wimbledon since Jack Kramer beat Tom Brown in a 1947 matchup of Californians.

Ashe, 1 to 6 with the village bookmakers when the match began, and 1 to 14 at the start of the fortnight, said, savoring the words, "Yes, I intentionally wore my Davis Cup jacket (emblazoned with USA) when we came onto the court. I think Jimmy got the message. Yes, I did say he was seemingly unpatriotic for refusing to play Davis Cup for our country—and that's why, I guess, he's suing me."

The message Ashe had gotten from Bill Riordan, Connors's

manager, was a lot less subtle intimation of a $4 million lawsuit they're laying on Arthur, alleging that Arthur has libeled Jimmy in the Davis Cup brouhaha. There are two other suits, totaling some $50 million, against Ashe and others in the Association of Tennis Pros. Never has a match vibrated with so much tension on and off the court. There was more to it than two guys who don't like each other.

When he crashed a last overhead beyond Connors on match point, Ashe hurled his fist to the sky—an extraordinary gesture of defiance and triumph for the introspective Virginian.

"No it wasn't a black power salute," explained Ashe. "It was for all the guys on the ATP board that Connors has made miserable with all these unjustified suits."

Annie Kiyomura and Marty Riessen completed the most productive Wimbledon for the United States since 1947 when Americans last had a hand in all five titles. Billie Jean King and Ashe won the singles: Vitas Gerulaitis and Alex Mayer the men's doubles. Ann Kiyomura, of San Mateo, Calif., won the women's doubles with Japanese Kazuko Sawamtsu over Francoise Durr and Betty Stove, 7–5, 1–6, 7–5. Riessen, from Chicago, joined Margaret Court for the mixed championship over Stove and Allan Stone, 6–4, 7–5.

It was an Ashe crowd of 14,000 in Center Court, some of whom had paid scalpers $200 a seat. They were startled at first by his early mastery, cheering him to a big lead, suffering as he lost a service break edge in the third—and eventually the set—and when he fell behind, 0–3 in the fourth.

Connors was beginning to goad himself back into the match, rifling the groundstrokes that interred thunderbolt-serving Roscoe Tanner in the semis. He had earned Wimbledon's awe as a tremendous strokemaker and competitor. His vulgarities had frequently turned devotees off. Yet Ashe, finalist for the first time, had been respected since first showing up in 1963 for his poise and faultless behavior.

They were contrasts in everything but schools: Ashe a UCLA graduate, Connors a UCLA dropout, both winners of the national intercollegiate singles in their day, which was six years apart.

Ashe has been called a choker so often for blowing important matches, but he's hidden the lump somewhere else this year in winning the World Championship Tennis circuit and now Wimbledon.

"He played better than me," said Connors. "I'm not unbeatable like everybody thought."

Ashe said Connors might have choked.

"I never choked in my life," snapped Connors, when informed of the quote.

He didn't appear to. Ashe just went after him brilliantly and patiently, using Connors's lickety-split pace to his own advantage to block winning volleys. Arthur showed Connors's two-handed backhand to be vulnerable to a heavily sliced serve from the right court.

At thirty-one, Ashe has reduced thunder and increased thought. He'd not beaten Connors in three tries, but instead of suicidally trying to slug with the kid, Ashe, chipping his returns, forehanding chops and chips, kept the ball low on the grass. Arthur seldom muscled the ball to give Jimmy the pace he loves.

Connors led for only an instant by winning the opening game on serve. Ashe rolled up the next nine to seal two sets and was up a break, 3–2, in the third. Connors got tough and broke back, and Ashe began a streak of frustration, missing several break points and finally the set at 7–5.

Connors was on his lone run of the match—five games from 5–5 in the third to 3–0 in the fourth. His claque felt he had it going, just like always. He was strutting again, shaking his finger at Ashe. Arthur refused to look, going deeper into his concentration.

He began to knock the strut out of the departing champion with a running forehand down the line. Ashe swung and landed on his face, but it was too well hit for Jimmy to volley. That made the break to 2–3. They went to 4–4, and Arthur broke again with three superb backhands; one a sizzling drive, the others chipped returns.

"I knew where I'd serve the first two in match game," Ashe said. He went for the backhand, got one point, then lost the next on a miraculous swooping forehand.

Connors slapped his hip. He'd come out of it yet. He roared in to whack another forehand with Ashe out of position—but the ball struck the tape as so many of his forehands had. It was the stroke that didn't fire for him. Two more points were easy and Ashe was champion.

"Fantastic, but not as satisfying as winning the Davis Cup for the United States in 1968," he said. "That was all-time number one."

"I had my battle plan, to keep the ball low, use a lot of junk. I deserved to win."

That was exactly the feeling of those who had backed Ashe and Billie Jean King together with their bookies. An Ashe-King double paid 153 to 1.

"I've always thought I had the game to beat Connors," said Ashe, who lost the 1973 U.S. Pro and 1973–74 South African Open finals to Jimmy. "Today I just played that game."

Like a virtuoso. Last night he returned to his other game in the Casino. Regardless of what he may have won, the cards must have seemed anticlimactic to the guy who broke the bank—and the basher—at Wimbledon.

BOXING

THAT THRILLA IN MANILA

By Dick Schaap

From the Washington Star
Copyright, ©,1975, Dick Schaap

The blood was flowing from inside Joe Frazier's mouth and trickling from his nose. The skin was puffed under the right eye and both above and below the left eye, and as Frazier made his way back to his corner at the end of the fourteenth round, Eddie Futch, his manager, his trainer, and his friend, came to an immediate decision. "Let's call it a day," Futch said.

"Don't," Frazier said, "don't stop it." But there was no conviction in his words. Joe Frazier always listens to Eddie Futch, and now Futch was telling his fighter that his bid to become the third man ever to regain the heavyweight championship was ended, that once again, despite a display of courage that was awesome, Frazier had lost to the man he calls Cassius Clay.

Futch leaned over Frazier and pulled one of his strong fists toward him and took out a pair of scissors and began to cut away at Frazier's red eight-ounce boxing gloves. In front of the challenger, the referee, Carlos Padilla, Jr., saw Futch's action and waved his arms, signaling the end. Across the ring, Angelo Dundee caught the signal and shouted, "It's all over," and reached down and lifted his man, Muhammad Ali, off his stool.

And then as chaos broke loose in his corner, as the members of his entourage jostled for position the way they always do, Muhammad Ali lay down on the floor of the ring and caught his breath. He was still the champion of the world, the winner on a technical knockout in 14 rounds.

For the fourth time in this calendar year, he had successfully defended the title he took from George Foreman a year ago, but all the other victims together—Chuck Wepner, Ron Lyle, and Joe Bugner—didn't put up half the struggle Joe Frazier did in a magnificent prenoon battle in the sweltering heat of the theoretically air-conditioned Philippine Coliseum.

"I don't know how he stood up," said Ali after the fight. "I know I would have gone down under all those punches I threw. He is greater than I thought he was."

A few days ago, Ali was saying that the fight would end early, possibly even in the first round, that Frazier was slow and soft and finished, that the fight would not even be close. But this fight was close. There wasn't a knockdown, and even though all three officials, the Filipino referee and the two Filipino judges, had Ali ahead on points by a comfortable margin after 14 rounds, there were many at ringside who thought Frazier, the underdog, outweighed by about nine pounds, was leading or at least even.

A crowd of 25,000 that paid $1.5 million—both records for an indoor fight—watched a fight that began with pseudopsychological warfare and ended with street slugging.

Frazier entered the ring first, wearing blue trunks with a dull finish and white piping. By the time he reached his corner, he was already drenched with sweat.

Then Ali came in, his trunks a shiny white with black piping, the glitter of his trunks and the dullness of Frazier's a perfect symbolic contrast. There was not a drop of sweat on Ali. He did not sweat at all until the fight began.

Someone brought into the ring a handsome trophy, and the ring announcer said that the trophy would be presented by President Ferdinand Marcos, who was in the audience, to the winner. Ali didn't wait. He scampered into the center of the ring, grabbed the trophy, and lugged it back to his corner, looking at Frazier defiantly, as if daring the challenger to come take it back.

And then the fight began and in the early rounds, the first two or three, Ali seemed to be in complete command, almost toying with Frazier, giving a boxing lesson. In the last 30 seconds of the first round, Ali rocked Frazier with a left hook and a few seconds later, connected with a straight right. When the round ended, Frazier gave the champion a little tap on the rear and walked back to his own corner with a sort of goofy smile on his face.

In the third round, for the first time, Frazier rocked Ali with a left hook, and the sound and ferocity of the blow drew oohs from the crowd. Ali, responding more to the crowd than to the punch, turned and made a face, opening his mouth wide, as if to say that sounded a lot tougher than it felt. He was making fun, Angelo Dundee said later. But it hurt him. I saw his legs when it landed.

In the middle rounds, from about the fourth through the eighth, Frazier was in charge most of the time. He was the aggressor, and even when Ali flurried and pounded him with combinations, Frazier kept boring in, kept punching. The goofy look was gone.

And in those middle rounds, a strange thing happened: Ali lost the crowd. Before the fifth round, he led his followers in chants of, "Ali, Ali, Ali," but the men in Frazier's corner came back with chants of "Joe, Joe, Joe," and then the crowd, basically Filipino, started shouting, "Frazier, Frazier, Frazier."

The feeling was by no means unanimous, but enough of the Filipinos felt that Ali was too *mayabang*, too cocky, for their tastes, and so they wanted the underdog, the less boastful man to win. Apparently, Filipinos admire cockiness when two cocks fight—not when two men fight.

By the eighth round, the blood began to roll out of Frazier's mouth, some of it staining Ali's white trunks. But Ali was accomplishing little in those rounds, often allowing Frazier to back him into a corner and pound away at him. His corner yelled instructions, "Stay there," meaning in the middle of the ring, and "Don't hook" —you never hook with a hooker, Dundee said later—but Ali seemed to ignore the counsel.

By the twelfth round, Ali was definitely running the show again, manipulating Frazier, dictating the pace and the fury of the fight. "We had an extra gas tank in the corner," said Dundee later, kidding. Then he turned serious and said, "Nobody can suck it up like my man."

Ali sucked it up, found new strength, and sapped Frazier's. The thirteenth and fourteenth rounds were exercises in punishment. Several times, Ali landed six, seven, eight punches in a row, rights and lefts, shattering combinations that sent the sweat flying off Frazier's face, the mouthpiece flying from his mouth, but couldn't send him down to the floor.

In the thirteenth round, Frazier slipped—helped by a flurry of Ali punches—and almost went down, but regained his balance. His eyes were beginning to close, and in the following round, he was squinting at Ali, making out mostly the form of red gloves, coming at his face, bouncing off his nose and his forehead and his cheeks, pounding and pounding and pounding.

"No," said Frazier at the end, facing the press with sunglasses hiding his eye, "I wouldn't say I was hurt. No, I wasn't hurt. Just banged up. Tomorrow, I'll be all good."

Then Joe Frazier took off his glasses, and the bumps under the right eye and over the left looked enormous. They looked almost as big as Joe Frazier's heart.

WORLD SERIES

ROSE STICKS IT TO THE RED SOX
(World Series Game VII)

by Bill Conlin

From the Philadelphia Daily News
Copyright, ©, 1975, Philadelphia Daily News

The Gods went back to Mt. Olympus. Zeus hid the lightning bolts.

Game seven of the World Series belonged to guys with dirt under their fingernails, clock-punching nine-to-fivers with names like Pete Rose and Joe Morgan, Clay Carroll and Jack Billingham.

The Reds won the Series 4–3 with two outs in the ninth on a flared single to center by Morgan that was inappropriate and correct as Carlton Fisk's twelfth-inning homer in game six was majestic and dramatic. If the already historic game that set the stages for last night's Fenway climax was the *Mona Lisa* of the Pastime, then this was the *Picture of Dorian Gray,* an awkward, unlovely struggle filled with warts and blemishes.

Rose came out of it with two singles, a walk, a dirty uniform, and the ante that goes to the Series MVP. He probably didn't clinch it until rookie Red Sox left-hander Jim Burton pitched around him with first base open and Ken Griffey on second with two outs, the contest tied 3–3 and waiting to provide the cosmic drama that never came.

But Rose knows in his mind when he won the auto and possibly the game. It came on a play that showed up on the score sheet as "forced at second, error second baseman."

It happened in the sixth inning with left-hander Bill Lee protecting a 3–0 lead and mesmerizing the Reds with his collection of sinkers, screwballs, and humpbacked slow curves.

Rose led off the inning with a single to right. Morgan flied to right. The Reds seemed knee deep in quicksand, their running game shut down by the Sox lead. When Morgan stole second despite the deficit in the fourth it seemed more symbol than threat.

Now Johnny Bench stroked a double-play ball to Rick Burleson at shortstop. Double plays had taken the Reds out of rallies in the third and fifth innings.

Rose slid recklessly into second and Denny Doyle, who had wretched Series running and fielding, threw the relay into the Sox dugout. It was a sliver of daylight and the Reds ran to it.

Three pitches later, Lee looped that Eeephus curve to Tony Perez. Perez double-hitched and fired an awesome two-run shot over the Green Monster. Still alive at 3–2.

"Sparky Anderson hugged me in the dugout," Rose said in the wet and wild Reds clubhouse. "He said, 'You got us two runs with a hard slide.' And I wasn't even on base. I was an out. But I gave one of our big hitters a chance to swing the bat and that's what it takes to win, the way the Reds came back to win all year.

"I tried to break it up. I knew it was a double play if he makes a normal pivot. I didn't even touch him on the slide, but I made him go too high in the air to clear me and he threw it away."

Lee threw that lazy pitch to Perez in game two. Once.

"I wasn't looking for the pitch," the Cuban veteran said. "He only throw it once. I swing and miss as it bounce in the dirt. I was embarrassed. I guess he think he can fool me again, but it was up high and I have time to adjust my swing. I just wait as long as I can and hit it hard. I love that home run. I can retire tomorrow if I want and say I am a World Champion, but the big play, the one that get me to the plate is Pete making Doyle throw to the dugout on the double-play ball. That is the game for us. It got us close."

Close wasn't always enough for the Reds against the tenacious Red Sox. They won three games by one run and had no right to believe their bullpen could prevent a repeat of the game six fireworks.

"We were tense, edgy," Rose said. "We were getting on the umpire (American League's Art Frantz) on some pitches. We were squirming, getting upset when we hit into those double plays. We could have folded it up when Merv Rettenmand hit for Don Gullett in the fifth and hit into a double play. But we hung in there."

Lee left after walking Griffey with one out in the seventh. He was too involved to tell Darrell Johnson about a blister on his left thumb that kept him from gripping his sinker properly. Rogelio Moret, the skinny left hander, waded into the pressure and wobbled like a whooping crane in a high wind.

Moret walked Ed Armbrister after Griffey stole second and looked into the squinting eyes of Rose, peering out of that contorted crouch. Rose tied it with a single to center.

"I worked hard during the rainouts," said Rose, who finished the Series 10 for 27 (.370).

Burton was pitching the ninth because Johnson said he was the man for the hitters coming up to the plate. Don't knock it. That kind of logic got the dour manager to the ninth inning of the seventh game of a World Series with a 3–3 tie.

Burton walked Griffey—"Ball four wasn't close," the left hander said—and Cesar Geronimo bunted him to second. Dan Driessen hit for winning pitcher Clay Carroll and bounced out to Doyle.

"Darrell came out and said don't give Rose a good pitch to hit," Burton said. "I threw a strike on the outside corner but I wasn't really trying to make it that good. He said we'd take our chances pitching to Morgan."

Great pitch, feeble hit, terrible result for Boston. Fred Lynn was playing deep in center. He never had a chance for a patented diving catch. Griffey scored, Rose dove headfirst into third while Morgan took second, the third time in the game Boston gave the trailing runner an extra base.

The Boston heroes of game six faded into history. Bernie Carbo played left, doubled in the first, and gunned out George Foster trying for two bases with a perfect play off the wall in the second.

Carlton Fisk struck out three times and was hitless. Dwight Evans and Lynn were both 0 for 2 with two walks.

The Gods went back to Mt. Olympus, Zeus hid the lightning bolts. And, finally, Pete Rose could sense what all the scuffling years of headfirst slides and dirty uniforms were all about.

"I just feel now that the other 12 years were wasted," he said, "because I never felt any feeling like this."

He reeked of sweat and souring champagne, the way it should be when an honest working stiff reaches the top of the mountain.

HOCKEY

BERNIE PARENT MISSES THE BOAT

By Stan Hochman

From the Philadelphia Daily News
Copyright, ©, 1975, Philadelphia Daily News

Are the fish biting off Barnegat Light? Are they nibbling? Does the five-day forecast include small-craft warnings? Is there enough beer in the cooler?

"You gotta relax," Bernie Parent explained last night over the bedlam of another Stanley Cup championship. "You can't go out there tight. So, I think about other things. Mostly, I think about my boat."

His boat. His ever-loving 33-foot boat. Beer in the cooler and bait in the buckets and gas in the tanks.

Gerry Desjardins, the other goalie, was so seasick he couldn't see straight. So Buffalo went with Roger Crozier, whose nerves have been known to twang like too-taut guitar strings.

And Parent? Parent ate a steak, took a nap, drank a cup of coffee, and went out and rode the roller coaster that is a Stanley Cup game.

He stopped 32 shots, which is how many Buffalo took. He stopped them with his glove, his stick, his chest, his arms, his skates. He stopped them from up close and from far away. He stopped the ones that came hurtling toward him straight on, and he stopped the ones that ricocheted off sticks and skates and darted in new directions.

"You ever see him play bad when it's a big game?" Bobby Clarke was asking people in the madhouse that was the Flyers' clubhouse afterward.

"It was just like last year, the last game against Boston. We could have played all night, and I don't think they could have scored."

It was a lot like last year, against Boston, when the Flyers snatched their Stanley Cup with a sixth-game shutout.

"This time," Parent said, between television charades, "I enjoyed it more. Last year, we were in the clouds. This year, we played the system."

Enjoyed it more? Desjardins was telling people before the sixth game he was beginning to hate the sport. Crozier was too grumpy to even express his feelings. Somehow it is beyond imagination's gloomiest reach to visualize Parent saying he "hated" the game.

"Bernie loves life too much to say that," Terry Crisp said, clutching a bottle of champagne by the throat. "The day he hates it, he'll quit."

Hate it? It is possible that Parent's love for the game explains his fantastic success, capped last night by the Conn Smythe Trophy that goes to the most valuable player in the championship series.

He takes the game seriously and himself lightly. A "big game player"? "Hey," he said, slumping into a corner of his locker. "Does that mean if you face 30 shots, instead of stopping 27, you have to stop 30?"

Parent was coming down now, out of the clouds, out of the giddy joyride that is the roller coaster. Making small jokes, because that is his nature.

"Fun?" he pondered the word lovingly. "Sure, it's fun when you play for *this* team. You only face 26 or 27 shots a game. It's fun."

That is the equation for measuring fun. Play for a team that scraps and hustles and bumps and thumps and keeps the other team at a distance, and it can be fun. Even if the other team gets 32 shots.

"Yeh," he said, "but we kept them from good angles. You don't win with one guy. During the season I only faced 26 or 27 shots a game. That's a team effort.

"The [Smythe] trophy has got to go to someone. But this is a team game. They say it's not the same, the second time. They're wrong. It's twice as good.

"This is what the whole game is about."

And last night, unexpectedly, the end of May, the wearying, skate-dragging end of May, and both teams unfurled a brilliant effort, etching it on fog-free ice.

The Sabres swarmed around Parent, testing him. They resembled hornets trying to sting some knight through his armor. He turned away 13 shots the first period, and 13 more in the second, withstanding power play after power play.

And in the end, his teammates had trouble sorting out the best of what they had seen. "He was beautiful," Clarke said, fidgeting with a cigarette. "He must have had 15 great saves."

"He plays good every game," said Ed Van Impe, blood thickening in a cut on the bridge of his nose. "Good every game and great some games. Tonight, he was great."

Parent talks about "anticipation." He has trouble articulating just what it is he does. Van Gogh had the same trouble explaining his paintings.

But he will not let his nerves turn his arms and legs to stone, and that might be his greatest asset. "You're tight," he said, "and you make mistakes.

"If you're tight, you can't make the moves. Hey, you get ready and then you go out there, and it's just like Doris Day sings, 'Que Sera, Sera.' "

Sure, Bernie, sure. But there must be some days when that afternoon nap is elusive as some nagging bumblebee, buzzing through the room. Some days when dreams come fitfully, full of shots that emerge from dark closets. Or does he make every save in the afternoon dreams?

"I don't dream about stopping shots," Parent said, smiling under that sweat-soaked moustache. "What you want me to do? Get tired *before* the game?"

The dreams can wait. Besides they have trouble matching the reality of another Stanley Cup championship. "Geez," Parent said over and over, "that is what the game is all about."

TENNIS

VIRGINIA WADE: WHATEVER BECAME OF HER "BRILLIANT FUTURE"?

By Catherine Bell

From Tennis Magazine
Copyright, ©, 1975, Tennis Magazine

Virginia Wade occupies a special place in the hearts and minds of the English people. She is an institution, almost a fixation. She exasperates and obsesses. She is sacrosanct.

Curiously, she won this singular status not on the lawns of Wimbledon but largely because of one glorious tournament on alien sod. At Forest Hills in 1968, she became the only Englishwoman to capture the U.S. singles championship since Betty Nuthall in 1930. She bought champagne for the press, tossed her hair, flashed her lopsided, shyly charming smile, basked in the attention, and flew home to general applause. She was twenty-three years old, attractive, rich, talented. A Brilliant Future was the popular opinion.

But a funny thing happened to Virginia's tennis career during the next few years. She became very famous in Britain without winning another substantial singles title. The more famous she became, the less she won. In 1969, it was Anne Jones—an unbeautiful, unsung, hard-working professional—who took the Wimbledon singles for Britain and hoisted the washed gold plate above her head. Virginia had lost somewhere in the third round. Whatever happened?

Looking back, it is easy to say simply that Virginia succumbed to the well-known infection of too much too soon; that she talked too much, believed too much in her image, colluded with the press in creating that image, and surrounded herself with people who kept her from self-criticism. She certainly accepts some of that now. In 1969, she believed she was the best tennis player in the world. "I've got an incredibly wide range of shots," she told a credulous reporter. These days she says, "I used to be conceited about it all. I used to think I was spectacular. Now I don't at all."

There's been a change. It may be that, at twenty-nine, she's grown up and that emotional stability has reached her toward the end of her career. Professionalism—in the sense of being in control of her game and her life instead of being controlled—may at last have found acceptance in the mind of the woman who was proud to think of herself as the last of the amateurs. "There's a different sort of satisfaction to be had out of winning," she observes. "If you play professionally, you train to play as well as you can and then you accept what happens. I'm no longer afraid of losing. I spend more time preparing and less regretting."

Yet for all that and for all the accompanying general improvement in her game, Virginia must have in retrospect plenty to regret. The hopes of 1968 dissipated in a series of high days and low days, of failures and excuses, of minor championships won and major ones lost. In front of her adoring and bemused English audience, Virginia acted out a morality play for which she wrote the script.

It could only have happened in Britain. A nation conscious of its own decline is desperate for heroes. Virginia not only won things in 1968, she had color, she was theatrical, she was exceptionally articulate for a sports star. The media devoured her, and the claws of the media were soft, like a sea anemone; it didn't even hurt, not at first. For a while, it was as if Virginia could see only through a glass that reflected faithfully her own constructed flawless image. The glass was smoky, but it shone so bright.

Virginia's temperament was suited to the flattering, glamorous and attention-filled life that swamped her after Forest Hills; her tennis wasn't. She was tempted, she fell and then it was too late, and she woke from fantasies to find that some people had turned against her, decided her tantrums were dull and her precious individuality a nuisance. Private hurt and bewilderment became public abruptness and obstinacy.

Physically, Virginia is taller than most tennis players, 5-feet-8, and not too heavy. Muscularly, she is well proportioned though her right shoulder is noticeably larger than her left and, like many athletes, she walks with a slight stoop. On court, she is generally considered graceful, but that is not really true. Her footwork is often clumsy and she cannot change direction very quickly.

Her serve is one of the fastest in the women's game, but her total action is slow and full of strain. She does not get as much flexibility or body into it as Billie Jean King or Rosie Casals or Evonne Goolagong, and she cannot whip her arm over as fast as Margaret Court. Her toss is sometimes so far astray that she wouldn't be able to catch the ball coming down. Virginia serving often gives the impression of someone doing something they know is observed and much admired. It is a performance in itself.

Virginia began life with a great deal, some might say too much. She was born in 1945 in Bournemouth, England, the youngest child and second daughter of moderately well-to-do parents, and spent her adolescence in Durban, the most English of South African cities, where her father was an Episcopal archdeacon. She grew up in the sun, more or less taught herself tennis, and returned to England with her family in 1961. She matured early in comparison to British girls her own age. She was strong, active, and full of energy. The serve-and-volley game came easily to her but, like many girls who play this brand of tennis from an early age, she had only minor success as a junior.

In 1963, Virginia entered the University of Sussex to study mathematics and physics. She never considered Oxford or Cambridge, although she would certainly have been admitted to either. Sussex in the 1960s was the Berkeley of Britain with new buildings at Brighton-by-the-sea and all styles of radical thought. It was a strange choice for someone with a strongly conservative background and who later admitted, "I'm incredibly unrebellious. I've got nothing to rebel against."

At Sussex, Virginia played a lot of tennis and took her final exams in the same week she represented Britain in the Wightman Cup. She lost 10 pounds in weight, won a third-class degree, and failed, with the rest of the team, to win the Wightman Cup. Nobody asked her to do all these things at once. She did it because, she said, "Somebody told me I couldn't."

Did Virginia think she could do everything? She tried. She came from a family and a social class whose aspirations were traditionally high. And Virginia could do most things well. Perhaps it was only by chance that she began to play tennis seriously. Certainly she was never dedicated to the game with the puritanical passion many great players possess.

She admits today her years of tennis have involved sacrifices that have come really hard. "Often you'd much prefer to be having fun at home," she confesses. "Some people play all the time because they haven't got anything else to do. Tennis isn't everything to me."

In 1966, Virginia set off on the international tennis circuit possessing a serve and a volley and, technically, not much else. Her service was good enough to take her a fair way in women's tennis by itself. No matter that as often as not she hit her way into trouble as she did out of it. She had presence, aggression, outward social poise, and that fateful thing: "temperament." She threw her racquet and swore. She already had the ability to attract others around her, not to advise, merely to be there. The English public began to chart her progress. In the wings, the press waited to pounce.

She pounded erratically through 1967, winning the Bournemouth hard court title from Jones and reaching the quarter-finals at Wimbledon. At twenty-two, this was as much as could have been realistically expected of her. She was not to reach even the last eight at Wimbledon again until 1972—and that was surely not expected.

The year 1968 began well; she again took the Bournemouth title and was runner-up in South Africa. But 1968 was the dividing year, the watershed, the decisive point at which the idea of Virginia as potentially the best player in the world was flung about and finally settled around her neck as heavy as any millstone. The press began making noises when she played a decisive part in Britain's Wightman Cup victory over a depleted U.S. team. At Forest Hills, Virginia whipped Francoise Durr, Casals, and King, all contracted professionals, and suddenly the individualistic amateur seemed better than the lot.

The press corps descended; Virginia had no chance. They slavered, they fawned. Her victory at Forest Hills had been admirable. The behavior of the British press was unconscionably irresponsible. The avalanche of adjectives rolled on—"sensuous, tempestuous, volcanic. . . ."

Virginia gave interviews here, there, and everywhere. She connived at the disaster. She was photographed and questioned almost everywhere but on the tennis court. The pulp press pulped her and left her with nothing. They talked to her about the wrong things, the silly superficial things that made spectacular copy and it was all written with a repellent intimacy designed to convey that this or that hack reporter was privy to the "real," the "true" Virginia.

With one or two notable exceptions, the British press gave her rope to hang herself and she obligingly did. Who could blame her? She was young, a bit naïve, and given to self-doubts that she couldn't express and were seldom guessed at. On the court, she clung to her own style, her independence. Only Maureen Connolly helped her much in her early, impressionable years in international tennis, but Maureen became ill and lived in America and was not able to be the consistent coach Virginia needed. Then, it's possible that in the heady days after her U.S. Open win Virginia really did think she was a complete player and that her No. 2 world ranking was a reliable estimate of her present and future ability.

Throughout the spring and summer of 1969, Virginia postured, the press slobbered and she began to lose matches. In truth, she was losing no more or less than she had done before or has done since. But now her wins were perceived as evidence of effortless brilliance and her bad matches as proof of the assumption that it was only "temperament," a momentary lack of self-control, that held her back.

The inevitable slide began that year and for the next couple of seasons it seemed downhill most of the way. The danger signals were there clearly enough but nobody paid much attention. Here she was talking in 1961 when she had already been playing the circuit for three years: "The number of times one doesn't care if one wins or loses is frightening." It's doubtful whether a King or a Court could ever make such a statement. Later, Virginia said, a bit peevishly: "If only everyone hadn't been on my back all the time, I'd have grown up sooner."

Her losses became more agonizing. In Italy in 1969, she went out fuming to Peaches Bartkowicz; at Wimbledon she lost to Pat Pretorious; and in the Wightman Cup at Cleveland she surrendered the opening and decisive rubber to Julie Heldman.

The more perceptive tennis writers began to refer to Virginia's "depressing limitations" as a player; the rest still told themselves that it was only a "psychological thing." Few paused to look, with clear-headed kindness, at the leg-end of Virginia's temperament and the complex pattern of her behavior. She always seemed so self-assured, so very much knowing the right way to say and do things. But beneath it all lay oversensitivity, timidity, and desperate fear of failure. The hard nugget of certainty and the all-excluding tunnel vision essential to consistent competitive success had never been part of her character. Intellectually, Virginia could accept her failures; emotionally she could not.

Such conflict forced her into seeking excuses for her losses outside the area of simple lack of skill. Her temperamental difficulties did not consist so much in the practice of her tennis as in an unwillingness to admit there was anything wrong at all. Yet a corrosive doubt was always there. As late as 1972, she admitted, "I would like to have more supervision when I'm practicing. I feel I need someone to make sure I don't get into bad habits." She was twenty-seven and still looking for someone to lean on.

The two or three years after Forest Hills were a bad time in her life. She suffered a lot and only those closest to her will ever know how much she suffered. Her game deteriorated and so did her temper. Her personal life, she says, was a mess.

Watching her became a distressing occupation for those who

admired her style of play and sympathized with her problems. The year 1970 was mostly bad; you can measure the true quality of a player by how they lose as much as by the way they win. Virginia's losses were obsessively horrible. After a debacle against Fay Moore in Hamburg, she shouted: "Oh, I just can't play this game!" "Frankly," wrote the reporter from the *Daily Express*, "I give up."

So did Virginia. For the first time in her career, she talked seriously of leaving the game. At Forest Hills, she flopped to Casals, wept, complained, threw her racquet, and abandoned herself to misery. Rosie looked on in some surprise and gratefully took the match that was handed to her. Throughout 1970, Virginia's behavior became so bad that a patent medicine company whose product she endorsed began to have second thoughts about their choice of player. "Virginia," said the press, "you're a bore."

That was unfair. Paradoxically, in her worst moments on the court she was more deserving of consideration and even respect than she had even been in her finest victories. At times of great unhappiness, a person can connect with reality, become integrated and coherent because the defenses are gone and they are truly alone.

On such occasions, flat on her face on Forest Hills grass, stumbling and slithering around European clay, buffeted beyond endurance by North of England gales, shouting hopelessly (Paris, 1974: "I don't know why I go on playing this horrible game!"), Virginia met her inner self. The affectation, the pretense, the façade, they all destroyed themselves because they were no longer necessary. Only out of this kind of trauma can grow calmness and self-knowledge. And Virginia has her own strength and resilience. After confrontations with humiliating defeat, she has always picked herself up, faced her trouble, and gone on playing.

She's inconsistent still, and will be; the public in Britain feel let down because they expected her to change her personality in some way, as if anyone ever does, and the public pressure became at times unbearable. She's a better tennis player now, though, without a doubt.

Three years ago King cast a cool glance at her game and said: "People talk about her being so unpredictable. I don't think she's that unpredictable. I feel most of the time Virginia is tending to go one way eight out of 10 times. I believe the way she flings herself at the ball makes you think she is unpredictable. But basically, she always hits the same shots in the same situations and doesn't seem to realize it."

She does now. Her rivals recognize that there is far more variety to her tennis. The pattern of her wins and losses has not altered very much—there are bad days and good days—but a more balanced attitude to publicity and a sense of security about the future has helped to relieve much of her former conflict and tempered her disappointments.

Years of playing the circuit produce strange conditioning, addictions, and habits, but stringing together titles is a habit Virginia won't have to lose because she never acquired it. She is probably not title-chasing anymore—that's a game for the young and ingenuous. She's earned a lot of money in her career and wants to earn more because she now has definite ideas about the thing she wants to do with it. And she'll accept and play according to a purer professionalism: winning well is winning well even if it means beating Billie Jean in Phoenix rather than at Wimbledon, that fortnight of distorted reputations.

She'll accept, too, if even only to herself, that she may never win Wimbledon unless everybody else stays away. The year, after all, is full of matches worth remembering and Virginia's finest moments will probably now be counted in individual matches against those players who bring out the best in her. She's been playing well in the United States this spring and it's one of the paradoxes in Virginia's nature that so strongly British a person reserves her best performances for transatlantic audiences.

Her game has leveled, without losing its original pounding, aggressive style. She keeps the ball in play longer nowadays for tactical reasons and not simply because she can't get rid of it. She reserves her strength because, at nearly thirty, she has to and this means in a match situation she considers things more carefully. She has developed her lob, her topspin, her dropshots, her discipline, during the past couple of years, though such is the organization of the circuit now that English crowds are denied the chance of appraising her late-maturing talent.

In any case, she's looking ahead now to other things. She says she may retire in a couple of years because she'll be thirty in July and doesn't "want to go on playing until I need crutches." Virginia is reserved about her plans; they are, after all, her own business. But her patriotism is deeply felt and she would very much like to do something for British tennis. Leading Britain to its Wightman Cup victory over the United States in 1974 pleased her a great deal and it was generally agreed that she made a good captain.

Militancy has never touched her—she won't see any significant connection between women's tennis and social reform, which is why she has stayed apart from involvement in politics, radicalism, and the women's movement. The other players take this for granted.

Virginia is herself, does her own thing and, if her actions sometimes seem contradictory (signing with World Team Tennis, for example), well, what the hell? There's plenty of room in tennis for personalities.

There will be a dreadful gap in the British game when she's gone, although it is not possible to say of her, as one can say of King, that she changed anything in the world. That's the true measurement of greatness and, measured against that, Virginia can only appear as excessively talented.

We can be grateful for that and grateful, too, that her career—after much turbulence, personal pain, and misdirection—is now drawing more peacefully to its close. "I've always believed," she once said, "that I play more beautiful and exciting tennis than most of the others. I'd rather do that than win. I'll be happy if when I retire, people say 'she was exciting, she gave pleasure.' "

BASEBALL

A ROOKIE LEAGUE

By Dave Kindred

From The Louisville Courier-Journal
Copyright, ©, 1975, The Courier Journal & Times

Pete Estep comes to all the games played by the Elizabethton Twins
professional baseball team. A fat man who sweats a lot, Pete drives
a taxi and when the police aren't looking, he sells whisky out of the
car trunk. Not long ago, alas, the cops were looking. "Caught me
with 56 pints," Pete said. "Fined me $150 and gave me six months'
probation." He sighed. "Goldarn it, what's wrong about providing
for your fella man?"

As is his custom, Pete stopped by the visitors' dugout, this night
occupied by the Kingsport Braves, the last-place team in the Southern Division of the Appalachian League. It's a rookie league, the
first step in a journey of a thousand miles to the major leagues. Of
250 players, maybe 20 or 25 will ever finish the trip. The others
dream. Pete Estep said, "Anybody who hits a home run tonight, I
got a $5 bill. Just come to the screen behind home plate, I'll give
it to you."

"What about for a shutout?" Rick Rhodes said. He would pitch
for Kingsport an hour later.

"Sure, $5 for a shutout," the taxi driver/whisky runner said.

The Appalachian League has teams in the eastern Tennessee
cities of Elizabethton, Kingsport, Johnson City, and Bristol and in
the Virginia cities of Marion, Covington, Bluefield, and Pulaski. The
biggest place is Kingsport, with about 40,000 people, and the smallest is Elizabethton, with 7,000. The cities are within 200 miles of
each other. It is a "bus league," baseball's way of saying all travel
is by bus.

Riverside Park in Elizabethton is a neat little baseball field next
to the Watauga River. A sign on the green wooden outfield fence

promises a case of quart-size beer to the accurate slugger who hits a ball over it. On this night, 586 people paid to sit in the new concrete bleachers. The loudest customers were under a sign reading, "Sexchun 8." The army discharges mentally disturbed soldiers according to Section 8 regulations. That gives you an idea of what the Sexchun 8 inmates are like. "Bunch of rednecks who are strong on goofy sayings," Rick Rhodes said. "But if you're going to make it to the bigs, there'll be verbal abuse all the way. So you might as well get used to it."

Rick Rhodes is a left hander from Louisville. He's twenty-two years old, a graduate of Westport High School and Vanderbilt University. Offered $15,000 five years ago to sign a professional baseball contract, he said no. Offered $8,000 two years ago, he again refused. This summer he signed for nothing.

"Well, I got a three-figure bonus," Rhodes said with a smile. In days when high school basketball players get seven figures—meaning a million dollars—a three-figure number is proof no one considers you a hot property. Rhodes passed up the earlier offers to stay in school, where he pitched well but not remarkably. No major-league team chose him in this spring's draft of maybe 500 players. Then a scout for the Atlanta Braves called and asked if he wanted to sign. Rhodes said sure.

Kingsport is not the bigs. The Braves' clubhouse is in a high school football stadium. Only four showers work. "We take turns soaping up," Rhodes said. The team uniforms are flannels, which are out of date in this age of double knits. "We look like hicks," Rhodes said. For a salary of $500 a month, plus $6.50 a day in meal money on the road, why does a college graduate play in the Appalachian League?

"I've wanted to play major-league baseball since I was seven years old," Rhodes said. A kid's dream. The kid is twenty-two now, and he knows the Atlanta Braves, alone of the 24 big-league teams, wanted him. For a three-figure bonus. "It's kind of a silly thing, to be here." Rhodes said, "Silly, if you don't love it. For some of the guys, it's like a job. Not me."

Thirty years ago, 20 years ago, a kid went into baseball and stayed until they threw him out. The game was life itself. For Rick Rhodes, it's a dream and, if the dream isn't made real, he'll go on to something else.

"This is temporary here in Kingsport," he said. "One way or the other, it's temporary. At my age, Atlanta will take a look at me next spring and either keep me or let me go. If they like me, they'll send me to Savannah. But if they send me to Greenwood. . . ."

Savannah is the Braves' second-best minor-league team, two notches above Kingsport. Greenwood is only one step up. "A lot of guys make it to the majors at twenty-seven, twenty-eight," Rhodes said. "But if I don't make it in the next two or three years, I'll get out for sure. I've got a lot of things I can do. What keeps you going, I guess, is that other guys nobody wanted have made it. Like Dan Driessen at Cincinnati. Nobody drafted him, either. But if it looks bad, I'm not going to knock around in a bus forever."

Kingsport's gasping, smoking bus lurched to a stop outside Riverside Park in Elizabethton. The Braves immediately began their search for quarters. Manager Gene Hassell gives out the $6.50 in daily meal money as a five, a one, and a 50-cent piece. But it takes a quarter to operate the soft-drink machine by the clubhouse. "Anybody got two quarters for a half-dollar?" Don Young said.

Young was Atlanta's No. 1 draft pick this spring. He's eighteen years old, 6-feet-3, 195 pounds. The Braves gave him a $60,000 bonus. Life in Kingsport has been a revelation for the man-child from Santa Barbara, Calif.

"The way they talk," Young said, rolling his eyes. "Especially the telephone operators. It's like a foreign language. And for entertainment, you know what they do in Kingsport? They get a glass of ice water and sit on the front porch. Really."

A crisis arose just before game time.

Trainer Gene Lane, a high school student, said to Hassell, the manager, "Is Johnson City long distance?"

"Yeah. Why?"

"Our towels are still in the laundry."

"Too late now," the manager said. "They're closed."

"You know how many towels we got? Five."

"All we need is one—for me," Hassell said.

Sheet King, a pitcher, said, "We can pass it around." They have lots of towels in the bigs.

Gene Hassell, forty-seven, left Flat River, Mo. (pop. 5,401), at age sixteen to play professional baseball at Elmira, N.Y. A month and a half later, he deserted the team, lovesick. "I went home, fiddled around, and got married," Hassell said.

Five years later, he was back in the minor leagues and has been a player, coach, and manager ever since (with the exception of four years when he ran two gas stations in Kansas City). A 5-foot-7, 140-pound infielder with speed, Hassell worked his way up to the Yankees' top minor-league team, Denver. But he never made the bigs. "I was always buried behind Gil McDougald and Billy Martin and Jerry Coleman and Bobby Richardson," he said, "Yeah, it hurt, not making it."

The only son of O. L. Hassell, a farmer who'd been a pitcher, Gene grew up playing baseball. "I wore out the covers of balls throwing 'em against the concrete foundation and catching 'em on the rebound," he said. Hassell grew strong tossing hay and milking cows. "I still got a helluva grip," the manager said.

Hassell is a friendly man, quick to smile. He likes today's players. "I can't say we were hungrier back then. If I was so damned hungry, I'd have never jumped the Elmira club. None of these guys ever jumped the club on me. And the players today are bigger, stronger, and better."

Hassell wouldn't call Rick Rhodes a major-league prospect. "You can't say that about anybody," he said. "Nobody knows who is going to make it. Rick is intelligent. What he needs right now is control of that curveball."

The first month of the 65-game season, Rhodes pitched poorly, losing three of four games. His best pitch is a big-breaking curveball. His fastball, by his admission, "is less than medium big-league velocity." To win, Rhodes must throw strikes "70 percent of the time with the curve, and I'd been getting about 33 percent."

If Rhodes is to be a major-league pitcher, he must throw that curveball precisely where he wants it, "There are pitchers with medium velocity and real good control of the curve who make it, like Whitey Ford, Freddy Norman, Tommy John, Ross Grimsley," Rhodes said.

"As of now, I don't have that control. If I can somehow find that —find that certain release point where I throw strikes consistently —then I can move up quickly."

Gary Cooper, the center fielder, wanted to put tape on his bat handle. "This is the only roll of tape we've got," said Lane, the trainer. "Come on, man, I gotta have tape," Cooper said. "It's for injuries," the trainer said. "Whatta we do if somebody gets hurt? Use glue?"

In the fourth inning, Kingsport's Dave Stevens hit a home run. It was the first of his professional career.

"Is that ball lost?" Stevens said to Lane.

"Why, you want it?"

"Sure. Take the $5 from that guy and give it to some kid to find the ball."

Rhodes pitched well after a first inning in which his own throwing error helped Elizabethton score two runs. Kingsport led 4–3 in the seventh when manager Hassell thought to give an outfielder some advice. "No doubles," he shouted.

Then he remembered the outfielder, one of four Latin-Americans on the team, didn't speak English. So Hassell turned to a Latin reserve, his interpreter, and said, "Tell him no doubles." The interpreter-bench warmer shouted something. Life is amazing in the bushes.

Rhodes and his wife, Sharon, also a native of Louisville, live in a two-room apartment in Kingsport. They pay $160 a month. Sharon works in a department store in Bristol, 20 miles away, and when asked how she likes life in a rookie league, she said, brightly, "It's only for two and one half months."

In the last of the ninth inning, Elizabethon put a man on first base with one out. Kingsport led 4–3. The next hitter doubled, and Rhodes was in trouble with men on second and third.

"That's two," Hassell screamed at Rhodes when the left hander threw two strikes to the hitter. "Gut up out there, Rhodes."

Rhodes came sidearm and the hitter took a called third strike. Two out. The next man, on the third pitch, sent a tall flyball to right field. As it dropped into the right fielder's glove, Rick Rhodes leaped in the air, celebrating.

It was his fourth victory, the most on the pitching staff. "Helluva game," Hassell said. Rhodes took congratulations from his teammates and then walked toward the team's elderly bus. He stopped by the soft-drink machine. "Anybody got two quarters for a half-dollar?" he said.

TENNIS

ORANTES'S TRIUMPH: PORTRAIT OF ECSTASY

By Barry Lorge

From The Washington Post
Copyright, ©, 1975, The Washington Post

It should be forever frozen as the definitive portrait of ecstasy, the joyous expression that flashed across Manuel Orantes's face moments after his last forehand whizzed past Jimmy Connors this afternoon, giving him the men's singles title of the U.S. Open tennis championships.

As a crowd of 15,669 roared and chanted its approval, Orantes —a softspoken twenty-six-year-old son of a Barcelona optician— lobbed and softballed, drop shotted and passed Connors repeatedly in a stunning upset, 6–4, 6–3, 6–3, to complete one of the most remarkable triumphs in the 95 years of the U.S. national championships.

Orantes was seeded third but had been given little chance to beat the twenty-three-year-old defending champion and No. 1 seed, especially after Orantes's emotionally and physically draining semifinal victory Saturday night over second-seeded Guillermo Vilas of Argentina.

In that match, the Spaniard with the elegant left-handed strokes had resurrected himself from 0–5 and five match points against him in the fourth set to win, 4–6, 1–6, 6–2, 7–5, 6–4.

The semi-final did not end until 10:30 P.M. By the time Orantes had dressed, eaten dinner, called a plumber to fix a leaking faucet in his hotel bathroom, and gotten to bed, it was 3 A.M. But now that he has overcome a chronic back ailment, he considers himself generally resilient—and he proved it by outclassing Connors with a strategy reminiscent of that Arthur Ashe used to upset the left hander in the final at Wimbledon in July.

The 5-foot-10, 160-pound Orantes is the first Spaniard to win the

U.S. title since Manuel (Manolo) Santana in 1965. "Santana was here earlier in the week, and I talked with him," the champion said. "He was my idol. When I was a junior, he called me 'Manolito— 'Little Manolo.' "

Orantes's victories in his last two matches provided an artful and emotion-charged conclusion for the first U.S. Open played on Har-Tru, the slow claylike synthetic surface that has replaced grass at the West Side Tennis Club.

Historians had to go back to 1927 to find a more amazing final two rounds in one of the traditional grand-slam tournaments. That year, Henri Cochet of France rallied from two sets and 0–5 down in the third to beat Bill Tilden in the semi-finals at Wimbledon, then again rallied from a two-set deficit to beat countryman Jean Borotra in the final.

Orantes has won 22 of 23 matches and eight tournaments this year. In the last five months he has won the German, Swedish, and Canadian opens, and the British and U.S. clay court titles. This was his first grand-slam title; he was runner-up to Bjorn Borg in the 1974 French Open after winning the first two sets of the final.

Connors, who won the Australian Open, Wimbledon, and U.S. Open crowns last year, finished as runner-up in all three events this year. John Newcombe dethroned him at Melbourne on New Year's Day, and Ashe did likewise at Wimbledon.

Connors already is scheduled to play another of his ballyhooed "Heavyweight Championship of Tennis" challenge matches at Las Vegas next February 28, but he now must be considered a somewhat diminished attraction. Orantes was asked if he would consider being the as-yet-unnamed challenger.

"I think now," he grinned, "he has to challenge me."

Connors did win one title today, teaming with Ilie Nastase to take the men's doubles over Tom Okker and Marty Riessen, 6–4, 7–6.

Margaret Court and Virginia Wade won the women's doubles for the second time with a 7–5, 2–6, 7–6 thriller over Billie Jean King and Rosemary Casals. King, who did not play singles this year as Chris Evert won the title, also was a runner-up in the mixed doubles as she and Fred Stolle were beaten by Casals and Dick Stockton, 6–3, 6–3, 6–3.

Orantes won $25,000 for his victory today.

Orantes had beaten Connors only once in seven previous meetings. But he had definite ideas about how to play the relentlessly aggressive "Brash Basher of Belleville."

"He is very fast and goes for the shots all the time," Orantes said. "He takes the ball very early and hits so hard, I said to myself, 'If

I give him the speed, he's going to kill me.' So I was trying to give him soft balls so that he had to do everything himself, make his own power. That's the way I planned it. . . .

"There is no way you can try to play him the way he plays. If you hit hard to him, he hits back so hard you don't have time to get in position, so I was slowing down, slowing down all the time. It is very difficult to play him stroke for stroke, because that way he takes advantage of your strength."

Like Ashe at Wimbledon, Orantes not only knew how he wanted to play Connors, but executed his plan perfectly. He stayed in the backcourt instead of coming in for slashing volleys and overheads as he had against Vilas. He drew Connors in with dropshots, and drowned him in a rain of topspin lobs. His passing shots were extremely effective, both down the line and cross-court, which surprised Connors.

Charging the net as frequently as possible, as he always does, the top-ranked American was frequently caught leaning to cover a cross-court shot, only to find Orantes passing him cleanly down the line.

"I think somebody told him that I pass all the time cross-court," Orantes said. "He was looking always for that, so from the beginning I was hitting down the line." Orantes's forehands were especially difficult for Connors, who has a slightly restricted reach on his backhand because he hits it with both hands.

Orantes said he was tired when he awoke at 11 A.M. after his long Saturday night—though even the deluge in his room when he tried to draw a bath before going to bed couldn't dampen his spirits after his victory over Vilas.

"I hit for 10 minutes when I came to the club, and I felt fine," he said. It didn't matter to him that "experts" were saying he had no chance to stand up to Connors's power just 16 hours after his marathon with Vilas. He recalled saving those five match points—three on his serve at 0–5 in the fourth, two on Vilas's serve at 1–5.

Reliving that fourth set in the semi-final, he admitted, "I thought my chances were none, but I kept trying to see what would happen. I said before that to win a big championship you have to play well and be lucky, too. I was very lucky."

Against Connors, he was more good than lucky. He lost his serve in the first game of the match and fell behind 0–2, then won four consecutive games to go 4–2. Connors drew even at 4–4, but Orantes held and broke Connors on his second set point with a brilliant forehand down the line.

The crowd that jammed the ancient concrete horseshoe stadium was vocal, involved, and all for Orantes. As pockets of Latin spectators chanted in Spanish, Orantes jumped to a 3–1 lead in the second set, then lost his serve from 40–0 in the fifth game.

On his second break point, Connors put away a twisting overhead smash off a second lob over his right shoulder. It was a great shot and Orantes smiled, as he always does throughout a match, and acknowledged it.

But the nimble Orantes continued to stroke away, mixing his shots and never giving Connors the pace he prefers. Orantes broke through again in the eighth game, floating another winning topspin lob at 15–40. Connors, caught in the forecourt, could only turn and watch as it landed on the baseline.

Other than his entourage—mother Gloria, manager Bill Riordan and wife, doubles partner and friend Nastase and wife, coach Pancho Segura and son—Connors seemed to have only a handful of fans pulling for him. But one woman in a courtside box was particularly vocal. "Come on, Jimmy," she bellowed as Orantes went out to serve for the set.

"I'm coming, baby, don't worry," Connors retorted, but from 30–30 he knocked a service return out and a forehand approach shot long to fall two sets down.

Connors lost his serve in the first game of the third set, after yet another winning lob got Orantes to 30–40, and during that game he gave the butt end of his racket to the crowd in the rudest of the obscene gestures for which he is noted. Orantes held his serve with an ace for 2–0, won the first point of the next game, then suddenly lost 13 points in a row.

Connors was suddenly more savage and accurate with the approach shots that he had been missing with maddening frequency, and exploded outright winners from the backcourt. When he got to 3–2, 0–15 on Orantes's serve, it seemed that a reversal was still possible. After Orantes-over-Vilas, wasn't anything possible?

But from 30–40, Connors made three bad errors—netting a forehand return, banging a cross-court backhand long, popping another forehand approach beyond the baseline. The tide was stemmed, and Orantes went on to get the crucial break in the next game.

He shoved Connors to 15–40 with a hard forehand, cross-court this time, that forced a lunging forehand volley error. The break came on a thrilling exchange, Connors at the net furiously punching volleys, Orantes absorbing them in the backcourt and firing back passing attempts. The agile Spaniard finally won the duel, passing Connors cleanly with another forehand, a perfect preview of the eventual match point, that scattered dust inches inside the sideline.

For the first time, Orantes allowed himself to applaud one of his own shots. His fist came up as he willed the ball in, and he smiled broadly with self-satisfaction. He wiped his palm on the yellow towel he kept in his shorts, over his left hip, and looked for the first time as if he was sure he was going to win.

BASEBALL

ALL NEW ENGLAND FEELS FEVERISH

By Thomas Boswell

From The Washington Post
Copyright, ©, 1975, The Washington Post

Red Sox fever broke the thermometer this weekend. More than 50,000 Boston maniacs mobbed scorching Fenway Park for two days to sit in a human barbecue pit where the temperature never dipped below 98.6.

"Get your cup of water here," cried the vendors as the mercury bubbled between 99 and 104. "Only 35 cents."

The lukewarm water in paper cups sold better than soft drinks. At least the water could be poured on the head.

The scene under the bleachers of the Fens was perhaps the most unimpeachable testimony to the torrid irrational love affair now going on between the first-place Sox and all of New England.

The caverns under the stands looked like a prison scene from *Les Miserables.* From 3,000 to 4,000 people at a time fled the burning bleachers to collapse under the stands between innings, lying on the concrete or standing in lines 40 long to suck a little water from fountains whose pressure had dropped to almost nothing.

A brace of galley slaves in full chain could have been driven with whips through the sweaty, bare-chested baseball mob with hardly an eyebrow raised.

Many of the folded and fried fans who had arrived two hours early after long drives from points all over Maine, Connecticut, Vermont, New Hampshire, Rhode Island, and western Massachusetts, only left their shady underworld to dash up the ramps into the stands when the Sox got men on base.

The bleachers seemed to breathe, inhaling and exhaling thousands of human specks, as Boston threatened to score or made the last out of an inning.

Even the Red Sox organization can no longer grasp the hold it has on the public mind. "I think these people have gone crazy," said the Sox' public relations director, Bill Crowley, whose job is not to say such heretical things. "Why don't they stay home and watch it on TV in some sort of comfort?

"Here we're in the bottom of the eighth [Saturday], five runs ahead and nobody's left the park. They're all chanting, 'We want a hit.' If that old Chicago writer Warren Brown were here, he'd just look at these screaming kids and growl, '5,000 more good reasons for birth control.' "

The Sox' rampaging attendance, which ticket manager Arthur Moscato says "should easily go over 1,800,000" to give Boston the lead in American League attendance for the sixth time in eight years, is hardly a youth movement. In New England adults are the rabid fans.

"I drove three and one half hours from Albany, N.Y.," rumbled an almost furious Bob Hipwell, standing at the Sox ticket window, "and you say you don't have my tickets."

"Please, sir. Please," begged the seller. "We'll get this straight."

"I don't mind driving all day. I don't mind the temperature being 100. Not if I can see the Red Sox," said the middle-aged Hipwell. "But I do get mad when they chase me out of my seats."

The Sox do their darndest to foment such devotion. Boston now televises 95 of its games on a 73-outlet cable-TV system that reaches all of New England and parts of Canada. The independent UHF channel has a new slogan ("Keep Your Sox On") and the envy of large stations.

"We're killing CBS, NBC, and ABC all over New England," claimed the station's sports director, Bill Flynn. "One Saturday last month 63 percent of the people who had their TVs on were watching this silly game."

Bostonians are already acting like midseason 1975 is late September 1967, when the Impossible Dream came to pass. After a successful road trip, a crowd of several hundred fans greeted the Red Sox at the Boston airport last week in the middle of the night. "This is only July," laughed flattered manager Darrell Johnson.

Already forgiven is the Sox collapse of last year, when a seven-game lead on August 23 turned into a sour seven-games-behind third-place finish in October.

In the bars around Fenway Park there is little of that big city cynicism one hears in New York. "They won't blow it again," said Waltham policeman Joe Piacentino, who once signed a minor-league contract with the Detroit Tigers the same day as Al Kaline.

"This year the Sox will win with Rice and Lynn."

Without a doubt Jim Rice and Fred Lynn, the two Red Sox super rookies, are the reason Boston's normal midsummer low-grade fever has turned into an epidemic. "They ought to give a dual rookie of the year award," said Piacentino's fellow officer, Don Waidy, as the two sipped a beer in Gemelli's, a tavern on Jersey Street with a giant Red Sox cap for a front awning. "People are excited 'cause they know that pair is going to be batting fourth and fifth for the next dozen years."

Gemelli's is really more a Red Sox shrine than a bar. Life-size color photos of players cover the walls. Every gizmo seems to be made from a bat, ball, or glove. Who should the guy at the bar next to Piacentino be but Stan Sohaski, a Sox third-base coach in the 1950s. (Sohaski, still a fan, often follows the club on the road simply to root.)

"The fans here are like nowhere else," said Carl Yastrzemski, the man who revived Boston's baseball madness when he played better than mortals should in the closing weeks of 1967 to produce Boston's first (and only) pennant since 1946. "My father lives in Prescott, Maine, and he asks me for 10 tickets to nearly every game for people who are glad to drive seven hours to get here."

"I'm hearing from people I haven't heard from since 1967," said ticket manager Moscato, "They say, 'I haven't bothered you for a couple of years.' I tell 'em, 'Well don't bother me now.' "

One college-age worker in Moscato's office rediscovered an uncle that the family feared might have met with foul play in some remote region of the earth, he had remained silent so long. The uncle surfaced to ask for tickets to Monday's and Tuesday's big two-game series with the Baltimore Orioles, the Red Sox' closest challengers, nine and one half games behind.

Moscato is ready for the shenanigans of a stretch drive. "I've polished off my, 'Too bad, the early bird gets the worm' line," he said. "And we've taken down the cranes that the kids used to climb up to the top of the left-field wall. This all makes my job simple. When the team's going good, it's easy to sell the bad seats."

When Fenway opens each day it is as clean as a living room with its blood red and deep blue seats, its freshly painted monster wall, and its manicured grass. "Fans feel comfortable here," said Flynn. "Shea Stadium in New York is a zoo. Here, if you cause trouble, you're out and in jail before you know it."

FOOTBALL

TRYING OUT FOR THE JETS

By Mark Jacobson

From New York
Copyright, ©, 1975, by the NYM Corp.
Reprinted with permission of *New York* Magazine

On the Greyhound up from North Carolina, Luther Carter, Jr.'s, palms were sweating so badly they almost rubbed the print off his return-trip ticket. Luther had read all about it in the Charlotte *Observer.* About how Broadway Joe was "seriously considering" a $4 million offer to play with Chicago in the resurgent World Football League. And how with Namath gone, the New York Jets would be hard-up for a winning quarterback. Fourteen hours on a bus gives a man plenty of time to think, and to Luther Carter the logic was irrefutable, as simple as "find a need and fill it." Hadn't he been All-Conference three years in a row at Johnson C. Smith University? Couldn't he throw a football 60 yards, like a rope? It didn't matter that Johnson C. Smith was a small black school with a poor team. Wasn't Johnny Unitas a $35-a-week semi-pro player before the Baltimore Colts gave him a try some twenty years ago? Anyhow, just suppose Namath decides to stay. How many more years can those gimp legs carry him? These were all questions with hopeful answers, Luther Carter thought. And to him the idea of playing with the big boys, even taking the place of Broadway Joe, the symbol of an age, the most famous athlete this side of Muhammad Ali, didn't seem so crazy. Still, by the time Luther reached his grandmother's house in Harlem, he was so nervous he had a hard time downing her best chicken and ribs.

Hempstead, Long Island, is a strange place to put the fantasy of a lifetime on the line. Out here, even the Golden Arches look limp. But today the suburban strip of gas stations and tract houses leading to Hofstra University, where the Jets hold their annual "free agent" tryout, is a ribbon of dreams. The hopefuls come from all over, paying their own way, looking to latch on to glory. There are pig farmers from Iowa with orange hair and aggressive hands; Kansas City schoolteachers who know the down-and-out verbatim; quarter-back-eaters from Arizona who go to 6-foot-4, 245, and still think they're too small; car repossessors from Philadelphia who claim to kick field goals, and a violin-playing golden boy from Flushing who'd rather be a free safety. Most played ball for their colleges and felt cheated by the draft, but in the crowd are semi-pros, nonpros, and a few guys who lost their shirts last year in the WFL. There is even a reporter—me—6 feet, 187, who once ran track for his high school, still reads Young, Roswell, Merchant, and Smith every day, and has fantasies of his own.

Last year the Jets had only 90 "free agents" at their tryout; now about 350 of us are getting into our sweat suits in Hofstra's Comet-clean locker room. Perhaps the depression makes dreams more urgent. Locker rooms are for boisterous macho, talking "locker-room talk" and spilling RC colas on each other. But there's no horseplay here. Free agents don't have any team spirit; they know they're on their own. Almost everyone is in super shape, not an armchair beer belly in the room. It's easy to tell which bodies go with what positions. The tight, close-together bums of the running backs and receivers protrude haughtily from the back ends of their jockstraps. Linebackers' rears droop a little, but that's allowed, provided the tops of their torsos are like triangular rocks. Every calf is full of ripples, every forearm a potential hammer. It's intimidating; you figure these guys aren't even being paid to keep taut like this. Obsessive health makes me guilty, so I gravitate toward the kickers. All kickers do is swing their legs—many of them have never made a tackle in their lives. They have puffy arms, soft tummies. Jeffy Gambaradella, who says he's "a crazy hippie house painter from Boston," even has pimples.

As more hopefuls arrive, the air becomes heavy with braggadocio and anxious BO. Ronald Thompson is waving his catcher's-mitt hands above his head and howling like an unfriendly coyote. "I'm 6-foot-5, 265, and I'm mean and mellow. I hear the Jets are looking for defensive ends. That means they're looking for me . . . ooo-eeeee!" (Actually the Jets just traded for Billy Newsome, a hard case from New Orleans, and are not particularly looking for defensive ends.) Ronald says he once tore up the Astroturf for Eastern New Mexico University, but hasn't been able to find a handle since. A few weeks ago he was down for the Redskins tryout and was "the mean-est, hard-hittingest mother in the camp," but George Allen, the

Skins' coach, "only looks for vets and they didn't even give me a chance to get out and hit." Just in case things don't work out here, Ronald's thinking of talking to the Giants, who he's positive need defensive ends. If they don't, there's always the meat-packing plant in New Haven.

Down the stained bench is Gregory Norman. Gregory, about twenty-one, didn't knock any heads in college. He got his football experience playing basketball in Bed-Stuy. A would-be defensive back, Gregory says he's 5-foot-11, 180, but since he's four inches shorter than me and much slighter, 5-foot-8, 155, seems closer to the truth. Figures like that make him virtually useless to a pro team. Besides, the pros aren't interested in any kid without college coaching. "I'm the Ed Bell type," Gregory says, referring to the Jets' mini pass-catcher. Then he asks me if I could talk to coach Winner for him because "they got to take me, they just got to take me."

Charley Winner says everyone should just be patient and they'll get their chance. Some people snickered last year when Charley was appointed Jet head coach by his father-in-law, the team's patriarch, Weeb Ewbank. The critics got progressively nastier as the Jets lost seven of their first eight games, but Charley shut them all up when, led by Broadway Joe, the team won its last six games. Today none of the 343 true believers in the Hofstra wrestling room are snickering at Charley Winner; they all hope they'll do something to catch his eye. "I wish I could have had the chance you're going to get today," Charley says in his flat voice. "I was always too small, but if you're big enough and fast enough to play ball in this league, you'll get a contract." Then he goes into the Johnny Unitas story. The few in the cavernous gym who haven't heard it gasp, and the room is full of naked ambition.

Charley says all he's looking for today are "athletes." There will be no pads, no tackling, no animal scenes. First you'll run the 40-yard dash, and then, if you make that, you go work out with an assistant coach who'll test your skills at your position. I'm on the 40 line with the running backs, and it's like a lawn party. Everyone's talking about how the Jets might not sign Anthony Davis, the USC star who is their second draft pick. The rumor is that Davis would rather play baseball if Broadway Joe isn't going to be around to tuck the ball into his belly. It's a good rumor; another opening, another chance. The question is, "What time do they want?" The answer comes back: "4.5's and 4.6's for guys without significant size, 4.7's for power runners." It may be just another rumor, but immediately everyone becomes a power runner. "Damn," says Richie, a twenty-two-year-old wrestler from Illinois, "I do 4.5's on the cinder track back in Springfield all the time; this is going to be a piece of cake. Piece of cake!" He runs his first heat and does 4.8. Second is another 4.8. Close, but no cigar.

The 40 is a mean race. If you don't get off the line quick, don't even bother to show up for the finish. Hundred-yard-dash swifties don't always score in the 40; it's a race you've got to muscle, a race you've got to take by the throat. First time out I blasted off the line, looked good, but didn't get to stretch out until well past the finish; hit 5.2 and felt satisfied that my body wasn't a lump of scrap. Next time, though, it was sad. Probably didn't even leave the go position for two seconds and lumbered across in turtle time, 5.6. Assistant coach Ken Shipp, a humorless man with a southern accent who wears Ban-Lon shirts, pronounced my death: "Boy, speed-wise, you ain't got what it takes to make this team." He must have said that same phrase a hundred times during the day. Didn't even get started and I was gone. It was like the chorus girl who gets told, "Thank you" at the open call before she gets a chance to go into her dance.

After my second heat I looked up and the field was half empty. Most of my locker-room cronies were heading for the Long Island Rail Road. Gregory Norman did the best 40 he ever did in his life, a 4.7, but it still wasn't good enough. Ronald Thompson is raging around making holes in the turf with his size fourteens. He did 5.1's in the 40, not bad for a man his size, but his 10-yard (a reflex test for linemen) was bad news. "All I got was a goddamn look-see; if they let me hit somebody, then they'll look-see something," he says with malice. Jeffy Gambaradella got three chances to punt the ball; two went off the side of his foot, and the one that traveled far didn't have the hang-time (time remaining in the air that enables proper downfield coverage to develop). All Jeffy said was, "Three hundred miles is a long way to come and kick crappy."

What started like a groove is turning to desperation. "If you're so good, why aren't you playing with some other pro team?" Charley Winner is saying to James Mathias, a twenty-two-year-old running back from Tennessee. Mathias says he was "terr-i-ble" in semi-pro last year, but only ran 4.8's this morning. "I got recommendations from my coach and even the president of my junior college . . . just give me one more chance. I know I can play," James pleads. "Nothing I can do for you right now, son," Charley says matter-of-factly. "But listen," James says, "all I been thinking for 10 years is football. I worked hard; it's not my fault I didn't go to a big college. I ran for 7.2 yards a carry in semi-pro last year, and where am I going to go now? I got nowhere to go." "I'm sorry, son," Charley says in his best Robert Young voice, "put yourself in my shoes." "Yeah,"

James sneers and walks away, pausing to turn around and say, "I'll be back, you'll see." "He'll cool off," Charley says. "You know, I'm glad people like that come out for these things. I really am. Because if they didn't, they would always think, 'If I'd only had my chance I could have made it.' This way they come out and find out the truth: 'I wasn't big enough. I wasn't fast enough.' It's better than living with an illusion."

Meanwhile, Luther Carter has a chance. The morning heats are over and a big knot of people have gathered around where Luther and the other QB's are pitching hooks and curls to the receivers who survived the 40's. Everyone is scratching his chin and grunting at the good passes. They know the quarterback is the nerve center of the team, the man who makes it happen, the hero. And this is no ordinary quarterback spot to fill; this is the great Broadway Joe's slot. Suddenly these guys sailing the down-and-outs are more than a bunch of dreaming free agents. Matt Snell, the great runner who, along with Broadway Joe, led the Jets to the shock they've never quite recovered from, the 1969 Super Bowl win, is also on hand. "Who knows," Matt says, "maybe the answer is here. The Jets got to stop depending on Joe. He can't do everything forever. Hell, even God died once." Mr. Shipp, the quarterback coach, is in charge. He's looking for "a good setup, quick release, gun arm." He watches each quarterback drop back and fire, then he rates them on his clipboard. Almost everyone has a line of "P's" (for poor) next to his name. There are a couple of "Avg's." Luther Carter has an "OK."

Luther's got what they need: he's better than six feet tall and can see over the paws of the behemoth linemen who'd try to mangle him in the NFL. He can throw long bombs and short bullets. He's got unscarred, twenty-one-year-old knees that can take him out of the pocket when things get hot back there. And Luther's got more. He's a "leader of men." Last night his stomach was going crazy, but this morning he woke up serene and confident. You could see, back in the locker room, that he had a special bearing, a certain athletic sense that tells him which players need to be coddled and which ones should be screamed at. Luther says, "I just like to know who I'm working with." Now he's quietly pulling the receivers aside to correct them on their patterns, showing them a better way. No one knows who he is, but they're listening.

Also dropping back 10 and pumping is Frank DiMaggio. Frank isn't "talking it up" like Luther; for him, the pressure's too great for that. Frank DiMaggio's youth is on the line. Last year Frank played for the WFL's Philadelphia Bell. The Bell started off like a house afire and drew 65,000 people to see their first home game. Later it was announced that the Bell management had "papered" the attendance figures with free admissions, and the paid totals were more like 7,000. Things went downhill from there. The Bell still owes Frank DiMaggio about $10,000. The Bell may be back in business next year if Broadway Joe decides to save the league, but Frank DiMaggio probably won't be there. Today's tryout could be Frank's last gasp as a football player before becoming a full-time insurance agent. It will be painful because Frank's got heritage. "My thing . . . is," he says, "to bring the name of DiMaggio back to New York. I'm Joe's third cousin, you know. That's why I got number five on my jersey. He knows about me. And if I make it here today, we're going to get together. I'd really like that." Frank's in trouble though. Mr. Shipp thinks he sets up sloppy.

Shipp makes short work of those "who can't cut it," and by the time Charley Winner comes over only a few are left. The atmosphere is charged, like before a fight when you know something's got to give, someone's got to go. After throwing more than 500 passes, Luther's getting tired. His spiral's getting flabby, his buttonhook flat. But Burt Cornash, a tall kid from Jersey, has been saving him with some incredible diving catches. People are whispering that Burt's "a young Barkum" (meaning Jerome Barkum, a classy Jet receiver). You can see that Burt wants it badly; he's sweating torrents through his corn rows. On his next "fly pattern," Luther uncorks a monster, maybe 60 yards, prodigious but way beyond the prescribed pattern. Nevertheless, Burt manages to get under it and makes the nab, tumbling like a stunt man in a kung fu movie. Back at the huddle, Luther slaps Burt on the butt and says, "Beautiful, homeboy, beautiful." Burt looks over to Winner and Shipp, who are laughing about something. It's apparent they didn't see his catch. Burt says, "Yeah, beautiful, but now it's nothing."

Moments later, Charley Winner calls for the ball. He reads off a few names and tells those called to meet him at the Jets headquarters (named Weeb Ewbank Hall in keeping with the academic surroundings). Luther Carter is called. Frank DiMaggio and Burt Cornash are told "Thank you for coming." Burt kicks the dirt. Frank stares at the sky for a few minutes and says, "Life is funky."

Luther is bouncing on the balls of his feet, calling everyone "homeboy," and smiling like his mouth is going to bust. A pudgy Jet assistant puts him on a scale to be weighed. "Wow," Luther says, "I didn't expect that in a million years, I didn't expect nothing." Someone says that most of the guys who showed up probably did expect something. Luther says, "Really? That's sad, man. That's real sad." Then the Jet man pushes him against the wall to be measured. Seven other guys are waiting for the same treatment. Out of 343, the Jets have offered contracts to eight.

In the Jets' "player personnel room," where the walls are covered with the name, height, and weight of every player in the league, it takes Luther about 25 seconds to sign a contract. The pact calls for a little more than the rookie minimum of $15,000 a year, not a bad starting salary for a business-administration major. It also entitles him to bang shoulder pads with the rest of the Jet rookies at Hofstra on July 15.

Fifteen thousand dollars is a long way from $4 million, and Charlotte is light-years from Broadway, but Luther's trying hard not to be too impressed. "Well," he says, going into a modified aw-shucks stance, "I hear old Joe was a country boy when he first started."

EDITOR'S NOTE:

A brief announcement appeared in *The New York Times* a week after this article was published to the effect that Luther Carter and four other unsigned Jet players had been dropped from the roster.

GENERAL

PLAY-BY-PLAY BEFORE ITS HEYDAY

By Hubert Mizell

From The Floridian
Copyright, ©, 1975, The St. Petersburg Times

Back when Howard Cosell was childishly humbling his way about the crowded avenues of Brooklyn and little Curt Gowdy was still riding Shetland ponies at the Wyoming State Fair, broadcasting of baseball games had already developed a handsome if somewhat bogus flair.

Home games were, as today, broadcast live from the major league, but when the 16 National and American League teams in pre-World War II times hit the road, it was something else.

Games were "re-created."

It was often masterful, at the same artistic plateau of such radio soap opera contemporaries as "Ma Perkins," "One Man's Family," and "Stella Dallas." Although based upon the sporting truth, baseball re-creations were sometimes embellished strictly through the imagination of the announcers.

It wasn't until New York Yankees owner Larry McPhail sent Mel Allen on the road in 1946 that a major-league team did "away" games on live radio. Before that, 99 percent of road broadcasts were done through re-creations.

Here's how it worked.

Let's suppose the Chicago White Sox were playing Boston in the late 1930s. Bob Elson, the Sox' venerable announcer, would have remained back in Chicago while his ball club traveled east.

The Red Sox take the field.

A Western Union operator in the Fenway Park press box begins to tap out dots and dashes on a Morse Code ticker. He watches the game live and sends coded messages to Chicago.

In Chicago, a second Western Union operator tunes his ears to the signals from Boston. He reads the dots and dashes as deftly as if someone was whispering in his ear and translates them into English on a typewriter.

Announcer Elson peers over his shoulder.

The descriptions from Fenway, or any major-league ball park, were extremely sketchy. It became a challenge to the re-creating announcer to transform such minimal reports into complete and hopefully exciting action broadcasts for listeners.

It might go like this:

Western Union report: Jones up, Bats L. Smith pitch. Throws r. 4–5, 2.98.

Announcer: First up for the White Sox will be Brad Jones, a .269 hitter with 12 homers and 34 RBIs. On the mound for Boston is Fred Smith, a big right hander with a 4 and 5 record and 2.98 earned run average.

Western Union: B1, Lo.

Announcer: The outfield is shaded to the right side for Jones, who can hit 'em a mile. Smith winds up, pumps, and delivers. It's a curveball, low and inside. Count of one and oh on Jones.

Western Union: S1, Foul.

Announcer: Jones digs in and taps his bat on the plate. Smith steps up on the rubber, wipes the perspiration from his brow, and begins his motion. It's a fastball and Jones fouls it back against the screen. The count is one ball and one strike.

Western Union: Out. Fly deep right. Johnson gets it.

Announcer: Jones steps out of the box and rubs his hands with a rosin bag. Smith does the same out behind the mound. Now Jones is back in the batter's box and we're ready to go. Smith pumps and pitches. Jones hits a line drive to deep right, Billy Johnson goes back near the warning track, reaches up, and spears it. What a catch by Johnson! The Fenway Park crowd is going wild. Man, how that Johnson just robbed our guy Jones!

That's the way it was. Take an extremely small amount of information and make it into a dramatic happening, taking whatever liberty was necessary to create realism and excitement for the listeners.

Many listeners never did catch on.

Not only in the major leagues, but throughout the then-vast minor leagues, the re-creation broadcasts of road games were as common as flannel uniforms and spiked shoes. At the major-league level, the Western Union ticker service from any of the 16 ball parks was for sale at $27.50 a game.

If you mention the term "re-creations" around baseball old-timers, you are almost certain to be tossed the name of a gutsy Texan who used the technique to build a financial empire.

Gordon McLendon's time, oddly, didn't come until after World War II, when most major-league teams had finally sent announcers on the road to provide live broadcasts of every game on the schedule. But what fascinated McLendon, a Dallas man, was that 50 percent of the United States west of St. Louis had no major-league baseball teams in the late 1940s.

The $27.50 Western Union price also fascinated him.

Lindsey Nelson, who has since developed into a national sports announcing figure and who currently does New York Mets games on television and radio, was hired by McLendon to come to Dallas and join a makeshift network that specialized in nationwide baseball re-creations on radio. Nelson had been doing minor-league games of the Class B Tri-State League in Knoxville, Tenn.

"McLendon was a Yale graduate who had a variety of talents including being a wartime interpreter in Japanese," Nelson said. "His dad bought Gordon a radio station in Palestine, Tex., and then got him KLIF in Dallas.

"McLendon was fascinated that so small an area, really only the northeastern corner of the country, had major-league baseball in the late forties," Nelson continued. "He came up with the idea of buying one $27.50 ticker-tape report a day from Western Union and turning it into a nationally broadcast game from our studios in Dallas.

"The Liberty Broadcasting System was born."

A Western Union operator named Jack Marshall received the signals for McLendon, Nelson, and Co. The Liberty network was soon alive not only with the highly embellished reports of major-league baseball games, but with sound effects and gimmicks that made it as realistic as most live broadcasts.

McLendon sent a sound man to each of the 15 major-league ball parks—the St. Louis Cardinals wouldn't cooperate with Liberty since they had a large network in the western United States. At each site, the various noises of the crowd and stadium were recorded for McLendon's use. So was the local rendition of The Star-Spangled Banner.

"When the Liberty network said the game was at Ebbetts Field in Brooklyn, you actually heard the famed Gladys Gooding playing the National Anthem at the Ebbetts Field organ," Nelson said this spring while recounting his days in the re-creation business.

McLendon, who called himself "The Old Scotchman," was actually only in his late twenties when he put the Liberty network into action. Soon, it moved out of Dallas when Oklahoma City bought the baseball re-creations for $10 a game.

"The young network mushroomed and there were over 300 stations involved after the first season," Nelson said. "McLendon offered the same deal to each station, $10-a-game fee with the station paying its own line charges. Add it up, 300 stations at $10—that's $3,000 a game for re-creations from a Western Union tape that cost McLendon $27.50."

Also on Liberty's staff was a young announcer named Jerry Doggett, who now has been a member of the Los Angeles Dodgers' radio-TV team with Vin Scully for about 20 years.

"To get sound effects, McLendon would go to any degree of creativity," Nelson said. "He decided to create the sound of a public address announcer in the background of the baseball broadcast, the way it would be in a live stadium.

"To achieve such an effect, McLendon needed an echo chamber. So, the young guy who was supposed to make the PA announcer sounds was sent to the radio station's men's room for each game. I might be doing the game while, in the background, this echoed voice would be saying, 'Welcome to Yankee Stadium and today's game. . . .'

"Our main worry was that somebody might miss the little sign that said the men's room was off limits during ball games. Anytime, we could have heard the sounds of a toilet flushing and we'd probably have to tell our listeners, 'The game is now being played in a downpour.' "

The sound effects included such gimmicks as rapping two sticks of wood together to create a "sound of the ball hitting the bat." Liberty's announcers might say, "There's a foul ball, fans, and it's coming right back toward our booth. . . ." Somebody would then bounce a baseball off a studio wall to create the sound of the ball "hitting the front of the press box."

There were several factors that killed McLendon's Liberty network after a few seasons. First, the Mutual network came on with its "Game of the Day," a true live broadcast from major-league parks, which was offered nationwide. Then, Liberty tried to go big dog, competing with the total broadcasting concept of NBC, CBS, and the other giants.

"We had soap operas, game shows, a staff orchestra, and the other things," Nelson said. "But, the expenses—mainly costs for telephone lines—ate the Liberty network alive. It finally went under."

Liberty was only a segment of the whole re-creation scene. Some of the more memorable happenings were in the minor leagues where sophisticated equipment and well-paid announcers were few.

Dick Stratton, who used to re-create Jacksonville Braves games in the old Class A South Atlantic League, recalls a humorous night when his embellishment of a game cost a player $25.

"Ben Geraghty, Jacksonville's fine and tough manager, had stayed off the road with the flu," Stratton says. "I was doing a game that was being played in Montgomery, Columbia, or someplace else. I suddenly noticed I'd fouled up . . . I had said there was one out when there were actually two.

"To correct my problem, I had a Jacksonville runner, a pitcher, picked off first base. Geraghty heard it on the radio and immediately fired off a telegram to the player, fining him $25 for being so dumb as to be picked off first base."

The minor leagues' use of re-creations was healthy until the 1960s when Western Union service waned and interest in baseball was generally satisfied by live broadcasts or telecasts of big-league games.

I recall seeing Dave Martin in 1962, re-creating games of the Jacksonville team, which by then had advanced to the Class AAA International League and changed its nickname to "Suns." Martin would strip down for action, sitting at a radio station control console bare from the waist up and without shoes or socks.

By then, tape cartridges were the thing. Martin had almost every baseball sound hidden someplace in his dozens of tape cassettes.

There was general background crowd noise and the constant rumble of people in the grandstand. Only problem was that, around the sixth inning of every re-creation broadcast, the same voice would say, "Cold beeeer. Get your cold beer right here." In the eighth inning, the same bellow each night would say, "Get that bum outta there. . . ."

Martin, as did most of his counterparts, had tapes for loud crowd noises, to be used when a player hit a home run. He also had triple noises, double noises, single noises, and wild-pitch noises. One tape provided the crack of the bat hitting a ball. He had another with a booing mob.

Long before the McLendons, Strattons, or Martins got into the business of re-creating baseball games, a variety of characters did road games in the major leagues. Their personalities and styles were as different as Jean Harlow and Ma Kettle.

"I never believed in fooling anybody," says Red Barber, now retired and writing books in Tallahassee after a fabled career as broadcaster for the Dodgers and Yankees. "I never pretended. On re-creations, I told my New York audience that I was in a Western Union office, looking over the shoulder of an operator who was getting reports from whatever ball park the Dodgers were playing in that particular day."

Sounds of the Western Union Morse ticker and the operator's typewriter were plainly heard over Barber's station. "If our machine went out, we just said so," Barber says. "We didn't have to make up stories about it raining or any other such nonsense."

There was a mild problem about the Western Union ticker sounds being heard over the radio. It was not uncommon for old Western Union operators to sit in saloons and listen to baseball re-creations. They would know what happened before the announcer said it, having "read" the dots and dashes coming over the ticker. A guy might bet a fellow bar-sitter that the next batter would hit a home run, fully knowing from the ticker noise that it was a sure thing.

Barber's heyday began in 1939. For the five previous seasons, there had been a ban on all broadcasting of New York baseball. Ed Barrow, owner of the Yankees, talked the Giants and Dodgers into the idea. "We refuse to give our product away," Barrow said.

"Larry McPhail took over the Dodgers in 1939 and refused to go along," Barber recalls. "That soon broke up the ban and baseball broadcasts resumed in New York."

Baseball owners were extremely powerful in those days. Players were at their mercy, so were fans. Sam Bradon, owner of the Gashouse Gang of St. Louis, banned radio broadcasts in 1934, which happened to become the most famous season in the Cardinals' history with Dizzy and Paul Dean, Joe Medwick, Leo Durocher, and the others.

As for re-creations prior to the 1934 St. Louis ban, an announcer named Thomas Patrick Convey did the Cardinals' games. The Western Union reports came into the Chase Hotel and Convey invited an audience of 50 to 100 fans. As he did the Cards' road games, the studio audience cheered, booed, and yelled. Convey's sponsors distributed ice cream, Cokes, and other goodies to add to the ball park atmosphere.

Jack Buck, the modern Cardinals' broadcasting voice, did re-creations beginning in 1950. His first job was with the Columbus, Ohio, team in the Class AAA minor leagues. "I auditioned for the job and the Columbus team's owner, Hal Bannister, knew that half my games would be re-creations," Buck says. "He put me in his office chair, turned on the intercom system, and went to an adjacent office. Bannister gave me the play-by-play report from the previous World

Series and made me do an entire game, making up everything as I went. Whatever, it got me the job."

Buck had a personal rule involving re-creations. "I would never mention how the weather was," he said. "There was always a chance the Western Union machine might get unplugged or something. I would suddenly have to tell the audience that it was raining at the ball park where Columbus was playing."

Professional radio men weren't the only ones re-creating games in that now-disappeared era. Back in the 1920s, a newspaper makeup man named Tommy Jenkins would get the play-by-play reports off the United Press wire in Jacksonville and relay them to a crowd gathered in front of the *Florida Times-Union* building. He used a megaphone and mainly worked World Series games.

In Tampa, a one-time pitcher for the Tampa Smokers did games in Spanish for workers at cigar factories. Manny Lopez, now vice-president of the Flagship Bank of Tampa, worked from a radio repair shop called Radio Center on Fifteenth Street.

"We were hooked up to six cigar factories for the World Series games," he said. "I listened to the live broadcasts in English. Had earphones on my head. I would then give reports in Spanish, which went over PA systems at the six factories. That was just after World War II and most cigar workers were old-timers and many didn't speak any English."

Dave Rush, a retired Western Union operator, did thousands of games from Chicago's ball parks. Now a St. Petersburg resident, Rush tells an amusing story of how Western Union was barred from the Cleveland ball park in 1873 because "they thought the publicity would be injurious to the game." Rush says, "Western Union rigged up a wire in the upper branches of a tree just outside the outfield wall at the Cleveland park. The operator squirreled up there and copied scores every half-inning from the stadium scoreboard, transmitting to a regional Western office for distribution to the entire nation."

One announcer who bought Western Union reports from Rush was a young Des Moines sportscaster named Ronald Reagan. "Although most Western Union reports were skimpy, I tried to dress up the background stuff over the wire," Rush says. "I was barnstorming with the Cubs after spring training in California and was providing ticker reports back to Chicago for broadcast by the late Pat Flanagan over WBBM. I described some ball park in Texas, telling of the Indians, cowgirls, and cowboys on hand. It was 1941 and I gave him anything that caught my eye."

Perhaps the most colorful, most creative, and most illegitimate of major-league radio re-creators was Albert K. "Rosy" Rowswell, who did the Pittsburgh Pirates' games until the Bucs' current announcer, Bob Prince, took over in the mid-1950s. Rowswell was at his nutty best when the Pirates were on the road, giving Rosy a chance to try his crazy stunts that became legend with Pittsburgh listeners over station WWSW.

"Rosy didn't use crowd noises, just two microphones at a desk," says Prince, who was Rowswell's assistant at the time. "He didn't believe in the usual sound effects. You could hear the Western Union ticker over the air."

Rowswell became famous for his own set of sayings. He always called a strikeout a "Dipsy Doodle." When Pirate followers heard Rosy say it was a "Doozey Marooney," they knew a Pittsburgh player had just slammed an extra-base hit.

The Pirates were lousy in the late 1940s, except for a home-run slugger named Ralph Kiner who now lives on Snell Isle in St. Petersburg. Kiner was just this year named to the Baseball Hall of Fame and is now a broadcaster himself, on the Mets' announcing team with Nelson and Bob Murphy.

Every time Kiner would hit a home run, Rowswell would shout to his radio audience, "Raise the window, Aunt Minnie, here comes another one!"

About that time, Prince would be standing in the studio with a bus boys' tray loaded with nuts, bolts, ball bearings, cowbells, and broken glass. On Rosy's signal, Prince would dump it on the floor to make an incredible noise.

Rowswell would then say, "She never made it, she tripped over the garden hose," to indicate his mythical Aunt Minnie couldn't get the window raised before Kiner's home run busted the pane.

Honest truth, folks. There was a time. . . .

"Rosy used to say the bases are F-O-B," Prince said. "That meant, to all his listeners, that the bases were Full of Bucs. If you listened to Pirate games, you knew. There I was, a dropout from the Harvard Law School, throwing trays filled with garbage to a radio station floor."

People attempted to talk Rowswell into doing games Gordon McLendon style, complete with sophisticated sound effects. He refused to the end. He had his own style and refused to budge.

"Although we never knew what the pitches were, we'd say they were fastballs, curves, sliders, etc." Prince said. "One day I got so damned excited that I said something over the air that I just knew would cost me my job.

"Whitey Lockman of the Giants, I found out from the Western

Union operator, had just hit a homer to beat us in a game at New York. I yelled out over the microphone, 'That son of a bitch just hit a grand-slam homer.'

"Rowswell was taking it easy that inning, snoozing on a couch in the studio. He came up with an instant excuse. He told the listeners, 'We have some painters working in the studio today and you'll have to excuse their language.' It worked. I didn't get fired."

For a variety of reasons, most of them obvious, baseball re-creations have almost disappeared. Even in the minor leagues, they are rare due to prohibitive costs and the fading of such service by Western Union.

But, while it lasted, it made life interesting.

FOOTBALL

SWARTHMORE FINALLY HAS CHAMPAGNE

By Frank Dolson

From the Philadelphia Inquirer
Copyright, ©, 1975, Philadelphia Inquirer

Widener College's unbeaten football team was on the way home after beating Ursinus on Saturday when the shocking news was first reported.

"One of the kids said, 'Hey, big upset. Swarthmore beat Muhlenberg,'" Widener coach Bill Manlove said. "'Yeah,' I told him, 'and the moon's green. . . .' I thought there was no way Swarthmore could beat Muhlenberg. . . ."

But there WAS a way. Swarthmore, beaten 34 in a row, scored 16 points; Muhlenberg, stopped an inch or so from the goal line in the final minute, scored only 12. "That HAD to be the biggest news in the area," Bill Manlove said.

And to the 30 or so young men who play football for Swarthmore, that HAD to be an unforgettable experience. There will be bigger football games played this season. But not even Ohio State-Michigan or Oklahoma-Nebraska or USC-UCLA will produce happier, more emotionally drained winners than the members of this Swarthmore team. . . .

A new week had started, but the memory lingered on. Especially in room 282 in Roberts Hall, where Bruce Leinberger and Bill Wheatley—two of the three seniors on the 1975 Swarthmore football team—live.

The game ball was there. It would take an act of Congress to get that battered-looking football away from Bruce Leinberger. And two jagged pieces of the goalpost that once stood on Clothier Field were there.

And, above all, the thrill of victory was there. A victory so long coming it must have seemed it would never arrive—at least not in time for seniors Leinberger, Wheatley, and Phil Hyde to be part of it.

Funny. This was the week CBS showed up with a camera crew to film Friday's practice and Saturday's (presumably) inevitable defeat. "They were doing a story on 'winning isn't everything,'" Leinberger said.

Instead they found out that winning, while not everything, was something that these young men wanted very much and had worked for very hard.

"Lou Lupin and Chris Brigham brought champagne," Leinberger said.

Before the game, they brought it. Think of that. Thirty-four straight defeats, five years without a victory, and two Swarthmore juniors brought champagne.

"Lou said, 'You guys better win,'" Leinberger said. "'We can't afford this too many weeks.'"

And they did win. . . .

It came down to this: Muhlenberg, trailing by four points, had fourth and goal inside the Swarthmore one.

"One of the (CBS) cameramen standing on the sideline said, 'They score, it'll be 18–16. That's a good story,'" Wheatley said.

"Don't you have faith?" asked an injured Swarthmore player who was standing alongside.

Sure, he had faith. Faith that a team with no victories in 34 tries would make it 0 for 35.

Leinberger had heard all the bad jokes, experienced most of the defeats. He had caught a helmet in the thigh earlier in the game, but the pain didn't bother him now. The next play bothered him.

"Actually, I was afraid they scored the play before," the Swarthmore captain said. "Somebody caught a pass on the one. . . ."

But the guy was stopped, maybe a foot and a half short, and it was up to Leinberger—a fullback on offense, a linebacker on defense—to call the right defensive signal on fourth down.

"I just get feelings sometimes," he said, and this time the feeling was that Muhlenberg would try to pull out a last-minute victory with a quarterback sneak. "I lined up a little bit closer," Leinberger remembered. "I hit him, and he bounced to the next hole, and he got hit again, and he bounced to the next hole and my brother Jeff hit him. . . ."

A big pileup. Bodies sprawled everywhere. Either it was a touchdown and Muhlenberg 18, Swarthmore 16, or it was Swarthmore's ball, and Swarthmore's ball game.

"They (the officials) took a long time," Leinberger said. "Then they made a decision. They put the ball down, and it couldn't have been this far from the goal line. . . ."

He held his two index fingers less than an inch apart. That's how close it was. So close that one of the Muhlenberg players protested so vigorously the referee slapped on a 15-yard penalty.

Now it was Bill Wheatley's turn to savor the final seconds. How could a quarterback who had lived through all those losses at Swarthmore, a quarterback who played for a high school team that won three and lost 21 while he was there, possibly forget the feeling as those last seconds ticked away?

"That's what I'll remember most," he said. "Being in that huddle, knowing all I had to do was fall on the damn ball. . . ." He smiled. "Brigham had already started crying . . . I'll remember that, and the people coming at me when the game ended, and my father coming up and putting his arms around me. . . ."

And opening the champagne in the locker room. And seeing the president of the college there, joining in the celebration. And so many other things, etched in their memories.

"Winning to me was not so much beating Muhlenberg," Bruce Leinberger said. "It was a group of guys here at Swarthmore proving we can do enough things right to win a game. Somebody like Chip Veise (last year's football captain), I feel sorry for him. Now I have a game ball. That's something Chip doesn't have. . . ."

A game ball. A couple of pieces of a shattered goalpost. A victory celebration.

Not the most important things in the world. Certainly not in the world of Swarthmore College. But there's still a place for them. Even there.

FISHING

FISHING WITH MY FATHER—
AND OTHER OUTLANDISH PARTNERS

By Nord Riley

From Outdoor Life
Copyright, ©, 1975, Times Mirror Magazines, Inc.

I may be the only North Dakotan around who learned how to fish from a black man whose father and mother had been slaves. We had more than enough red men up there on the northern Great Plains; I played basketball against the Sioux all through high school, and they lifted our hair every time. But black men were hard to come by in those days. I never knew why Tom Miller decided to live in Wyndmere, a village of 521 people, mainly Norwegians. The cold, windswept prairie where it was often 40 degrees below zero must have been rough for a man from magnolia-and-grits country. We were proud to have him; he gave the town some style. He was the only black man anywhere in the county.

Tom was about 50 when I knew him, a broad, powerful man with a face limber from smiling and hair going gray. His neck was uncommonly short and his head round, so that it looked like a cannonball sitting on a shelf. I don't remember ever seeing him in anything but bib overalls, heavy shoes, and a hat. Tom made his living performing odd jobs about the village. He turned gardens in the spring and cleaned out furnace clinkers in the winter.

On those still golden mornings in summer when school was out I lolled in bed until I heard Tom coming down the alley with his wheelbarrow and Cutter, his affable black water spaniel. He came down the alley whistling. He was a first-class whistler with a wide repertory. He moved ponderously, like a calliope.

His residence was just off the livery barn. He shared it with seven buff Orphington hens, each with a Norwegian name. Visiting Tom in his digs was a major privilege in my life, but at times unsettling.

"Watch out where you sit yourself down," Tom would say. "I heard that Sigrid cluckin' and braggin' about a new egg not more than two minutes ago."

Everyone liked Tom. My father, the village banker, admired him for his honesty, his sound work, and his savings account. He told me that Tom was the best shoveler he had ever seen.

"That man makes a badger look incompetent," he said. And it was true, Tom had a gift for digging. He went through loam and clay with a smooth grace that men from the pool hall would break off rummy to watch.

When my father heard that Tom liked to fish it gave him an idea. In our village a boy who didn't like to hunt and fish might grow up to be a piano player. At eight I was a fair shot on tin cans and street lights with a BB gun, but because of the scarcity of water I was a dud at fishing. My father figured Tom could teach me.

It was a three-mile hike to the nearest stream, Elk Creek, where the cemetery was. If we had a wet spring, Elk Creek held a few fish, a family of mallards, and a multitude of mud turtles. Tom walked right on by those mud turtles.

"Nothin' you can do with a mud turtle," he pointed out. "He won't play, and he's low on flavor." So he led me on two more miles to the Wild Rice, a thin river sauntering aimlessly across the prairie. I always felt a little sorry for the Wild Rice; the land was as flat as a floor, with no place for the stream to work up any momentum; there was no place it could go, like other rivers, so it just lay there on the prairie like a sleeping python.

We carried two eight-foot bamboo poles armed with green line, sinker, and single hook. Most people fished with corks, but Tom was against them. They interrupted intimacy with the fish; they deadened communication.

"Corks lead to a slack line," he said, "and a slack line is bound to keep you ignorant about what the fish is doin' down there. You got to keep them vibrations comin'." So I fished without a bobber, and I kept my line to the hook straight. And I still do.

The fish were chubs, somewhat like trout in appearance but without a trout's highfalutin tastes. Chubs have no name at all as gourmets. Worms were plenty good enough for chubs, but Tom wouldn't use just *any* worm. Mine came from the rich soil under our apple trees, but he turned them down as being pale and short on zip. He grew his own, back of the livery barn. Tom wouldn't put up with a lackadaisical worm, and his weren't. He bred them for durability and irritability, and I have not seen their like since; lissome, pink, extremely fit, and irascible.

"See those red rings on this worm? Those are breedin' rings and the toughest part of a worm. Just run the hook through them, and that worm is not just goin' to stay on the hook, he's goin' to kick up a fuss half the afternoon."

He kept the worms in a Copenhagen snuff can with just enough "snoose" in it to keep them turned on.

Once in a while the chubs weren't interested, even in Tom's worms, but he was ready. If nothing bit in 10 minutes he took a bottle from his bib pocket, a bottle about the size iodine used to come in. It held a liquid about like corn syrup in color and viscosity. It wasn't corn syrup; corn syrup *couldn't* smell like that. It didn't smell like a dead horse upwind in August, but it was of the same magnitude. This was his fish lure, a secret formula, privately brewed, for jaded chubs. One drop on a worm changed it from hog jowl to porterhouse. Not always, but often enough to keep Tom proud.

When he had as many fish as we wanted, Tom spread himself out on his back, slid his hat over his eyes, and, with Cutter at his side, slept. Not me. No eight-year-old kid can sleep in a pasture full of gophers. North Dakota had millions of gophers: flickertails, grays, striped, pockets. Send a whistle out over a North Dakota pasture on a sunny day, and a hundred of them came to attention beside their holes like a battalion of tent pegs. Farmers detested them for unspecified crimes, but the gophers enchanted me. I liked their dumb, jaunty ways, the way they romped and wrestled and visited with each other. Not the pocket gopher, of course—he was wary and withdrawn; I never saw another gopher play with him. Tom had shown me how to snare gophers with a length of binder twine: put a running noose over the gopher hole, stand back about six feet with the other end of the twine, and wait until the gopher stuck his head up to see where everyone had gone. As a general thing I tried to make a friend of the gopher I snared, and as a general thing he bit me.

Chubs are never going to push trout off a menu. Tom ate them, though and so did I, out of noblesse oblige. My mother would fry up the chubs, but that's as far as she would go. My father wouldn't go anywhere with chubs. We all knew where he stood: if it wasn't a walleyed pike, to hell with it—he'd have pork chops.

I would like to be able to say that Tom and I remained friends and that when I grew up he and I were made honorary members of the Sons of Norway, but the truth is that when I was about nine Tom left Wyndmere for another small town 40 miles away. My father kept tabs on Tom through a banker in the new town. When Tom died a couple of years later he left instructions that the money in his bank account should be blown on a fine funeral. A lone black man on the lone prairie was going out in style. I was a little hurt that he hadn't left any bequests. I could have used that stuff he put on worms to make them voluptuous.

With Tom gone, my father took over teaching me to fish, although it wasn't a very broad education. He wouldn't eat anything but walleyes, and he wouldn't catch anything else either. He claimed that a walleye looked as a fish should look: clean and shapely. He preferred the walleye's expression, particularly those guileless eyes. To catch these fish we had to drive 60 or 70 miles to the lakes near Fergus Falls, Minn. He fished with a bamboo pole and a minnow for bait when everyone else used a rod and reel. That mortified me no end, as did the clothes he wore when he went fishing. He wore what he wore at the bank: conservative suit, stiff white collar, tie, and neat black ankle-high shoes made of kangaroo.

He caught a lot of walleyes, more than anyone else, but I couldn't stand the square way he did it, so my mother and I pooled our resources and bought him a fine steel rod and a reel with an antibacklash device. He accepted it with his usual good manners. He used it too, because he understood how I felt. It really didn't improve matters much, because he couldn't get the hang of casting. He didn't use his wrist or his arm. He coiled up all 134 pounds of him and, starting with a decapitating backswing, whipped the rod around low over the boat like he was cutting hay. His casts never went far because he had so many snarls from backlashes. His plug sailed about 20 feet, then was stopped in midflight like a roped calf.

Worst of all, he stopped catching walleyes; instead he caught great northern pike, a fish he despised. He found their serpentine figures and the slime on their bodies and their evil, underslung jaws intolerable.

"Damn!" he'd say when he caught one. "Another snake!" And he'd drop the slippery, snapping fish at my feet as if I were responsible—me and the confounded antibacklash mechanism.

He stayed with the rod and reel until we made a long trip with our great friend, Doc Olson, into some remote lakes along the Canadian border. We went in by boat, guided by a man named Justis, the only human being I ever saw with round incisors.

We were way hell and gone out on Lac la Croix, three days from a tackle shop, when my father wound up with one of his terrifying casts and heaved the whole outfit—rod, reel, line, and lure—75 feet into deep water. It was the longest cast he ever made.

He always said it was an accident, and that the bamboo pole back at our camp was a surprise to him. But when he began to use the bamboo he once more began to catch his beloved walleyes. And it finally dawned on me that he was absolutely right about the capabilities of the bamboo pole in catching walleyes. It's simple, trouble-free, and fun. It is unsurpassed for holding a shiner a foot off the bottom.

It has additional virtues, the bamboo pole: its 10- or 12-foot length is just right for measuring depths, and it has a kind of built-in sonar—it reports back to the surface what kind of bottom you're over. You can feel mud with it, and you can determine rock from gravel, which sends up vibrations. Gravel's best for walleyes my father said.

Dr. Carl T. Olson believed in the latest and finest equipment when he went fishing: big fast cars and a tacklebox fat with spare reels, lines, plugs, and the surgical devices he used for removing hooks. A rather short, stocky man, Doc had a fine intelligence and a compulsion to go fishing. We had no hospital in Wyndmere; fortunately the nearest one was to the east of us about 25 miles, at Breckinridge, Minn., right on the way to the lakes. About once a week, when Doc was overcome by desire to fish, he picked me up and we drove down to the hospital, where he saw his patients. Then we went on 30 or 40 miles more to a lake.

Being a surgeon, he had great wrist action and he cast with precision; being impatient, he preferred casting to stillfishing. Consequently he didn't catch many walleyes, but he caught a lot of northerns, which like a moving bait. He taught me all I know about catching fish with plugs and spoons and spinners: depths, rates of retrieve, and the wonderful truth that no matter how many lures a man has, three or four do all the catching—the rest are deadheads and drones.

Unlike my father, Doc liked great northerns and their wicked, savage ways. When they struck they struck to kill: there was none of the gentlemanly nibbling of a walleye. A great northern is in constant bad temper, which gets even worse when he finds out he's been swindled by a piece of wood dressed up as a minnow, and hooked and lifted into a boat with strangers. He snaps away until the end, hoping for a finger or thumb. Though a great northern from cold water is good eating, we never took any home: Doc left them off for the nuns at the hospital for use on Fridays.

One day in July Doc came out of the hospital with a man who had his collar on backward. This was Father Rosenthal, a German Jew who had been converted to Catholicism. He was a jolly man with an early Henry Kissinger accent. He was also the first priest I had ever been closer than 40 feet to.

Father Rosenthal, Doc said, knew where there was a lake full of fish and was going to take us there. He led us to a small, shallow, weedy lake; on its shore was a country store and a spavined dock with one rowboat for rent. Father Rosenthal went into the store. When the proprietor saw who it was, he rolled his eyes and got wearily to his feet.

"Same, Father?"

"Ja, only more, please, I haf two friends mit me."

The proprietor got out a big smoked ham, oddly lacerated, and began to slice off lengths of the white fat.

"Ham fat?" said Doc. "For *bait?*"

"You vait," said Father Rosenthal. "Ham fat is driven the pickerels crazy." He thanked the proprietor and took out his wallet, which made the proprietor roll his eyes again and appeal to Doc.

"He keeps wanting to pay. Now how am I going to charge a guy named Rosenthal, no matter how he wears his collar, money for pork fat?"

"I like dot man," said Father Rosenthal as he changed from his clerical garb into a pair of brown overalls.

The lake was only about eight feet deep, hardly enough to keep the mob of great northerns wet. The ham fat really turned them on. They weren't big—two-footers mostly—but they were mean. Doc laughed and slapped his leg with joy; Father Rosenthal chortled and cried out things in German.

My job was putting the fish on the stringers and keeping count. The daily limit then was 10, and it was a problem counting the slithery, slimy fish hanging over the side of the boat on stringers.

"That's the last one," I said after a couple of hours. "Thirty."

"So ve quit. How about dis fishen, Doctor—is not so bad, yes?"

As we drew the boat up to the dock I heard Doc mutter: "Watch it, here comes trouble."

A tall, scrawny, somber man shambled toward us. Binoculars dangled from his neck; a game warden's badge was pinned on his shirt.

"I think that's old Orrin Gast from the look of him," Doc said. "Nastiest warden in the country."

It was Gast. He asked for and inspected our licenses. "How many 'snakes' you got there?"

I told him 30 exactly, and he said, kneeling to count them, "You're sure about that, are you?" He lifted aside each fish as he counted. "Now I get 31."

Doc gave me a look and counted; *he* got 31. So did Father Rosenthal.

"Turty-vun is right. Der boy makes the mistake. Dot's easy, ja?"

"You've got one over the limit, and that breaks the law. You people are coming along with me to see the justice of the peace."

Father Rosenthal said, "Vun minute, please." He went up to the car, changed from overalls into his priest's outfit, and came back. His crucifix swung back and forth over his chest as he walked.

Gast flinched, and I figured the priest had him, but this was a tough warden. "Oh no you don't! That doesn't cut any ice with me. My wife's Catholic, but I'm not, so you can stop waving that cross at me. As a matter of fact, you aren't all that holy and pure. I got proof of that right here." He tapped his binoculars. "I've been watching you all afternoon through the glasses, keeping count. And you know something? *You caught twelve!*"

This time Father Rosenthal flinched.

"Which is two over your limit," said Gast, getting his enthusiasm back. "And I'm wondering what the JP's going to say about that."

I felt low; I felt so low at being responsible for a priest getting thrown in the slammer that I couldn't speak. I wanted to tell them I was willing to take the rap for the crimes and to absorb any punishment, including the rope, but I couldn't. Doc, a short-fused man, wasn't at all tongue-tied.

"Dammit all," he roared, "you can't arrest a priest and an eleven-year-old kid!"

"Is that a fact? And who are you besides being Carl T. Olson?"

"*Doctor* Carl T. Olson!"

Adding a physician to his bag seemed to make the warden feel good all over, and I think he was going to smile when a blue sedan pulled up. Two men got out. The red-faced, red-haired one with the big bushy red eyebrows like an autumn hedge was a priest; the tall, dark one smoking a cigar and wearing a long brown robe, a black rope around his waist, a skullcap, and sandals was a monk. Doc let out a whoop and slapped his leg.

"Rosenthal's called in the cavalry!"

A beaming Father Rosenthal introduced us to Brother Joseph and to his old friend Father Murphy, who had driven over to the lake to invite us to the parish house for dinner. "Und this is der game varden, Mr. Gast."

"I know Orrin," said Father Murphy. "He's in my parish. How's Millie?"

The warden's eyes were closed, his teeth clenched; he seemed to be enduring internal pain and disorders. "The wife's fine."

"Ve haf by mistake caught vun fish extra," said Father Rosenthal, "und Mr. Gast vants to take us to jail."

"Not *jail!*" cried Gast, clearly struck by what he thought was a foul blow. He appealed to Doc and me, "Did I say one word about jail? Did I?"

Doc said nothing, and I couldn't. The two priests and the monk regarded the warden with sorrow and disappointment. "Orrin," said Father Murphy. "Orrin."

Gast broke. He couldn't face that wall of clergy. He backed off. "All right. All *right!* Forget it! The boy could have made a mistake. I can see that." His hot, humiliated eyes fell on me. "You better learn to count, sonny, or you're going to wind up in real trouble." He left us then.

At eleven years of age I had learned some of the lore of angling. I knew about tight lines and aggressive earthworms, about bamboo poles and plug casting, about chubs and walleyes and great northerns, about ham fat. Now I knew one more thing: when nothing else works, call for divine intervention.

FOOTBALL

DEFENSE, THE OLD EQUALIZER

By Blackie Sherrod

From the Dallas Times Herald
Copyright, ©, 1975, Dallas Times Herald

Nineteen zillion wild-eyed leather-lungs in red coats and red hats and blouses and maybe even underpants stood in the baking sunlight and chanted DEE-fense, DEE-fense, until the old gray Cotton Bowl concrete quivered in protest.

On the simmering green run below, their sweaty and worn Oklahoma idols were girding for a last-ditch repulse of the equally sweaty and worn Texas offensive troops. As in almost all titanic struggles—and this was one of the giants—the game had come down to defense, ye olde equalizer.

The eventual 24–17 score doesn't sound much like a defensive epic, but here was the moment of truth. The favored Sooners were clawing to regain their No. 1 national ranking and prolong their 24-game win streak. They had shot suddenly ahead on a stunning 33-yard bolt by Horace Ivory deep in the final period, and now it was up to the Sooner defense, all those Selmon brothers and their cousins and whatnot, to have and to hold.

And here was Texas, with five nervous minutes left in the Bloody Mary afternoon, still alive with an attack that had shown ability, even tendency, to score from afar. Rigor mortis had not threatened, nor would it. Tension in the jammed saucer was at its highest.

The Longhorns were the leading attack in the nation, right? True, they had not slashed their usual 465 yards on this day, but this was no ordinary defense they faced.

Texas, with nifty Marty Akins in charge and massive Earl Campbell in constant collision with the Sooner middle, launched its drive from its own 20 after Ivory's scoring spurt. DEE-fense, etc. Leroy Selmon, one of a dozen brothers who seemed stationed in the

Oklahoma defense, mashed Akins like an offending bug on the first play. Zac Henderson, a sophomore safety, rolled off Jimmy Walker's block beautifully and nailed Gralyn Wyatt on the next snap. Akins, still shunning the pass even though now there were but four minutes left, tried a keeper at left tackle on third down and there was Jimbo Elrod, Oklahoma's great defensive end. Hello, walls.

The Longhorns were forced to punt as the Sooner defenders were escorted off the field by a deafening ovation from their frothing supporters.

Texas got the ball for yet one more shot, after a brilliant Sooner sidewinding quick kick by jittery Joe Washington, this time with 2:25 remaining. There was enough time, but Akins would have to, excuse the expression, pass the football. Oklahoma knew this. On first down it was defensive end Mike Phillips dropping the Texas quarterback for a six-yard loss as he tried desperately to throw from deep in his homeland. Lineback Bill Dalke chased Akins out of bounds on the next play as the Texas senior looked vainly upfield for an isolated friend. And then on third down, the entire state of Oklahoma, students, senators, bootleggers, whatever, came from the stands and banged Akins out of bounds again.

That was it, Whiskey River had run dry. The Longhorns had no choice but to punt from their own seven and pray for a fumble. It was not to be. The upcountry invaders ran out the clock and Oklahoma had its fifth victory of the season and its fifth straight triumph over Texas in this historic rivalry.

"We ran our guts out," said Akins. "I couldn't have taken another step."

"I'm proud of our defense," said Sooner coach Barry Switzer. "They came through when they had to perform."

This was a game that had some of everything—even mistakes. Admittedly, it was a grudge meeting between the two coaches, young Switzer and his elder, Darrell Royal, who have clashed openly over recruiting practices. It was a collision between two almighty offenses, two gluttonous Wishbone T attacks. It was a confrontation between perhaps the two best running backs in America: Washington, the Port Arthur mongoose, and Campbell, Texas' sophomore landslide.

Yet not all of this materialized. The two coaches met at midfield before the game, shook hands, patted shoulders; heck, Royal even fixed an overlooked button on Switzer's knit sport shirt. And when the day was finished, there were no back-alley challenges en route to the mutual tunnel. Campbell, the day's leading rusher with 95 brutal yards, congratulated Ivory, a fellow Texan who attended

Navarro JC before migrating cross-river. Steve Davis, the winning quarterback, shook hands with Paul Jette, the Texas defensive back. And so on.

"They were class people," said Davis. "They had compliments for us after the game. It would have been difficult for me to have been that nice if we had lost."

Those high-geared offenses were held to 335 for the winners, 289 for Texas, highly respectful but not the usual gaits. Campbell and Washington were factors, but they were not monopolistic. Campbell manfully strove to bash his brains out against the big Oklahoma middle, and did manage 95 yards in 23 carries, despite having to retire twice for sideline repairs. Washington scored a touchdown, had an 80-yard punt return score canceled by clipping calls. But they had to share the afternoon with defenders like Phillips, Anthony Bryant, Elrod, Dalke, Dewey and Leroy and Tom and Dick and Harry Selmon for Oklahoma. And Brad Shearer, Lionel Johnson, Rick Fenlaw and, at times, Tim Campbell and Raymond Clayborn for Texas.

Mostly, the game was crammed with phases and stages of suspense. The players and the crowd of 72,000 lived it one play at a time. Seemingly, the tide could have turned like a dervish, as befits a meeting of unbeatens, ranked second and fifth in the nation. However, the afternoon did get off to a rather ragged beginning.

Oklahoma converted two Texas fumbles (and overcame one of its own) into a 10–0 lead in the first quarter. First, the starting Longhorn center, Billy Gordon, received an eye injury on the opening kickoff. His replacement, Jim Wyman, and Akins had coordination trouble right off. There were a couple fumbled snaps and Dewey Selmon plopped on the second to give Oklahoma ownership on the Texas 46. This recovery led to a 45-yard field goal by Tony DiRienzo.

Shortly after, an 80-yard punt return down sidelines by Washington was nullified by two—count 'em—two Sooner clips on the play. Then Washington messed up a subsequent scoring bid by losing the ball on the Texas two-yard line. This gift was quickly returned by the Steers, when an Akins pitchout, a blind toss to Wyatt, arrived at the same time as Sooner safety Scott Hill. The ball bounced off a flank, dribbled into the Texas end zone where Phillips outraced Akins to cover for an Oklahoma touchdown.

The Longhorns mounted a 90-yard drive in the second quarter, capped by a 38-yard touchdown pass (that's right, touchdown pass) from Akins to Alfred Jackson, who backtracked to take the pass on the Sooner two as Sidney Brown, defending on the goal, searched helplessly for the ball.

Texas began the second half with aroused defensive fury, perhaps refreshed by the rest. (Oklahoma had just finished two close games and its regulars might have been in somewhat better condition for the 93-degree heat and the accompanying pressure.)

Campbell fumbled away good Texas field position on one occasion, Bryant recovering. Oklahoma stabbed quickly. A Davis pass to Billy Brooks, one stride behind little Joe Bob Bizzell, gained 54 yards to the Texas 14. Three plays later from the nine, Washington zipped over right tackle, swept through Bill Hamilton's grasp, and exploded into the pay zone for Oklahoma's 17–7 lead.

In the fourth quarter, Akins pulled his patented specialty. After Tinker Owens's punt sailed straight up at midfield, Texas again had good field position for one of the few times all day. From the Sooner 37, Texas scored in five plays. The 30-yard scoring play saw Akins spin around left end and after a 10-yard gain, flip a lateral to Walker who sped unheeded down the sidelines.

Once again, back came Texas, back into serious contention; back in truth, to the point of winning. Royal's attack moved to the Oklahoma 15.

This again was fourth down and only two needed, when Royal surprised everyone with a pass call. Akins shoved a low toss behind Jackson in the right flat and he somehow twisted and dived and caught the flutterball on the Oklahoma 21.

However, a Texas delay penalty and a Bryant sack of Akins for a six-yard loss, shoved the Steers out of touchdown territory and on the fourth down, Russell Erxleben booted a 43-yard field goal to tie the proceedings at 17-all.

That's how it stood until Oklahoma put together its clutch drive, moving slowly but certainly, helped early by a face-mask penalty against Texas, to the Longhorn 33. On first down, Ivory—a natural halfback transplanted to fullback only last week—shot quickly through left guard and one step behind the line of scrimmage, there was no Longhorn around. He was across the goal before some Steers could locate the ball.

Then, it was left up to the Big Red defense to repel the last Texas efforts and it was equal to the task. And the series domination remained across the border, as it once camped out with Texas. Ain't it funny how time slips away?

GENERAL

HE'S NOT AS SIMPLE AS ABC

By Paul Hendrickson

From The National Observer
Copyright, ©, 1975, The National Observer, Dow Jones & Co. Inc.

"Quarterbacks and tight ends," Alex Karras once told author George Plimpton, staring moodily at New York's East River, "die comfortably, in big beds, and the Irish Setter is whimpering on the other side of the door. . . . But the linemen give it up in these little rooms in poor sections. They wake up on a cot in a room the size of a closet and they look at their pushed-in kissers in the little mirror, and they pull their old football jerseys with the number on the back out of the bottom drawer of the beat-up dresser, and they put them on and go up to the bridge there . . . and they drop off. . . ."

Another football Monday, this week in Dallas, and Alex Karras has the motel blues. Sockless and sleepy-eyed, he sits in a shaft of harsh afternoon light, squinting at a newspaper. A plate, smeared with dried catsup, is at his elbow.

The Mad Duck, as his teammates used to call him, has just gotten in from Hawaii. He arrived at 9 A.M., hustled to a meeting with ABC brass, then slipped off to bed. In two hours he will be dressed and on his way to Texas Stadium for a "Monday Night Football" battle between the Cowboys and the Chiefs, which he'll broadcast with Frank Gifford and Howard Cosell. He will be "up" by then, full of his old sass and sarcasm, ready to take apart the phenomenon of grown men trying to hurt each other. But now, at 3:30 P.M., looking out on a Marriott parking lot, Alex Karras, funnyman, is not very funny. He is tired.

"Yeah, it can be a drag sometimes," he says, pinching a cigarette between two massive fingers. "This thing about being funny. I mean, I don't like booze, okay? But all my life someone wants to shove a Scotch and water at me. I walk into a room and people start laughing—and that's all right, 'cause that's my image. But why doesn't somebody ever ask me about politics, or about music? I mean, Christ, I was once elected president of the Bloomfield Hills, Michigan, PTA. . . ."

This last is not said with any sense of boast—just frustration. He seems ready to say something else, but lapses instead into silence. So the subject changes—to acting.

"Yeah, I see myself primarily as an actor now," Karras says, holding in his smoke. "In fact, 'Monday Night Football' is just a hypo needle to get me exposure. I've been acting off and on since the middle sixties, when I was in *Paper Lion*. That hooked me, I guess. I don't know . . . I like it for a lot of reasons. I like to move around. I like to make a lot of money—and there can be heavy money out there. It's also a form of release. In the last picture I did—the one about Babe Zaharias—I had to do a crying scene that made me feel terrific."

Babe, a made-for-TV movie that aired in October, was unquestionably Karras's big break. Before that he had done mostly minor parts and comic roles. (In Mel Brooks's *Blazing Saddles* he played a brute named Mongo who cold-cocks a horse.) Karras's agent, Tom Vance, says the two of them spent months negotiating for the part of George Zaharias, husband of the late female athlete. Now the scripts are coming in faster than they can read them.

But what about football? Wouldn't you miss it? Don't you sort of, well, *owe* it something? "Are you kidding?" Karras snaps, coming forward, his eyes suddenly flinty behind lenses thick as Coke bottles. "I'm forty years old, and I've been playing football in one way or another for 22 years. I mean, enough's *enough*, for crissakes! Sure, I love the game. But I don't owe it a ——ing thing. I'm sick of hearing that. You know what football gave me all those years? A big ——ing headache, that's what!"

He has begun to salt his talk with the most explicit cuss word in the language; he applies it with locker-room ease. "Look, my son is sixteen, okay? He's been in organized sports since he was nine, okay? Well, you know what? I don't think he's having any fun. I don't want him or my other kids to have to go to college, like I did, and have some ——ing coach point at him and scream, 'You run until you faint!' I mean, that's criminal."

So Alex Karras, All-Pro defensive tackle for the Detroit Lions, wages now and yesterday a love-hate relationship with the game he played so well for so many years. To understand the quicksilver nature of this relationship, you must know about the lower-class neighborhoods of Gary, Ind., where as a fatherless teen-ager he worked summers in the steel mills and made All-State in the fall. (He had more than 100 scholarship offers, in several different sports, by his senior year.)

You must know about the University of Iowa and four tormented years under head coach Forrest Evashevski. (Karras says Evashevski kicked him off the team seven times and he quit six—doubtless an NCAA record.) You must know about a year-long banishment from pro football, in 1963, for a gambling scandal. (Karras says he bet on three games, none involving his own team, and contends the national press wildly distorted the story, pressuring National Football League Commissioner Pete Rozelle to suspend him.)

And, of course, you must know about his old buddy and teammate, Joe Schmidt, who as coach of the Lions called him up one fine fall day in 1971 and told him he was through, that his lateral movements were gone, that he couldn't—to use the lingo of linemen—"play the piano" anymore. (Karras, by then in his fourteenth season with the Lions, had gone through the entire summer and six exhibition games with no warning that the front office wanted him out; he was let go a couple of days before the opening game.)

"Those sons of bitches in Detroit," Plimpton later quoted him as saying. "What did they mean, taking that thing away from me?"

He is on the phone now, his mood abruptly changed. He is talking to a sports writer in Florida who was with George Zaharias the night *Babe* aired. "Geez, he really loved it, did he?" Karras says softly, his meaty brown face screwed into a boyish, almost babyish smile. "Wow! That's really great. I mean, I don't think I've ever done anything so satisfying as that film. And George thought it was okay, huh? Wow!"

Off the phone, jingling the change in his pockets, he is suddenly buoyant. "My dad was a doctor and had this little office in Gary over a theater," he says. "I'd run up to see him and he'd flip me a quarter and I'd go down to the movies and invariably the Eyes and Ears of the World would come on, and there'd be ol' George and Babe Zaharias, going to some golf tournament. I fell immediately in love with both of them—he because he was a wrestler and a Greek, like I am; she because she seemed everything a woman would want to be—free, active, even kind of beautiful."

The reverie, not all of it happy, goes on—how his dad died when Alex was thirteen; how he worshiped his high school coach, substituting him for a father; how he chose Iowa because he was afraid of following his big brothers, Louie and Teddy, to their schools. (Both were standout collegiate football players—Louie at Purdue,

Teddy at Indiana; both also had pro careers.)

And then almost without transition, he is into the Iowa stories. They are nearly legendary in football circles—told and retold in NFL training camps to the point where Karras himself probably wouldn't recognize some of them. There's the series about him and his roomie, Big Mesho, forever scaring the bejesus out of the dorm proctor. ("The guy was a Mister Peepers type, about 5-feet-1, and weighed 33 pounds.") There's the one about Phil Lawson, a horny Sigma Nu, whom Karras once talked into taking a math test for him. ("I told ol' Phil I'd get him straight with this forty-year-old barmaid. When they caught us, my paper had rabbits and ticktacktoes all over it.")

But the most celebrated story concerns the time he went to a school dance (supposedly because Evashevski was worried about Karras's social life), stumbled through a waltz with the biggest girl in the place, then blurted, "You sweat less than any fat girl I've ever seen."

"Yep, I really said it," he says, grinning in spite of himself. "I wasn't trying to be mean or anything. It was just all I could think of. I bet she didn't even take offense."

A little later, toned down a bit, he talks about his sense of humor. "In 1961 I was a guy totally devoted to football because I needed it as an instrument—it was all I had. I went to Iowa in the first place with a chip on my shoulder—the poor kid from Gary. I can't get along with the coach. I start hating my teammates because I feel they're not good enough for us to win every time. I was a very unhappy guy. I guess I was on the verge of losing my personality altogether. Well, by 1966, after the suspension, I knew I had to change. And somehow I did. Ever since, when I feel myself losing something, I get away for a while. That's what I was doing in Hawaii last week. Once, in 1971, I jumped off an airplane and went up into the mountains of Arizona with some Indians for a few days."

And then: "When you come right down to it, I'm just a paper cup. All my life I've been living by my wits. I never thought, hanging around those street corners in Gary, banking those damn fires at the steel mills, I'd someday be doing this."

There is more to say, but we are out of time: The limo will be here in 45 minutes. "When they come to pick me up," he says, rising, "I always figure I'm supposed to drive." He shrugs, sticks out a paw, then cracks into an altar-boy grin. "Did you know," he says, "that Gary, Ind., is the only place in the world where the birds cough?"

Game time. Outside, Texas Stadium is a blur of creamy Caddies and Lincolns. Inside, an armada of Texettes (in white-patent go-go boots and polyester miniskirts) is directing oil and cattle barons to their private boxes.

In the ABC broadcast booth, Gifford—in tinted aviator glasses and Gucci loafers—is preparing lead-ins. Humble Howard, in pointy-toed cowboy boots, is ranting at reporters. He also wants a vodka. He is tight for this game, says everybody around him, because of remarks he made a couple of Monday nights ago about the abilities of Dallas fullback Robert Newhouse. The Dallas fans have been laying for him ever since—and Cosell knows it. (A local radio station has even sponsored a contest to see who could come up with the best anti-Cosell poster; during the game, whenever Newhouse gets yardage, hundreds of fans stand and raise clenched fists at the press box.)

Karras turns in an exceptionally good performance, never letting on to the game's 14 million viewers that he's going mostly on adrenaline. Though he gets off a dozen good lines, the best comes in the second half when Cosell is putting the rap on Dallas. By then the Cowboys have fumbled several times and been intercepted twice.

"Uh, Howard," says Karras urgently, "will you please say Dallas is awesome so we can get out of town alive?"

By 11:30 it is over; Dallas has lost, 34–31. Back at the Marriott, Cosell and Gifford briefly hold court at the bar. But Karras is nowhere to be seen. The next morning, before the sun has climbed high over Texas Stadium, Alex Karras is on a plane with his agent, bound for Hollywood and bigger dreams.

GOLF

"THE ONLY-NESS"

By Nick Seitz

From Golf Digest
Copyright, ©, 1975, Golf Digest Magazine

Hale Irwin responded to my leading question like a true champion. He coined a catchy word.

What, I wanted to know, sets a professional golfer apart from athletes in other major professional sports? What makes him unique?

The serious-visaged, bespectacled Irwin is as thoughtful as he looks. He briefly contemplated his navel in the locker room this day and then answered, "The only-ness."

I found it a marvelous reply. Golf often has been called a lonely game, but to speak of a player's only-ness is to add needed dimension. It is a word that comes from the stomach, the heart, and the head, speaking to us meaningfully on several levels.

"You're all by yourself out there in the center of the fairway with only a small ball and your psyche," Irwin went on. "It's a long way to the hole. There are no lines regulating play. You can rely on your caddie, but only one person can hit the shot—you."

Irwin contrasts only-ness with football, America's most popular spectator sport, which he played well enough as a defensive back at the University of Colorado to make All-Conference in the rugged Big Eight.

"In a team sport like football, there's always something to stimulate you. I wasn't very big, and I felt that every play was for my life. In golf you don't get stimulated by a whack in the kisser. Your stimulation has to come from little things . . . a good bounce, a good lie at a crucial time. Then you tell yourself maybe your luck isn't all bad after all."

The only-ness. Once stimulated, the professional golfer knows he must keep his emotions under tight rein. His sport provides no real emotional outlet.

Tom Weiskopf, by nature temperamental, has trouble selecting the correct club under pressure. "That adrenaline gets to flowing and I'll hit the ball 15 to 25 yards farther than normal," he says. "I've hit a 9-iron 175 yards coming down the stretch when distance is the last thing I want. In other sports you want to be fired up, but in golf you have to be in control of your emotions all the time. You have to discipline your imagination."

Says Irwin, "On the tour you almost never hit a full shot. Every swing demands a different degree of control. It's very wearing emotionally. I'm most relaxed late in a round, when I'm tired."

George Plimpton, the best-selling author and sporting dilettante, observes that in other sports tension is released once the game starts. But in golf the tension steadily builds throughout the round.

Bad shots are inevitable over a period of 18 pressurized holes, and there is nowhere for the golfer's frustrations to go. In tennis a disgruntled player can bash a ball over the farthest fence or berate the nearest linesman. In golf a disgruntled player can only swallow his anger and try to compose himself for his next shot.

It never ceases to amaze me that volatile men like Tom Weiskopf and Dave Hill can win on the tour. The effort it must take for them to subdue their explosive impulses and play this most disciplined of games so well has to be monumental, particularly since they are such perfectionists. Some golfers want to win major tournaments, some want to become millionaires, some want the glory only. As for Weiskopf and Hill, I am sure they would trade their kingdoms for a dozen perfectly struck shots.

(What appears to the gallery to be a sensational shot may be largely unsatisfactory to the man who struck it. He alone knows what he intended for the shot and how close he came to bringing it off. A good result does not necessarily signify success in his own mind, where the real game is waged.)

The pace of golf does nothing to ease this kind of psychological pressure on the players. A round usually lasts at least four and one half hours and demands, if not sustained concentration, a greater attention span than other sports. Golf often is played too slowly, but on the other hand it is an activity that cannot be rushed and played well. As Jack Nicklaus puts it, there is no way he can play a shot until he knows he's mentally ready to play it.

The only-ness. In a different way, the only-ness decided Nicklaus in favor of golf over football, basketball, and baseball, at which he also excelled as a youngster. He liked being able to play golf by himself in the summertime instead of having to round up enough players for a team game.

Jerry Heard is another pro golfer who was a good all-around athlete. At 6 feet and 195 solid pounds, he would look at home roaming center field for the Oakland Athletics or bringing the ball up the court for the Boston Celtics. Heard typifies the athletic young breed newly attracted to the riches of professional golf.

To him, the game's strongest lure is its ongoing challenge. "Unlike other sports, golf always offers you the chance to improve yourself on your own," he says. "It's exciting to improve."

The only-ness. Not only is golf a game of individual skill, it is based on individual integrity. For all the mass commercialism pervading sports today, including golf, golf remains essentially a gentlemanly activity with a bedrock honor system.

The professional golfer calls penalties on himself. If his ball moves in the rough after he has addressed it, he is expected to assess himself an extra stroke even if no one else saw the ball move. It happens almost every week on the tour. It would be naïve to assume that no golfer ever takes advantage of the code, but instances of fudging are so rare, they serve mainly as exceptions to point up the rule.

To Deane Beman, himself a good tour player until he moved upstairs into the commissioner's job, the honor system is golf's special quality. "Golf stands for what all sports are supposed to stand for," he says. "In the quest for winning and making a lot of money, athletes in other sports learn to cut corners. It becomes part of the game. If you're a cornerback in football and a wide receiver gets behind you and catches a pass for a touchdown, the next time he comes off the line of scrimmage you grab his shirt to slow him down. In golf a player doesn't want to win unless he can win fairly."

Beman makes another point about his game. "There are no specialists on the tour, no designated hitters. You have to be able to do it all, from driving to putting. If you have a weakness, you correct it in a hurry or you don't last."

That's a commanding insight from the smallish Beman, who as a player lacked power but was known among his peers as the best on tour with all 14 clubs in his bag. The fifteenth club in his bag was determination.

The only-ness. Not counting himself, the tour player's primary opponent is the course. In no other game, says Jack Nicklaus, is it so distinctly one man against the elements.

On every shot, the golfer must consider the lie of the ball, the air density and wind, and the condition of the ground where the shot will land. No two shots are the same, which imbues golf with bound-less variety—and also makes it unconquerable for even the greatest players.

Its diversity of venues gives golf an aesthetic advantage over other sports. A tennis court is a tennis court is a tennis court, whether in Vancouver or Venezuela. A football field looks the same in Wash-ington, D.C., as it looks in Tacoma, Wash.—and is probably laid with an artificial surface at that.

A golf course, by contrast, is a particular, fetching slice of nature, enhanced (hopefully) by the fine hand of man. If Thoreau were alive and well, I have to believe golf would be his favorite professional sport.

The only-ness. Because each player is competing mostly against the course and against himself, golfers are willing to share their expertise to an extent I have witnessed in no other sport. Visit the practice range at any tournament and you repeatedly will find one player sincerely trying to help sort out the gremlins in the swing of another.

Can you imagine Jimmy Connors offering well-intentioned advice to John Newcombe before they meet in the finals of a major tennis tournament? Hardly. And yet at the Masters tournament last spring Jack Nicklaus was giving intense counsel to Tom Weiskopf shortly before the tournament started. Weiskopf finished second in the Masters to Nicklaus, by the scant margin of one stroke.

The only-ness. A tournament golfer becomes virtually obsessed by the game, so complex are its demands on him.

"A golfer can't be a man of the world," says Steve Reid, a former tour player who now is pro golf's liaison with the television net-works. "The game requires total application. A golfer goes to din-ner with other golfers, and the dinner conversation is all about golf. One guy is going through his round shot by shot, and the other five guys are wishing he'd hurry and finish—so they can go through their rounds."

When Reid was traveling the tour and rooming with Frank Beard, it finally reached the point where he and Beard struck a pact agree-ing never to discuss their rounds in detail. "What'd you shoot?" one would ask. "A 71," the other would reply, and that would be that.

"Charlie Coody is unbelievable," says Beard. "He'll give you his entire round right down to the number of tees he broke. When I see him I say, 'I hope you shot 64, Charlie, so it'll take you only an hour to tell me about it.'"

The only-ness. The typical pro golfer is a staunch conservative. A casual sampling after the last presidential election turned up one player who voted for George McGovern—young Tom Watson.

"Actually, most of us don't follow politics closely, but if we did we'd probably be somewhere to the right of Barry Goldwater," says the vociferous Dave Hill. "Don't let the bright clothes fool you. We're conservatives about almost everything because we've worked hard for a lot of years at this damned game—hit thousands and thousands of practice balls—and we've learned that you get back from it exactly what you put into it, nothing more, nothing less. There are no shortcuts in golf. We have a definite sense of value."

Adds Arnold Palmer, whose future conceivably could include politics, "I keep hearing that golf isn't exciting enough for today's young people, that it isn't violent enough or doesn't relate to the society they're growing up in. That's nonsense. Golf is relevant today. It's a totally individual sport. A golfer pays his own way, pays to enter each tournament, and gets paid only if he performs and in direct proportion to the quality of that performance. Americans like to look on themselves as strong individuals. You can question the social significance of any sport. I think we professionals give a good many people considerable pleasure, and that's important to me."

Arnold also might have noted that golf is sufficiently violent when played with the robust aggressiveness that characterizes his game. If you've ever seen a stop-action photograph of Palmer at impact on a tee shot you have seen enough violence to get you through the day.

The only-ness. The professional golfer goes to work knowing he cannot kid himself about what he accomplishes. He will come home —or back to his motel—with a firm measure of his day's labor: his score. All the excuses in the world (and golfers have been known to contrive some highly imaginative ones) won't change it a fraction of a stroke.

If he fails, the golfer has to confront his failure, accept it, and overcome it. There's no one else to blame.

What sets a golfer apart from other pro athletes? The answer isn't simple; it has as many varied facets as the game itself.

But for a two-word summation it's hard to surpass Hale Irwin's. The only-ness.

The Other Stories of the Year

WORLD SERIES

IT WAS TIANT'S SHOW
(World Series Game I)

By Allen Lewis

From the Philadelphia Inquirer
Copyright, ©, 1975, Philadelphia Inquirer

An awesome performance by an incredible pitcher, and the Boston Red Sox may be on the verge of changing from underdogs to top dogs in the baseball world.

Luis Clemente Tiant, a pudgy Cuban with a Fu Manchu moustache who is thirty-four going on forty, shut out the heavily favored Cincinnati powerhouse on five hits in the first game of the World Series yesterday before 35,205 at Fenway Park, 6–0.

Despite an upsetting and controversial balk called against him in the fourth inning with the game still scoreless, Tiant kept the clamps on the heavy-hitting National League champs for the full nine innings and became the first starter to complete a World Series game in four years.

He did it with his variety of motions, a wide assortment of pitches and masterly control. And he did it despite the fact that his fastball wasn't as swift as it sometimes is.

The final score doesn't indicate the tension of the duel that suddenly erupted in the seventh inning when the Red Sox scored all their runs and chased Cincinnati's best pitcher, left-hander Don Gullett.

As in the American League playoffs, it was captain Carl Yastrzemski who made the big defensive play and got the winning hit. The thirty-six-year-old left fielder kept the Reds from almost certainly taking the lead in the top of the seventh with a diving catch, then singled home the only run Tiant needed. A walk, two more hits, and a sacrifice fly scored the other runs.

"I thought that Yaz won it for them," said the beaten manager, Sparky Anderson, "and Don's slip lost it for us."

Gullett's slip occurred when Dwight Evans bunted after Tiant had led off the big seventh with a single. Gullett's foot gave as he turned and threw to second. Both runners were safe and the rally was on.

"The turf went out from under him," Anderson said. "We warned him about it but he's used to Astroturf instead of grass."

Tiant, credited with his first hit since 1972 because AL pitchers don't get to bat in regular-season games, grounded a fork ball to left and slid into second when Gullett's throw, both low and late, skittered into center field.

Former Phil Denny Doyle, who made two fine defensive plays, fouled off a bunt, then swung and missed before grounding a single through the hole to left field, loading the bases.

"I was glad I didn't get the bunt sign again after popping the first one up," Doyle said. "I was just trying to go the opposite way and keep the ball on the ground, and I was fortunate enough to do both."

"As far as I'm concerned," Yastrzemski said, "the key hit in that inning was Denny Doyle's to left field with men on first and second. It's tough to hit with men on first and second and none out; it's easy to hit with the bases loaded and none out."

Of late, everything seems to come easy for the pride of Boston. After missing a fastball with a vicious swing, Yaz hit the next pitch to right for his all-important single.

As the ball left the bat, Tiant darted back to tag up at third because it appeared Ken Griffey might rush in to make the catch. But the ball fell in front of Griffey and Tiant scored—although he overran the plate and had to go back and tag it.

"I thought he hit it real good," Griffey said, "and I took a step and a half back. Somebody said we had a shot at Tiant, but I didn't even see Tiant until he came back to tag the plate."

Griffey's throw died 20 feet from home and first-baseman Tony Perez cut it off as the Sox ended the scoreless tie—and Gullett's stay on the mound.

Right-hander Clay Carroll relieved and walked Carlton Fisk on a 3–2 pitch to force in a run, then gave way to left-hander Will McEnaney, who promptly struck out left-handed Fred Lynn.

Right-handed Rico Petrocelli, the only remaining—besides Yaz—of the 1967 Red Sox pennant-winners, grounded a two-run single to left and the rout was on.

Rick Burleson, who had three hits and a walk, grounded another run-scoring single to left and Cecil Cooper hit a sacrifice fly to deep right before Tiant, who'd begun it, ended the inning by fouling out to first.

Despite all the running the aging Tiant had to do, he had more than enough of a cushion and retired the last six batters in order.

After the game, soaking his right elbow in ice and puffing on a big cigar, Tiant said, "This was my biggest game. . . . My biggest day in baseball in 11 years. I've had better stuff, but I got outs when I needed them. . . . Always I want to be in a World Series, and now is my chance."

Tiant helped himself get that chance by not only winning 18 games during the regular season, but also by beating Oakland in the playoff opener a week ago and not allowing an earned run in the 7–1 victory.

"I don't like a week off," Tiant said. "I like to pitch every fourth day. That way I have better control. This week, though, I throw hard twice in between, which I don't do when I pitch every fourth day."

In the early going the Red Sox kept wasting scoring chances. They had runners thrown out at the plate in the first and sixth innings, and stranded eight before finally breaking through.

Tiant's biggest jams came in the fifth and seventh, the only innings in which the Reds put more than one runner on base.

George Foster singled at the start of the fifth and, after Dave Concepcion struck out, took second on Griffey's slow roller to third. Here the Sox elected to walk Cesar Geronimo and pitch to Gullett, who homered in the playoff game last week. This time the pitcher fouled out to third.

Foster also opened the seventh with a single to left and Anderson, again disdaining the bunt, let Concepcion hit away.

That looked like a good move when the shortstop hit a looper to short left that appeared to be dropping in for a single—until Yastrzemski came racing in to make a diving tumbling catch.

"I play right behind shortstop in this ball park," Yaz said. "I usually don't dive straight in because of the chance of injury. I usually dive sideways, but this time I had no choice."

The catch kept Foster on first, and he was thrown out trying to steal on the 1–1 pitch to Griffey.

WORLD SERIES

THE OLD CAT-AND-MOUSE GAME
(World Series Game V)

By Si Burick

From the Dayton Daily News
Copyright, ©, 1975, Dayton Daily News

In the sixth inning, when the score was still 2–1, Cincinnati's tricky
Joe Morgan drew a walk from Boston's Reggie Cleveland, then drew
16 throws to first base. Obviously, the pudgy Red Sox right hander
had determined he would not allow Morgan to do his normal thing
by stealing second base again. Joe had filched the base earlier after
a first-inning single.

It was the old cat-and-mouse game. Although Morgan did not
steal, he, as The Mouse, changed the entire course of the contest
by splitting Cleveland's, or The Cat's, concentration between himself and the hitter, Johnny Bench.

Reggie lost the byplay; lost Morgan; lost Bench; lost the next
hitter, Tony Perez; lost, in a manner of speaking, his second baseman, Denny Doyle; lost the ball game; and, maybe, lost the 1975
World Series. Before the inning was over, the Reds scored three
times on Perez's second homer of the night in one monstrous act
of destroying his 0-for-15 World Series slump. Tony's explosion
blasted Reggie Cleveland out of the box, and the Reds went on to
win the fifth game, 6–2. This sends them back to Boston for Saturday's Series renewal at cozy Fenway Park, leading by 3 games to 2.

It was the walk to Morgan and the agitation he created in the
pitcher's mind because of his threat to steal that swung the issue in
favor of Cincinnati and evened Don Gullett's fall tournament record
at 1–1.

Pitching ever so carefully as Little Joe, the Reds' 5–7 stick of
dynamite, led off, Cleveland finally passed him on the 3-and-2
count.

And here the cat-vs.-mouse game began. Bench was the next batter. Reggie threw seven times to first-baseman Carl Yastrzemski before delivering a single pitch to Bench. Morgan took off on that pitch, but Bench, seeing a fastball that was to his liking, fouled it off.

Then Reggie threw four more times to Yaz, but Morgan kept getting back in time from his stealing stance, his right foot on the turf, his left foot barely in the dirt.

Cleveland pitched to Bench again. It was ball one, but this time, Little Joe didn't run—to the surprise of both the pitcher and catcher Carlton Fisk, who was poised to throw to second.

Next, four more throws to first; four safe returns. Three times, Cleveland made Joe dive back. Several throws almost picked Yaz off.

On the Reds' bench, Manager Sparky Anderson turned to Coach Ted Kluszewski and said, "Is he pitchin' to the plate or first base?" Sparky was beginning to feel sorry for Yaz, "jumpin' and divin' for the ball."

The record baseball crowd in Riverfront Stadium of 56,393, while thoroughly enjoying the cat-mouse game, grew restless, and many booed.

After his sixteenth pickoff attempt failed, Cleveland delivered a called strike, a breaking ball, but Morgan did not move. Then, on a second consecutive pitch, Bench bounced a grounder directly at Doyle. "Double play," Johnny muttered, adding some choice expletives.

But a strange thing happened. As the ball approached the veteran second baseman, Doyle ran away from it, toward the base. That almost certain double-play ball—since Morgan had not broken on the pitch—continued into right field for a single.

Morgan raced all the way to third; Bench to second on the throw. When the thoroughly frustrated pitcher threw a fastball inside on the 1-and-2 count to Perez, "The Dog," as his teammates call the lovable Cuban Comet, lashed it high into the seats for three runs. And the happiest man in the park was Joe Morgan, who was responsible for it all.

Sure, Doyle maintained, undoubtedly with total honesty, he lost the ball "out of Bench's uniform." He expected Johnny to hit the ball through the middle. But to Morgan, the drama was created because he broke the concentration of all concerned.

"I enjoy what I do on the bases," Joe said. "Ted Williams loved hitting. I enjoy defense. I enjoy hitting. But I love base-stealing more."

Four times in this World Series, Morgan has drawn a pass. He's proud of the fact that run in front of Tony's homer was his third after walking. In every case, he helped upset the Boston defense.

"My purpose," he said, "is to make the pitcher change his rhythm. The infielders get jumpy. The pitcher gets jumpy. The catcher gets jumpy.

"How could this pitcher concentrate on me on first base—and on Johnny Bench at the plate, too? Everybody's reactions are different when the threat is there.

"That's the difference between having a runner on first and a slow man: the change in defensive reactions."

As a second baseman himself, Morgan felt a natural empathy for Doyle's wrong-way reaction. "Before John swung, I bluffed. I slowed up a little, then I went. I'm sure Doyle lost the ball when John swung, but he also was running for a throw from Fisk."

Sure, the game was won by Don Gullett's lovely pitching; by Perez's two homers; by the offensive production of the team's superstars—Bench, Morgan, and Pete Rose. But it was superstar Morgan's walk and his upsetting influence on the defense that put the Reds back in the Series lead.

Now they need to win one out of a maximum of two remaining games in Fenway Park to make them world's champions for the first time since 1940—or after 35 long years.

WORLD SERIES

PLAY THAT SERIES AGAIN, SAM

By Art Spander

From The Sporting News
Copyright, ©, 1975, The Sporting News Publishing Co.

Play it again, Sam. And Pete, and Dwight and Luis. And all those fans who clung to signboards and hope at Fenway Park, or splashed in the fountains at Cincinnati. Play it again on video tape or play it merely in the mind's eye, throughout the long, cold winter and throughout the decade as well.

This was a World Series to relish, to recall, to replenish, a fortnight of fun and games—and controversy—that proved the value and provided the entertainment that is the essence of baseball, indeed all sport.

Leaping catches and laughing winners, games that seemed to go on forever but still were too short, a nation caught up in the frivolity and feigned importance of an athletic event that has global designation but barely is understood beyond the continent.

So the name is totally pretentious. So it didn't solve the problems in New York or Belfast. So there are a billion Chinese who never heard of Pete Rose.

There are a hundred million Americans who have heard of him, and of Dwight Evans and Sparky Anderson and the Tin Monster and the idea that for a few days each autumn, you don't have to feel guilty about sitting in front of a television set and marveling at the grace and talent of grown men playing a child's game.

For a few days this October, it was 1910 all over again, when sport was as much fun for the participants as it was for the spectators, when headlines provided scores and not casualty numbers, when even winning and losing became secondary to the way the game was played, when cynicism hadn't yet punctured the balloon that was the Great American Dream.

The Cincinnati Reds won this World Series, but nobody lost it. Certainly the Red Sox were disappointed, their fans silenced. Certainly the gaudy trophy that professional baseball decided was obligatory to compete with pro football's will be the property of the Reds. Certainly people like Joe Morgan and Johnny Bench will now be identified with the exaggerated description, world champions.

But the play was the thing in this Series, not the outcome. A few years from now the recollections will be of Luis Tiant stuffing a cigar in his face, of Fred Lynn crashing into an outfield wall, of Tony Perez waiting for a pitch that seemed to have been thrown in a junior high game, of the Reds, at last, jumping and embracing in response to a victory they seemed destined never to achieve.

To be sure, there were aberrations. Red Sox Manager Darrell Johnson was determined to make sports writers believe he could be as churlish as Henry VIII. Anderson tried to convince a lot of people that proper grooming is the only method to save America. And some of the Cincinnati players talked as if they were the greatest thing this side of the 1927 Yankees—before play started in the Series.

But even the managers and the bragging could be overlooked easily—especially if you were intent on watching what was happening on the field or in the stands. And most people certainly were fascinated by what they saw on the field.

The most significant facet of the Series was the interest it aroused in a country that supposedly had lost interest in baseball, that was now said to be intrigued only by football or hockey—or worse, by nothing. No one lost interest. Instead people lost sleep and probably a great deal of betting money when the sixth game crossed into midnight—and into the twilight zone of fantasy.

Home runs that figuratively came at the eleventh hour but in reality were much later on the clock. Catches that would be conversation pieces for a generation. A general feeling of enthusiasm that affected everyone from the pitching mound to those illegally sitting on the billboard behind the park.

Attention and excitement created by that sixth game, by the entire Series was all-encompassing. High taxes and low wages had temporarily been replaced as coffee-break subjects. Teachers acknowledged Tony Perez's batting slump as a current event. Never have so many people outside Massachusetts asked about the weather forecasts for Boston and environs.

Sparky Anderson talked about the days when children would sneak radios into classrooms and teachers, bending the rules, would allow the World Series to be turned on. That, insisted Anderson, was what the Series used to be. And that was what it had again become, although because no games were on midweek afternoons, radios were unneeded.

Television, however, was requisite. It not only put a nation behind home plate, it did it with a mastery that made you forget all the malfeasance that had gone on before—and even to ignore the over-enthusiastic bellows of Joe Garagiola, who may have been the most impetuous man in either ball park.

One of the problems with baseball in recent years, if there were problems, was the game's display on a 21-inch screen. Television might stimulate the growth of football, but it could only hinder baseball, which because of its pace and area could never be presented properly in so confined an area as a picture tube. Or so we believed.

But NBC, with a maximum of cameras and determination, proved baseball could be as big on TV as Johnny Carson. If anything, the network was guilty of overkill, but you'll not get that complaint here. Watching Ed Armbrister step in front of Carlton Fisk, or Dwight Evans leap for a deep fly from a half-dozen different angles only added to the spectacle, reinforced the vision in the brain, provided insight into how the ump blew the interference call and Evans made the catch.

All the anxiety and joy of sport was epitomized in Fisk's elation when he hit that home run in the bottom of the twelfth in game six. And no one saw the play better than the millions in front of television screens.

GOLF

A LANDSLIDE IT WASN'T

By Furman Bisher

From The Atlanta Journal
Reprinted by permission

Well, as you might have expected, Jack Nicklaus won the Masters for the fifth time Sunday. But it wasn't on a TKO. He didn't destroy golf in the process. He didn't do it standing on one leg using one arm, or blindfolded.

He was standing around like the rest of the crowd watching two other very mortal fellows miss putts on the eighteenth green. Thus, the crusade to save golf for the rest of the world, preserve it from the blond Ohio scourge, was called off.

You remember the campaign to "break up Jack Nicklaus"? Well, he almost did, quite emotionally assisted by two other men of the trade. Johnny Miller and Tom Weiskopf. Each had his chance on the eighteenth green, and all Nicklaus could do was stand around like the target at a gunnery range. Miller missed a putt on the low side from about 12 feet, and Weiskopf missed one on the high side from about eight, and the thing was over.

That much of it, charged with tension and nail-biting denouement, became as it turned out, the only drab moments of the fourth round. Nicklaus had putted somewhat "commercially" on the fifteenth green, and again on the eighteenth himself. But Miller and Weiskopf had a chance to run the tournament into Monday, to bring it home for themselves. This is a time that electrifies men's systems. They missed.

This was for no $2 nassau. This was for $40,000 and a touch of immortality. A green jacket. A fellowship in one of the most exclusive clubs of America. This is when the supreme performer presents his soul to posterity on a silver service. They missed, and by that miss, Jack Nicklaus won once more the Masters golf tournament.

The throbbing question of the moment is, what does a man do with five green jackets? Does he open a men's clothing store in Ireland? Does he uniform the bellhops of the Shamrock Hotel? Does he donate his wardrobe to the Fighting Irish of Notre Dame?

Statistics show that beginning in 1963, Jack William Nicklaus has been winning the Masters golf tournament at a rate of one every two and a quarter years. That sets a record. It also brings the poor fellow to grips with the proposition that any time he doesn't win it, there's somebody wants to call an investigation. They also ask him if he has lost his zest for winning.

When he does win it, they want to talk to him about the Grand Slam for the late arrival from Yugoslavia, Samoa, and other foreign soils, which is a figure of speech that includes the four greatest golf tournaments in the world, so to speak—Masters, U.S. Open, British Open, and the U.S. PGA.

"Well, when we started here Thursday, 76 of us had a chance," Nicklaus said this time. "Now there's only one. So I guess you'd have to say I've got a chance."

Mainly, what I want to impress upon you is that it wasn't as easy as it seemed it was going to be after the second round, when Nicklaus was threatening to turn the tournament into a landslide.

There is no bookmaker who would establish odds that Nicklaus would leave six strokes to any field in a day. Saturday, he did it. He simply played like Terry Diehl or Phil Rodgers. You know, the average everyday touring American golf professional who may win a tournament when nobody else is looking.

By Sunday morning, the whole town was so excited people were lined up at the walk-in gates by 7:30, nearly four hours before Rich Karl and Jumbo Ozaki were to tee off. It wasn't a wasted display of fervor. By the end of the day, the crowd had become a stampede. The enthusiasm had lost track with reality. The fight had turned into a classic, matching the three finest players of the time, as it turned out, in a fight 15 rounds to a knockout. No dogs in this one. Class from scalp to toenail.

Nicklaus, Miller, and Weiskopf went around the brilliant acreage of Augusta National as if nobody else was allowed on the course. The U.S. Open champion tied the course record of 64 and made eight birdies and nobody realizes he's playing. It's lost in the milling about and the threshing around of the three leaders. Hale Irwin walks through the clubhouse after the big round and people ask, "Who's that?"

I will not subscribe to the insistence that this was a finish history will have to make room for. Hell, they're forgetting Gene Sarazen and the double eagle that tied Craig Wood. You can't simply sweep aside the finish of 1959, when Art Wall came stroking home with birdies on five of the last six holes and wiped out Arnold Palmer.

Give me Nicklaus sinking the putt on the fifteenth hole. On the seventeenth hole. And on the eighteenth hole, and you've got a finish that's like the cow jumping over the moon again.

This one was like three men trying to catch a greased pig. It was the fox and the hounds from the start, which Nicklaus bogeyed, to No. 18, where Weiskopf and Miller rolled fours. The front nine was a charge and a challenge. On the back nine, the charge and the challenge died in their throats.

Meanwhile, something of insignificance was taking place just ahead of their twosomes. An exercise in pathos, you might say. Arnold Palmer was within earshot throughout the day of all the vocal hysterics of the Nicklaus-Watson, Miller-Weiskopf twosomes. His army had deserted him. Only a few stragglers, dregs of other galleries, spillovers and aimless wanderers watched him play. Background for the scene was the shrieks, the yelps, the wild elation and exaltation of the galleries following the three contenders.

Perhaps Arnold Palmer has become used to this. I haven't. I recall the one moment of the week, brief and fleeting, when he led a Masters for the first time in years. What the excitement was, how the pulse of Augusta beat a little quicker, then how it faded, and one chided himself for ever having entertained such an absurd fantasy.

Once this course was Palmer's. Now it's Nicklaus's. The sentimental value is still there. Some look back upon Palmer as others look back upon Glenn Miller, first dates, the DC-7, homecoming games, and rumble seats. That was another age dismissed to the attic when Jack Nicklaus put on his fifth green jacket.

HORSE RACING

THE LADY IN RED

By Hal Lebovitz

From the Cleveland Plain Dealer
Copyright, ©, 1975, Plain Dealer Publishing Co.

The meeting will come to order precisely at 2 P.M. Friday.

Squeaky Highlow will be there along with Sour Krause, Dr. Zhivago, Dr. Cyclops, Berlin Gertie. The Birdman, One Track Tony, Won Numb, Jungle Larry, Belmost Brooke, and many of the other more colorful personalities of our town.

They'll be there when Wheez Rosenberg, fashioned like a fireplug at a fox hunt, blows his bugle to announce the opening of Thistledown.

The characters at Thistle easily rival Nathan Detroit, Nicely Nicely Johnson, and others traveling through those delightful Damon Runyon fables.

There's a story behind each of those nicknames. Jungle Larry has wild hair; The Birdman is said to be an off-track scientist. Whatever, he flits to the windows—hence, the nickname. Dr. Zhivago and Dr. Cyclops are real doctors trying to diagnose daily winners, and so on.

Too bad the "Lady in Red" is gone. She had become such hot stuff she eventually had to carry a second costume and change in the ladies' room.

On that you have the testimony of Junior O'Malley, a character himself who has worked the mutuel windows at Thistle for over 30 years.

The Lady in Red began her career around Boston tracks. Her husband owned a bakery and the two definitely had dough in common. They figured out a way to beat the horses. Hubby was the shy type so his missus did the betting and rather conspicuously, for she always wore red.

Sam McCracken, the turf writer for *The Boston Globe,* remembers her, but not her name. They never were formally introduced. He is prepared to verify this story, which rivals Damon Runyon's best, but until now has not been made public.

Her system was simple: Pick a huge favorite and play it to show. ("Show" means to finish third, for those who never have been to a track. If a horse finishes first, second, or third, the track pays off on a show bet.)

By law, even if there isn't enough money in the betting pool, the track must pay a profit on a winning ticket of at least 10 cents on the dollar. Thus, a $2 winning show ticket brings back at least $2.20 in Massachusetts. Also in Ohio.

That's a sure 10 percent return, figured the baker and his wife. On $2 it doesn't mean much. But on $10,000 it comes to a clear $1,000. Beats kneading dough, to coin a phrase, or so the baking couple decided.

The Lady in Red would head for the $50 or $100 window and start peeling out the big bankroll, buying her show tickets on the heavy favorite. In a reasonably short period, McCracken recalls, she put together about a dozen jackpots at Suffolk and Rockingham.

It got so that if the track saw her they sometimes would call off the show bets in a race where there was an overriding favorite. On other occasions the mutuel clerk somehow would manage to jam the machine. Becoming aware of these tricks and hoping to keep the odds as high as possible, she often would wait until shortly before the race was off to place her bet.

The dough was turning to a lovely golden hue for the Lady as she zeroed in on the Massachusetts Handicap of 1950. Assault, the famous King Ranch horse, which had won the 1946 Triple Crown, was running in a five-horse race. It was announced in advance "show betting" would be permitted. A cinch for this great horse to take a third to finish in the money, agreed the baker and his wife.

The Lady in Red put her entire roll, $30,000, on Assault to show, figuring on a $3,000 profit. Assault finished fourth.

Occasionally she was seen around Boston tracks after that, making $2 bets. Meanwhile, she saved up for a comeback.

This time she decided to try Thistledown, where the chalk usually is heavy. ("Chalk" is a racetrack expression meaning the favorites generally win.)

At Thistle she bet the chalk to show and she would win. The word got around and other bettors began to follow her to the window.

To avoid them she eventually had to take along a change of clothing and switch in the ladies' room from the red she loved to something more subdued.

But, alas, one day the heaviest chalk finished out of the money and the Lady in Red never was seen again.

In her place at Thistle has come "The Colonel," alias "Show Man," who has been using the Lady's identical system, wagering $10,000 at a crack on show tickets on Thistle's chalk.

Last summer, according to Junior O'Malley, Show Man put a bundle on a sure thing. The race became so topsy-turvy that the actual winner paid $6 to win, $3 to place, and $8 to show. Show Man's horse finished fifth. He was tapped out.

O'Malley has it on good authority. Show Man has come up with a new bankroll and has been waiting eagerly for Thistle to open again.

He'll be there looking for chalk Friday—unless perhaps he reads this.

There's a moral in it somewhere.

HORSE RACING

THE GREAT DICTATOR OF THE THOROUGHBRED WORLD

By Neil Milbert

From the Chicago Tribune
Copyright, ©, 1975, Chicago Tribune

Foolish Pleasure, a colt whose funny way of walking is remindful of Charlie Chaplin, became The Great Dictator of the thoroughbred world this gray Saturday afternoon.

He ran a masterful race.

The race was the one hundred first Kentucky Derby at Churchill Downs.

Rumbling down the stretch with the authority of a panzer tank, he blasted the last vestige of opposition to bits with an eighth of a mile to go and drew off to a decisive victory before 113,323 onlookers.

At about the same time Foolish Pleasure roared past, Avatar and Diabolo, who had been battling for the lead, collided.

But neither Bill Shoemaker, who rode Avatar, nor Diabolo's jockey, Laffit Pincay, felt the collision had any bearing on the outcome of America's premier horse race.

"I got beat by a better horse," said Shoemaker. "I might have been a little closer, but the collision certainly didn't keep me from winning."

Pincay concurred. "He just got tired," Pincay said of Diabolo, who two weeks ago ran the fastest California Derby ever. "My horse came in more than Shoe's came out. We got turned sideways when we hit, but I can't say it made a difference in the outcome."

Foolish Pleasure, who charged past Diabolo on the outside, cleared the collision with room to spare. In fact, jockey Jacinto Vasquez said he didn't even see the Californians collide.

The winner prevailed by two and one-half lengths over runner-up Avatar. Diabolo held on for third, trailing the place horse by another two and one-half.

Diabolo pulled up lame, bleeding badly from a gash just below his knee, and the stewards conducted an inquiry involving the No. 2 and 3 finishers. But they decided Diabolo was to blame and validated the order of finish.

Foolish Pleasure's time for one and one-quarter miles was 2:02 flat. (The record time is Secretariat's 1:59 2–5 set in 1973.)

The crowd made Foolish Pleasure the 19–10 favorite in the $262,-100 race. He overcame 14 adversaries and paid $5.80, $4.40, and $3.60. (There were 12 betting interests; Prince Thou Art and Sylvan Place ran as an entry, and Fashion Sale, Gatch, and Rushing Man were linked as the field.)

Many of the people at Churchill Downs and those who saw the race thought it was the highly touted Prince Thou Art when Foolish Pleasure made his stretch move. Announcer Chick Anderson erroneously called "Prince Thou Art," and didn't correct himself until just before the wire.

"I heard him call the wrong horse," said Vasquez, "and I looked around to see if he was coming. I didn't see anybody and I saw the wire coming up. I said, 'Let him call the other horse—he's going to need a jet engine to catch me, and I know he don't have one.'"

Foolish Pleasure, breaking from the No. 3 post position, was restrained by Vasquez and dropped far back.

"I was surprised because it didn't seem to me he broke too well," said trainer LeRoy Jolley. "When he went by the stands the first time it didn't look like he was handling the track too well.

"Then I saw the fraction of :22 go up for the first quarter and I felt better. I realized those horses on the front end (Bombay Duck and Rushing Man) were burning pretty hard.

"No, I didn't give Jacinto any instructions before the race. He has given a great deal of himself to the horse. He's been riding him since last year and he even comes out mornings to work him.

"It would really be pretty stupid to tell someone who knows the horse as well as he does what to do."

For about five-eighths of a mile, Foolish Pleasure ran in an unhurried manner. Then, he made his move, rushing along the inside and leaving horse after horse in his wake.

In the stretch, Vasquez steered the colt to the outside and there was no stopping them.

As they turned for home, Diabolo and Avatar were showing the way. But when Foolish Pleasure crossed the wire, both of these California-based colts were bent, spindled, and mutilated.

The victory was the eleventh in Foolish Pleasure's 12-race career. His only defeat came in the Florida Derby in March, a race in which he slashed the soft cushions of both front hooves. Even then he was able to salvage show money, finishing behind Prince Thou Art and Sylvan Place.

Foolish Pleasure is still being treated for the wounds he suffered in that race. But on Saturday, trainer Lou Rondinello's entry didn't even provide token opposition. Prince Thou Art finished an unimpressive sixth; Sylvan Place was ninth.

While the bettors remained steadfast in supporting winter book favorite Foolish Pleasure, there were skeptics galore going into the race. Writers and trainers here repeatedly questioned the pedigree of Foolish Pleasure, contending that his breeding (What a Pleasure —Fool Me Not, by Tom Fool) wasn't equal to the one and one-quarter mile test.

All along, owner John Greer, trainer Jolley, and jockey Vasquez dismissed the theory that Foolish Pleasure couldn't handle the Derby distance.

"Every time, he did everything I asked," said Vasquez. "The only time he didn't (the Florida Derby) he had a reasonable excuse—he was hurt.

"No, I can't compare him with Secretariat. I never rode Secretariat. But I know this. Secretariat got beat a few times (three times, once by disqualification) before the Derby. And he's supposed to be the horse of the century.

"My horse only got beat once—and that day he was hurt. Sure, I think we can win the Triple Crown."

Coming up next is the Preakness at Pimlico in two weeks, followed by the June 7 Belmont.

Saturday's triumph earned Foolish Pleasure $209,600 and he will go into the Preakness with a career bankroll of $673,515. The Florida-bred was acquired by Greer for only $20,000 at the Saratoga Sales.

The funny way he walked with his feet pointed out turned off the majority of those who saw him at the sale.

Earlier in the week, Jolley was asked if he had done anything to compensate for that funny way of walking. "I didn't have to," the trainer replied. "Horses are athletes. The ones with heart and desire overcome their disabilities. The others don't."

GENERAL

MUHAMMAD ALI TAKES ON HARVARD

By Larry Eldridge

From The Christian Science Monitor
Copyright, ©, 1975, The Christian Science Publishing Society
Reprinted by permission from The Christian Science Monitor

The ivy-covered walls and the bookshelves lined with Dickens and Thackeray looked formidable at first, but just like most of Muhammad Ali's foes in the ring they too turned out to be overmatched.

The world heavyweight champion's debut as a Harvard lecturer was a knockout from beginning to end. He took over the sedate faculty club as though he'd been born to academe, handled a jammed press conference with his usual skill, then wowed an audience of graduating seniors with an hour-long speech.

Introduced as "Professor Muhammad Ali," the champion held to a serious vein during most of his address, discoursing on life and love and the value of friendship.

"I had to let you know there are more sides to Muhammad Ali than you see on TV," he explained.

But eventually he gave his audience the showman's side too—reciting some of his famous poems and drawing whoops and shouts as he pranced around the stage doing the Ali shuffle and imitating Howard Cosell.

Ali was originally invited by the seniors to address their Class Day exercises on June 11, but after accepting the date he realized he'd have to leave the country before that to get ready for his June 30 title defense in Kuala Lumpur against Great Britain's Joe Bugner. He then agreed to come this week instead and waived his usual $3,000 fee, saying it was "a big, big honor" just to speak at Harvard.

Arriving on campus with an entourage including his wife and several aides, Ali was resplendent in a salmon-pink suit, blue shirt, and striped tie. He was right in his element at the beginning too, thrust into a huge auditorium for a noisy, crowded press conference like hundreds of others he's had over the years.

"Friendship is the hardest thing in the world to explain," he said in words he also later repeated to the students. "It's not something you learn in school. But if you haven't learned the meaning of friendship, you really haven't learned anything."

In a lighter vein, Ali regaled his audience with an excellent imitation of Cosell.

"After every fight he always says to me, 'Muhammad, you're not the same man as 10 years ago,' " the champion said. "That shows the extent of his knowledge. Who is the same man he was 10 years ago?"

When somebody noted that Cosell has predicted Ali will lose to Bugner, the champion shot back: "That must mean I'm going to knock him out." Ali wouldn't make one of his famous predictions about the round, however, or even a serious one about the outcome of the fight, saying only that, "Joe Bugner is a good fighter."

In answer to another question Ali said that while he likes to display his skills, he doesn't enjoy boxing as a whole—and never did. Asked why he has pursued it as a career he replied:

"It's not the action that makes a thing right or wrong but the purpose. My purpose is to help my people, and I can do it through boxing. My purpose is to be the biggest black man in the world, and here I am. No other person in the world is as well known as I am. Not Ford, not Kissinger. I have the most recognized face in the whole world."

When Ali, who confesses to "barely making it out of high school with a D-minus average," was asked to speak at this center of culture it raised a few eyebrows, and it did indeed seem an incongruous sight when he and his party first battled through the crowds into the faculty club for a prespeech reception and dinner. But the champion, relaxed and confident and in control of the situation as always, soon demonstrated that he wasn't about to be intimidated by the academic world.

"I was anxious to come here and match wits with these people," he said. "I do a lot of studying in my own way, but I don't give this side to the boxing world. People don't pay for that. They pay for foolishness."

Ali also noted with his engaging smile that "I can't read or write very well, but I can hire people who can."

With his speech, Ali held the audience of some 1,200 students and others spellbound for the first half hour with a straight, serious

discussion of his philosophy. Noting that he was probably addressing future leaders in many walks of life he advised the seniors:
"Remember what you are today, because when you make it you have
a tendency to forget what you were yesterday . . . I'm from Louisville, Kentucky; a little black boy who made $18 a week and wanted
to be Golden Gloves champ."

You don't ask Muhammad Ali who the greatest fighter is, of
course. That goes without saying. So one bright student phrased the
question in a way more appealing to the champion. Who, he asked,
is the second greatest fighter?

"That's a smart question," Ali said, "but do you mean for now or
for all time? The second best fighter of all time was Sugar Ray
Robinson. The second best right now is Foreman."

And how does Ali rank the great heavyweights of history—after
himself of course?

"The second greatest heavyweight was Jack Johnson, but in my
prime I would have been too fast for him. He fought like this (here
the champion adopted an awkward, stiff, stand-up stance a la James
Earl Jones in *The Great White Hope*). He could never have hit me even
if we went 25 rounds."

As for the upcoming Bugner fight, Ali indicated he was taking it
a lot more seriously than he had his recent bouts against Chuck
Wepner and Ron Lyle.

"I'm running twice a day—six miles every day. I don't have to do
much gym work anymore, you know. I know how to box! But I'm
building my legs and wind to move for 15 rounds if I have to.

"I can still move when I want to, you know. I did it for a couple
of rounds there in the middle of my last fight. I was beautiful—
moving, sticking. Float like a butterfly, sting like a bee. His hands
couldn't hit what his eyes couldn't see!"

Ali has a tendency to get carried away at times like this, rolling
his eyes and shadowboxing, but it's all an act, of course. And he
came right back when asked if he'd fight Foreman again assuming
he gets by Bugner.

"Frazier first," he said. "I've had offers from the Philippines and
also from Egypt. Maybe after whupping Lyle I'll get Frazier on the
Nile."

BASKETBALL

WAYNE ESTES'S FINAL GAME

By Harvey Kirkpatrick

From Sport
Copyright, ©, 1975, M.V.P. Sport, Inc.

Wayne Estes played his last basketball game 10 years ago. No one suspected it was going to be his last game, no one except, perhaps, Wayne Estes.

The leading scorer in college basketball 10 years ago was a University of Miami senior named Rick Barry. The third leading scorer in college basketball 10 years ago was a Princeton University senior named Bill Bradley. The second leading scorer, behind Barry and ahead of Bradley, was a Utah State University senior named Wayne Estes.

Going into his last game, against Denver University on a snowy night early in February 1965, Estes was averaging 32.9 points a game. He was 6-feet-6, weighed 225 pounds, and could shoot from inside or out. "Wayne Estes," said one enthusiastic sports writer, "possesses a touch of velvet."

But early in the game against Denver, Estes thought he had lost his velvet touch. He had no feeling in his hands. "Take me out," Estes suggested to the Utah State coach, LaDell Andersen. The coach refused. "Keep on shooting," said Andersen. "They'll start dropping."

Estes kept shooting, and soon his shots started dropping. He sank his last 11 shots before half time, and at the intermission, he had scored 24 points. Still, Estes insisted his hands were numb. "Go out and score 24 more," said coach Andersen with a laugh, "and we'll operate on you after the game."

In the second half, Estes scored 24 more, and when his last shot ever dropped through the basket, a jump shot from 20 feet out, near the right baseline, he had a new single-game scoring record for Utah

State's Nelson Fieldhouse and he had a school career scoring record of 2,001 points. Utah State won the game, and its happy fans carried Estes off the court. His average was up to 33.7 points a game; he had made 49 percent of his field-goal attempts for the season and 88 percent of his free throws. He was a cinch to be an All-America.

"I was just putting the ball up," said Estes, during a radio interview after the Denver game. "Somebody else was putting it in for me."

Within a few hours, he was dead.

Two months earlier, at the age of twenty-one, with a bright athletic future stretching in front of him, Wayne Estes had purchased a $10,000 life-insurance policy. He bought the policy from L. Jay Silvester, a former Olympic shot-putter and discus-thrower. Estes asked Silvester whether the triple-indemnity clause for accidental death applied to death by electrocution.

After the game against Denver, the Utah State trainer pricked Estes's finger with a pin. Estes, the trainer reported, failed to show the normal reaction. The team doctor said that Estes was probably overly keyed up; he said that if the numbness did not disappear, he would conduct a thorough physical examination in a few days.

Estes showered, got dressed, then telephoned his parents in Anaconda, Mont. "I've never played so well in my life," he told his parents. Then Estes and a few of his friends went to celebrate with a pizza.

On the way back to their off-campus apartment, cruising along the snow-slickened streets of Logan, Utah, Estes and his friends passed the scene of an automobile accident. An ambulance was already on hand, but Estes and his friends stopped to see if they could be of any help.

Everything was under control. Estes and his friends started to walk back to their car. A sagging wire from a bent telephone pole was swaying overhead, its lowest point almost six and a half feet from the ground. His friends passed under it. Estes's forehead brushed the live wire. Several thousand watts of electricity shot through his body.

"Wayne's hands started to smoke, and he fell to the ground," John Vasey, one of Estes's companions, said later.

Coach LaDell Andersen and his wife were on their way home from a victory party when they, too, passed the accident that had caught Estes's attention. They, too, stopped, and Andersen walked quickly toward the still body lying on the snowy sidewalk.

As Andersen approached, and was recognized, someone called out, "It's Wayne."

Andersen stopped. "Well, he's all right, isn't he?" said the coach.

Technically, Estes was already dead. A doctor, policemen, and ambulance attendants were working over him, trying to revive him, trying to bring some feeling back into his large body. Andersen and his wife, who had practically adopted Estes into their home, both prayed. Nothing helped. LaDell Andersen telephoned Estes's mother and father in Anaconda. He cried when he told them that their son was dead.

A few days later, the entire population of Anaconda lined the city's streets all the way to a small cemetery on a hillside. Youngsters who had spent their summers shagging shots for Wayne Estes cried openly. So did their parents.

Rick Barry was drafted by the San Francisco Warriors on the first round of the 1965 college draft. Bill Bradley was selected by the New York Knicks on the first round of the 1965 college draft. The Los Angeles Lakers, in the first round, selected Gail Goodrich, who was not their original choice.

The Lakers had planned to pick Wayne Estes.

GOLF

THE QUIET GOLFER FROM NASHVILLE

By Bob Addie

From The Washington Post
Copyright, ©, 1975, The Washington Post

Lou Graham, a thirty-seven-year-old journeyman, proved that, like the presidency, the U.S. Open golf championship is within the reach of the common man.

The quiet golfer from Nashville, Tenn., who once served in President Kennedy's honor guard, won the Open today with a par 71 in an 18-hole playoff at Medinah Country Club, two shots better than Houston's John Mahaffey.

Mahaffey, 10 years younger than Graham but growing older fast, finished second for the fourth time this year and the eighth time in his career. "Mr. Almost" had a cold putter today and that told the story.

Graham served in the army at Ft. Myer in 1960–61 and was part of the president's ceremonial guard, in addition to doing several tours as a sentry at the Tomb of the Unknown Soldier.

"Even then I played golf every chance I could," he said. "I played some on public courses around Washington and once in a while I got an 'invite' to a country club."

Upon his discharge from the army, Graham worked for a time at Ft. Meade and then was an assistant pro at Chestnut Hills, Baltimore, before going back home to Nashville and trying the tour.

Graham had a three-stroke lead coming down "Death Valley," the seventeenth and eighteenth holes. That was where this Diamond Open was decided.

Frustrated all day, Mahaffey used a 3-iron on the 220-yard seventeenth and was 10 feet above the hole. Meanwhile, Graham's 3-iron shot went over the green, he chopped out, and the ball slid eight feet past the pin. Mahaffey could have picked up two strokes with a birdie, but missed and got par. Graham missed his eight-footer for a bogey and now his margin was down to two strokes.

"I was calm on the seventeenth," Graham said, "I was talking myself out of thinking that this was the U.S. Open. I said, 'Lou, this is only another golf game, boy.' But after the seventeenth, that subconscious or whatchamacallit kept bugging me that this really was the U.S. Open."

Mahaffey put a perfect drive down the fairway on the eighteenth. Graham again had problems with the narrow, 406-yard hole that cost him the title outright on Sunday. He had bogeyed the hole three out of four times in regular play in his rounds of 74, 72, 68, 73 for 287. He used a 2-iron off the tee this time and ducked it into the left rough, in a cluster of spectators.

"I heard Bob Rosburg, who was doing the TV for ABC, say that the ball hit a spectator. I got to the ball and it was under a tree but only seven yards from out of bounds. That's when I said to myself, 'This golf tournament belongs to Lou Graham.' I then punched a 4-iron, low and running to the green."

Mahaffey also heard Rosburg (who must have been using a bullhorn). "That revelation by Rosburg [that Graham's ball had hit a spectator] didn't exactly tickle me to death," the Texan said.

P. J. Boatwright, executive secretary of the USGA, sent word that Graham's ball didn't hit a spectator. But it was hard to see how the ball could have missed the crowd, gathered five deep at the finishing hole.

If the ball had gone out of bounds, it would have meant a penalty of stroke and distance, sending Graham back to the tee where he would have been hitting three.

Instead, Graham was able to hit a low hook under and around the trees to within five yards of the green. He chipped within seven feet after Mahaffey hit his second shot within 10 feet. Graham made his putt for par after Mahaffey missed his birdie attempt.

Each man parred the first hole but the pattern was set on the second hole, a 187-yard par-three with carry over water. Both got on the green. Graham putted first and almost holed a curling putt on a break of at least three feet. He got his par.

Mahaffey, about 12 feet away, misread the green completely, the ball breaking below the hole and dropping three feet. He missed the comeback, took a bogey, and was one stroke down.

The stroke play went even again on the third when Mahaffey got his par four but Graham put a 9-iron shot over the green, came back 15 feet long, and missed.

Graham then got birdies on the fourth and fifth. He put a 7-iron

10 feet from the pin on the fourth and made it. He pitched to six feet on the fifth and made that, too. Mahaffey parred both holes and now was two strokes back.

Graham consistently outdrove Mahaffey all day. On the sixth, Graham cracked his longest drive of the tournament, 290 yards down the fairway. Mahaffey was 50 yards behind in the rough but managed to halve with a par.

Graham saved par on the 205-yard eighth when he put a 3-iron over the green, ran it past the cup eight feet, and made the putt to save par. "I think that was a key putt," said Graham, who had others. He turned in one-under-par 35 to Mahaffey's 37.

Graham picked up another stroke on the tenth when he hit a 4-wood off the tee down the middle for what he described as "my best shot of the day." He put a 2-iron in the rough and then hit a pitching wedge from 115 yards within three feet, making the birdie putt.

Graham had nine straight fours on the back and two of them cost him bogeys on the short holes—the fourteenth and seventeenth. But the fours were enough to win this twenty-sixth playoff in 75 U.S. Opens.

Mahaffey just couldn't buy a putt. He had something like seven opportunities for birdies within 10 feet and missed them all. He didn't have a birdie all day. He had 37 putts.

"I didn't hit too many bad shots," he said, "but I couldn't putt. I never got the ball to the hole. I threw away the golf tournament on the greens."

Graham seemed dazed by his achievement. What does winning the U.S. Open mean to a man who has been, except for one year on the Ryder Cup team, an obscure member of the gang? He joined the tour in 1964 and has won two victories in his career, both in tournaments since dropped from the tour. This year he finished in the top 10 four times.

"It's hard to say how I do feel," he said. "It's something you dream about. Few players on the tour think they'll ever win it. They hope they will and they hope they have the guts to win it. I don't feel like a U.S. Open champion. It's hard to get into my mind. It's a tremendous achievement—difficult to imagine."

Graham shot a 65 to lead the Philadelphia Classic in the first round last week and then faded. "A Philadelphia newspaper guy wrote that nobody would ever recognize my face," Graham said. "So all day today whenever anybody took my picture, I said: 'Do me a favor. Send a copy to that guy in Philadelphia so he might remember my face.' Maybe a few people will now."

GENERAL

CHINA THROUGH DIFFERENT EYES

By Will Grimsley

From The Associated Press
Copyright, ©, 1975, The Associated Press

Two young Americans struggled clumsily with chopsticks in the second-floor dining room of the modernistic Peking Hotel and groped for an insight to this vast country of 900 million people—one-fourth of the world's population.

"They are beautiful," said Terry Porter, twenty-three, of Wharton, Tex. "They don't have much by our standards but they all seem happy. If I didn't have some problems to clear up back home, I wouldn't mind living here for a while."

"But their life is so drab," said Roland Carter, twenty-eight, of Houston. "They all dress alike, the men and women both, with those blue and gray Mao jackets. They are pleasant enough but they seem so programmed. There seems to be no individuality or incentive to their lives."

Here were two men of similar cultures from the same Texas—and with a common competitive aim—to pole-vault in the 1976 Olympics. They spent two weeks getting a close look at the People's Republic of China, but they saw through different eyes.

"Achievement is the name of the game in this world," Carter argued. "I am reading a book about that. Man was put on earth to strive and achieve. I admire what the Chinese have done for the people generally but I think their lives are too patent. They are denied enterprise. All their efforts are funneled into the state."

"But," interceded Porter, "they have managed to keep 900 million people fed and clothed. That's something in itself when you consider how many people are starving in India and Africa and idle in the big Western countries like Britain and the United States."

Such discussions have been commonplace among Americans

who have visited China this year. They certainly were among the 94 Americans—64 members of a track-and-field team, coaches, managers, physicians, and other official personnel—who visited Canton, Shanghai, and Peking recently at the invitation of the Chinese.

Almost unanimously, the visitors were impressed by what they saw—masses turning red clay beds into green farmlands, once rusting factories into bustling enterprises, and cities that once reeked with dope peddlers and prostitution into metropolises of respectability.

"I can't get over how friendly everyone is," said Jane Frederick of Goleta, Calif., a high jumper whose father is a retired professor of political science at the University of California. "It's so different than the trip we made to the Soviet Union. The people there seemed so grim. I notice so many children playing in the streets here. I never saw that in Russia."

The Americans found an absence of red tape and a seemingly genuine warmth and hospitality in all of the three cities they visited. People lined the sidewalks and formed human corridors outside the stadiums, smiling and clapping as the visitors entered and disembarked from their buses.

Never during the trip did the Americans experience a feeling of being under surveillance. Army men, in their loose-fitting green uniforms, could be seen strolling the streets but few wore guns. They never presented themselves as a barrier, not even at the border where the group changed from a Hong Kong train to a clean, air-conditioned streamliner for Canton.

In Canton, a city of 2.5 million, the visitors were astounded to see the main streets swarming with bicycles, thousands of them as thick as ants.

They appeared to have right of way over the few buses and automobiles, which moved slowly through the morass only because the drivers kept their thumbs on constantly honking horns.

"There are 500,000 bicycles in Canton—one for about every five people," a guide explained politely. "It is our main means of transportation. No one is allowed to own an automobile—only the government for official business and taxicabs."

For the Chinese, a shiny bike is like an automobile to an American. A good one costs $75, about twice the average monthly salary of a worker or farmer.

Hundreds of the bicycles are parked at shopping centers or at the big stadiums where athletic events take place.

"Lock them? No, there is no need to lock them," the guide replied to an obvious question. "No one would ever think of riding away on another's bicycle."

China prides itself on the absence of crime. One sees no beggars or derelicts on the streets. During their two weeks in the country, the Americans saw thousands of Chinese but never a drunk or disorderly person.

Shanghai once was the sin capital of the Orient. Dens of iniquity beckoned sailors and vagabonds. Prostitution thrived. Slave peddlers, dope merchants, and smugglers operated openly. Today the city of 10 million is one of the cleanest and most sophisticated in the world.

The U.S. entourage visited a kindergarten school in Shanghai where deaf and mute children of preschool age were being treated with acupuncture.

Nurses with the long, sharp needles entered the room and signaled to the tykes to bend their heads over their desks. They responded in unison. Then the needles were applied. There wasn't a single whimper.

"This treatment has been successful in about 80 percent of the cases," a physician explained through an interpreter. Later the visitors were to witness a singing performance by some of those who had been cured.

As Chinese officials haul their guests by bus to various points of interest—a model commune, a factory, a children's palace, the Forbidden City, and the Great Wall—they follow a fixed routine.

First, the guests are brought into a large reception room and are seated at long tables with cups of green tea and small packages of cigarettes in front of them.

Then, through an interpreter, the director of the particular project, explains how the common people were abused by the land barons and rich owners before the revolution. Finally, he relates the great changes that have been made by Chairman Mao Tse-tung.

Always a giant picture of the chairman, with a mole on his chin, looks down from one of the walls. On an opposite wall hang side-by-side pictures of Karl Marx and Joseph Stalin, the father and one of the chief exponents of communism.

The Chinese continue to honor Stalin although the Russians refer to him as "a comrade who lost his mission."

A thread of militancy runs through China's doctrine of friendliness, selflessness, and honesty.

When a Chinese youth finishes middle school—equivalent to American high school—he or she must work in a factory or go to a farm for two years before entering upon a career.

"The purpose is to avoid the establishment of an urban class," a Chinese spokesman explained.

Even university students and professors are required to do farm and factory work periodically lest they grow fat and contented—losing concern for the ordinary worker—in their citadels of learning.

At Tsing Hua University in Peking, the Americans met a little electronics professor named Dr. Tung Shih Pai who had earned a Ph.D. at the University of Illinois in three years and had taught at Brooklyn Polytechnic Institute before returning to China in 1955.

An old Dodger fan, he was distressed to learn of the death of Jackie Robinson and the demise of Ebbets Field. He was anxious to hear about New York's teeming subways and fender-scraping taxicabs.

Someone remarked that it was marvelous that the professor could attain a Ph.D. in three years.

"That is easy," he replied solemnly. "Learning the truth is hard." He did not elaborate.

Then an American asked him if he thought capitalism and communism could ever be compatible.

"History will tell," he said.

BASKETBALL

LITTLE LOOIE

By Tony Kornheiser

From Street & Smith Basketball Annual
Copyright, ©, 1975, Conde Nast Publications, Inc.

Little Looie has his recruiting budget for the year spread out in front of him in little piles—100 subway tokens, 50 bus transfers, and two $5 gift certificates from Orange Julius.

He's on the phone, talking to his co-captains for next season: Solly "Rat" Pizzaroni, a half-Jewish, half-Italian point guard with boils on his neck, whose idea of a good time is drinking a six-pack of beer and then eating the bottles. Tough kid. And So-Sweet Cecil Robinson, a 6-foot-4, 150-pound forward who plays with a toothpick behind each ear and moves up and down the court like he's being chased by a street gang.

They're making plans to meet and Little Looie is giving directions. "You take the CC train to Utopia Parkway. Wait for the D bus, and take it to Union Turnpike. Then walk over to the deli on Avenue J. I'll be in the back booth eating a turkey and pastrami on club."

And right away you know we're not talking about Montana.

St. John's University (St. John's, N.Y., on your top-20 AP and UPI weekly polls) plays its home basketball games at Alumni Hall, which is something less than a palace but nothing to be ashamed of. It holds about 6,000 people, and at any given time 4,500 of them have sons or cousins or good friends who play or played for the team. It's a family place. Like McDonald's, only the food's worse. Little Looie Carnesecca, who coaches St. John's and would probably sweep out the gym if they asked him to, thinks of Alumni Hall as his home.

"My blood is down there on that floor," he says.

And if they'd wax it, they'd probably find his coat and his tie, too.

Looie doesn't so much coach a game as he orchestrates it. He scurries up and down the sidelines like a field mouse, barking instructions at his players and bellowing cross-examinations at the officials. Looie never sits in a chair, not since the time a few years ago when he sat down where he thought his chair was and ended up on his butt because his chair was in the stands, where he booted it 10 traveling violations earlier. You can lose weight just watching Looie coach. The only way to keep him reasonably close to his bench is to tie an elastic cord on his belt and jerk him back there on times-out.

"Before every game," he says, "I tell my assistants to hold me down. Keep an eye on me. But I just get so involved in the flow of the game. . . ."

Looie's style is controlled chaos, and who can argue with his results? In seven years as head coach—he did split shifts, taking off three years to coach and general manage the New York Nets—St. John's has won 145 games and gone to seven postseason tournaments, three NCAAs and four NITs. Granted, St. John's could go to every NIT from now to Doomsday because the Redmen sell more tickets than say, Lemoyne-Owen (Tenn.). Guaranteed that one of these years St. John's will go to the NCAAs, and the NIT will list the Redmen as a tournament team anyway, figuring people will buy tickets because they won't believe that there can be an NIT without St. John's.

But seriously folks, let's look at the numbers. In the past 69 years St. John's has won 1,070 games, fourth best in the nation. In the past 56 years the Redmen have had only two losing seasons, and since postseason tourneys began in 1938, St. John's has been to more of them—seven NCAAs and 23 NITs—than any other school. Say what you want about the NIT (but don't let the *New York Post* hear you); some pretty good teams have won that tournament. And four of them have been St. John's.

"We've got a basketball tradition," Looie says. "It's imbedded in the bricks here. You know how they breed the bulls for the ring? It's the same thing here."

Buck Freeman. Joe Lapchick. Frank McGuire. Kevin Loughery. Leroy Ellis. Billy Paultz. Tony Jackson. Alan Seiden. Bobby and Kenny MacIntyre. Johnny Warren. Joe DePre. Billy Schaeffer. Mel Davis. Sonny Dove. Mel Utley. Carmine Calzonetti.

Carmine Calzonetti?

"I beat him down the court once against Fordham," Looie says. "He had a breakaway lay-up, but I was really moving."

Not only great coaches and players, but such exotic names, too. St. John's never gets your run-of-the-mill Bill Smith. This year they've got one, and he comes with the nickname, Beaver. They get a common, ordinary Glen Williams, and he comes up from the Virgin Islands. Frankie "Flea" Alagia and Hernel Robertson are more like it. Carmine Calzonetti with the drive—yes, and it counts.

But let's not paint too romantic a picture. St. John's won't be competing for a national championship in the near future. Even though the Redmen have New York City to draw from, they rarely get the superior blue-chipper they need to escape the NIT. The plain fact is that most city kids would rather leave the city as soon as it's humanly possible. Cunningham. Hawkins. Archibald. Alcindor. Meminger. Grunfeld. King. The list goes on forever.

And since St. John's doesn't have any dorms to offer, Looie has to go after what's left behind after the cream has whipped itself off to cleaner air. He's a 50-cent subway token away from any playground in the city (except Staten Island—nobody plays any ball in Staten Island), and when he gets there, the pitch is always the overhand fastball. No sense in being subtle.

"If you're a great player and you wanna be a pro," Looie says, "this city is your stage. You're gonna get to play in the Garden, the mecca. You're gonna get the TV, the newspapers, the coverage. You go to a small town and 10,000 people will see you. You play here and 13 million people will know about you. Why do Jabbar and Erving and McGinnis want to play here? Because it's the only place to play. And maybe one day in New York is more of an education than one month in any other city."

Sometimes you eat the bear, and sometimes the bear eats you. Looie gets his share, but Wooden and Knight and Driesell and Smith and both McGuires get more. Looie's teams have to win with hustle and guile. They have to scrounge like rats and dive for loose balls like winos dive for spare change on the Bowery. And even if they make it, sometimes nobody's watching.

You got Nassau Coliseum to the east, and the Garden to the west. The Nets, the Knicks, the Islanders, the Rangers, the Metropolitan Opera, Broadway shows, first-run movies, the U.N., the Giants, the Jets, and more hookers than Idaho has potatoes. Fear city demands the best.

"You've gotta give it to them," Looie says. "They expect it. We get newspaper men who cover the Knicks one night and St. John's the next. You don't con them. You play like dogs and they write about you like Gravy Train. . . . But the toughest place to make it is in your backyard; the biggest critics are your friends. You make it here, and you can make it anywhere. It's a challenge."

It's a city day-hop school. The rest of the world thinks St. John's is on Forty-second Street, but it's really in Jamaica Estates, as pretty a place as there is in New York. You drive there, you bus there, you subway there, and you go home at night and your mama cooks you a good dinner. Nobody cons nobody. St. John's doesn't have to prove anything to anybody. And anyway, who's kidding who? You can't sell the Brooklyn Bridge to a kid who grew up selling it to you. City kids grow up with enough street sense to smell a rat before it bites them.

Little Looie knows all the angles. He's up there every season with the giants, and all he can throw at them is the shrimps. Not bad for a guy from the East Side who could have been slicing salami at his old man's deli.

And he sits in his office, surrounded by the split-pea green walls, talking about how much St. John's means to him. It's a 15-minute walk from his house, and every step of the way is like a stroll through his backyard. And as he talks about the future, he admits that there is one thing he'd like to do when all this basketball is over.

"I'd like to train bird dogs," Looie says.

AUTO RACING

THE INDY "FLOAT"

By *John S. Radosta*

From The New York Times
Copyright, ©, 1975, The New York Times Company
Reprinted by permission

In a motor race that has a history of oddball finishes, Bobby Unser won the Indianapolis 500 today as a sudden cloudburst cut it off at 435 miles, after 174 of the scheduled 200 laps.

It was the second Indy victory for Unser, a forty-one-year-old member of a distinguished racing family, who first won in 1968.

Johnny Rutherford, the defending champion, finished second after an inopportune pit stop for fuel toward the end. A. J. Foyt, who had been the heavy favorite, had to settle for third place after he was done in by a combination of tire and fuel problems and an ailing hip.

Indy always has a hard-luck story and today, besides the usual Lloyd Ruby jinx (he lasted only seven laps) it was also Wally Dallenbach's turn. Dallenbach looked like a sure winner until the one hundred sixty-first lap, when he slowed down a bit too much and burned a piston.

The race ended under an unusual combination of signal flags— red for stop and a checkered for end of race—that followed a long yellow for caution, during which no changes of position are permitted.

Before the red flag could be waved at the drivers, there was so much rain water that race cars were floating on the track surface of Indianapolis Motor Speedway like boats out of control in a strong current.

Racing tires have no tread—which is why they are called "slicks" —and no traction or adhesion. On a wet surface and especially when there is as much water as there was today, the race cars aquaplane on the film of water, with no contact between tire and pavement.

That is how Steve Krisloff, moving as slowly as though he were parking a car, spun and lightly tapped the wall and stopped near the start-finish line, facing the traffic.

As Krisloff frantically waved his arms in warning—he could not get out and run because his left ankle was in a cast—Unser and Foyt came boating along, at less than 20 miles an hour, around his disabled car.

At about the same time, 1,500 feet away and the head of the front straight, another three cars floated—not skidded—into one another and the retaining wall. They were moving quite slowly, really at a crawl, and no one was injured.

Altogether there were five accidents, but only one with serious results. Tom Sneva suffered first- and second-degree burns on 15 percent of his body and third-degree burns on his hands after a wreck with Eldon Rasmussen. Sneva was taken to the intensive-care unit of Methodist Hospital, where his condition was reported as good.

Unser drove an Eagle-Offenhauser built and prepared by Dan Gurney, who is one of America's racing greats.

As always, the results of the race remain provisional until official listings are posted at 8 o'clock tomorrow morning. Under the tentative results, Unser completed the 435 miles in 2 hours 54 minutes 55 seconds for an average speed of 149.213 miles an hour.

Unser's lead over Rutherford's McLaren-Offy was, unofficially, about 54 seconds. Foyt, driving a Coyote-Foyt of his own design and construction, and Rutherford finished on the same lap—one hundred seventy-fourth—as Unser.

Duane (Pancho) Carter, Jr., a son of an Indy racer of the 1950s, ran fourth, with 169 laps completed, in an Eagle that was rebuilt after a crash during fuel-consumption tests on Thursday. Roger McCluskey ran fifth in a Riley-Offy.

Unser led only 11 of the 174 laps, but they were the most important ones—the closing laps. Only six drivers held the lead, three for insignificant periods. The count was Dallenbach 96, Foyt 53, Unser 11, Johncock 8, Rutherford 5, Allison 1.

Thirteen of the 33 starters were running at the finish.

The day started hot and humid, with a festive crowd of at least 300,000 enjoying the preliminaries.

At the start Gordon Johncock, riding in the middle of the front row, broke out ahead of Foyt, sitting on the pole position, and Unser, who was on the outside of the front row.

Johncock led the first eight laps but then slowed down perceptibly on the ninth lap with ignition trouble. There had been an omen of that just before the beginning when, after the command, "Gentlemen, start your engines," Johncock's engine would not start.

Foyt, the crowd's favorite, took the lead on the ninth lap and quickly built up a five-second margin over Unser.

Rutherford took the lead briefly after Foyt pitted for fuel, and soon Bobby Allison took over for a couple of laps. Then Foyt retrieved the lead from the twenty-sixth through the fifty-eighth laps, and the crowd was delirious with delight.

But here comes Dallenbach, who's been working his way up from the back of the pack. Because of the way Indy's qualifying rules work, Dallenbach started from twenty-first position, in the seventh row.

Driving a bright-red Wildcat prepared by George Bigotti, Dallenbach simply carved his way through the field and by the fifty-ninth lap he had passed Foyt for the lead. Dallenbach led for 11 laps, relinquished it to Foyt for one lap while he pitted, and then recovered the lead on the seventy-first lap.

Dallenbach, a one-time New Jersey earth-moving contractor, dominated the race from the seventy-first lap through the one hundred sixtieth, relinquishing the lead only when he pitted for fuel and tires.

Sneva's accident on the one hundred twenty-seventh lap was to affect Dallenbach 33 laps later.

To evade the debris of the Sneva-Rasmussen wreck, Dallenbach drove into the grass margin for 10 laps or so. There he picked up a nail that caused a very slow leak. He nursed the car along, slowing down to avoid damaging the tire. But in reducing the boost from his turbocharger, the fuel mixture became too lean, and that in turn caused the burning out of a piston.

Dallenbach was dejected. "Without the grass business," he said sadly, "that sweet car could have run all day, a thousand miles."

Dallenbach had a lead of about 20 seconds on Rutherford when his engine quit on the first turn. Rutherford moved into the lead.

Soon Rutherford went into the pits for fuel. That was on the one hundred sixty-second lap, under the green flag. The pit stop took only 19 seconds but in that time Unser, who had taken on fuel on the one hundred fifty-ninth lap, cruised out in front.

Then the trouble began. Gary Bettenhausen, coming off the fourth turn, lost a wheel. With magnificent skill, he controlled the three-wheel car by bumping it along the wall to scrub off speed. When the car slowed enough, Bettenhausen steered it across the track to the grass margin. But it spilled a lot of debris on the track, and that brought out the yellow flag.

Under the yellow, no one can improve position. So there was Unser in front, with Rutherford next, while workmen cleaned up the track.

Quite suddenly the light rain exploded into a violent cloudburst, and it was impossible to race at all. The 13 cars still running were strung out all over the two-and-one-half-mile rectangular track, and they slowed down to a crawl.

Pat Vidan, the starter, pulled in the yellow flag and then waved the red and checkered flags together, an unusual procedure.

That was after the one hundred seventy-fourth lap had been completed by the leader, Unser, and while Unser was somewhere out there on the course. It seemed to take hours for Unser to find his way to the finish line through the downpour.

FOOTBALL

FOOTBALL TROPHIES: THEIR STORIES

By Ron Martz

From The St. Petersburg Times
Copyright, ©, 1975, The St. Petersburg Times

On a dreary October Saturday afternoon in 1903 the venerable Fielding H. Yost took his undefeated and unscored-upon Michigan Wolverines to Minneapolis to meet the University of Minnesota Gophers in what was to become one of the most important college football games ever played.

The game was significant not for its outcome, but for what came out of it. For from this bitter battle emerged a significant and lasting contribution to the game of American college football—the Little Brown Jug trophy.

The jug was the predecessor of all the other trophies awarded to winners of games between traditional rivals. And many of the trophies were conceived and dedicated at a time when the most important thing on campus was football.

In recent years the trophies have lost much of their significance. Nobody seems to have the time to worry about such trivialities. With their collective consciousness raised, college students now find it difficult to see the merit in rah-rahing the old blue and white to victory so they can recapture an old bucket, or jug, or shoe.

But in the days of Fielding Yost and his fabulous "point-a-minute" Michigan teams, nothing was quite so important on Saturday afternoons as football.

Under Yost Michigan had not lost a game in two years, going 11–0 in both 1901 and 1902, giving up only 12 points in those two years and 22 games. Going into the Minnesota game on October 31, 1903, Michigan was 7–0 and had outscored its opponents 437–0.

It was the tradition in those days for the home team to furnish the visitors with drinking water. Given the intensity of the Michigan-Minnesota rivalry, Yost did not put it past the Minnesotans to slip something into the Wolverines' drinking water.

So Yost instructed trainer Keene Fitzpatrick to make adequate preparations to supply the water. Fitzpatrick in turn sent student manager Tommy Roberts to a Minneapolis variety store where for 30 cents he purchased a five-gallon jug.

The game was a classic, ending in a 6–6 tie. As it turned out, those were the only points scored against Michigan that season and the only Michigan game in four years (including 1904) that was not a victory.

Minnesota fans swarmed the field after the "upset" and Roberts was unable to recover the jug. Oscar Munson, a janitor, found it during cleanup operations and took it to the Minnesota athletic department. There, it was labeled: "Michigan Jug 'captured' by Oscar, October 31, 1903."

Because of the brutality exhibited by both teams, Michigan and Minnesota broke off athletic relations following the 1903 game and did not play again until 1909.

At that time the Minnesota athletic department wrote to Michigan: "We have your Little Brown Jug, come up and win it."

And the Wolverines did, 15–6, providing the necessary second step in the creation of the Little Brown Jug trophy and the impetus for a spate of imitators.

The Old Oaken Bucket trophy, awarded to the winner of the Purdue-Indiana football game, was conceived by alumni groups from both schools and first awarded in 1925. The bucket itself is more than 100 years old and is believed to have been used by Morgan's Raiders during the Civil War.

But there is a host of lesser-known trophies, the histories of which far surpass the Old Oaken Bucket in charm but are not so well-chronicled as the bucket or the Michigan jug.

There is, for example, the Floyd of Rosedale trophy.

Floyd was a prize-winning porker who was the object of a bet in 1935 between Minnesota Governor Floyd Olson and Iowa Governor Clyde Herring. The two bet on the outcome of the football game that year between Minnesota and Iowa and when the Gophers won, Floyd of Rosedale was trucked off to Minnesota.

Floyd soon disappeared, however, presumably ending up as a pork chop repast on the governor's table or at the University of Minnesota dining hall. So, the following year, a trophy was cast in the likeness of the late Floyd and the 21-inch long by 15 1/2-inch high trophy is still presented annually.

The Kit Carson Rifle has one of the most interesting histories of all the trophies.

Initiated in 1938 by J. F. "Pop" McKale, head football coach at

Arizona, the rifle is presented to the winner of the Arizona-New Mexico game. According to McKale, he had captured the rifle from Geronimo when the great Apache chief was roaming through the Southwest.

No one thought the rifle was anything other than what McKale claimed it was. But on his deathbed McKale confessed that the rifle was in fact an old Springfield he had liberated from a well on campus just before it was to be buried with a number of other obsolete Springfields from the school's ROTC armory.

Even if the legend doesn't endure, the trophy does.

Indian artifacts used to be hot items on the college trophies' market. The Stanford Axe goes to the winner of the Stanford-California game, the Tomahawk to the winner of the Illinois-Northwestern game, and the Indian Skull to the winner of the Ohio Wesleyan-Wittenberg game.

Axes and tomahawks make great trophies. But a skull?

Seems the skull was unearthed during construction of Selby Stadium on the Ohio Wesleyan campus in 1929. Someone thought it a more than suitable trophy to be presented to the winner of the traditional Ohio Wesleyan-Wittenberg game. The skull has since been mounted on a plaque and after 45 years remains as the major trophy of those two schools.

Not all the unusual trophies have such a storied past.

The Illibuck trophy is nothing more than a wooden turtle (there used to be a real one), which was originated by honor societies at Illinois and Ohio State in 1925 to honor the winner of the football game between those two schools.

The Telephone trophy was started in 1959 by Northwestern Bell Telephone of Ames, Iowa. That company was responsible for putting in the field telephones for the Iowa State-Missouri game. But just before the game started it was discovered that each team could monitor the other's signals from spotters in the press box.

The Bronze Hat is a replica of a 10-gallon Stetson that was donated by the State Fair of Texas in 1941 to the winner of the Oklahoma-Texas game. Five years ago the hat was gold-plated but it is still called the Bronze Hat.

The Old Brass Spittoon is just that. The trophy started in 1950 at the urging of students at Michigan State and Indiana. The 125-year-old spittoon was unearthed from the ruins of a Michigan trading post and is supposed to signify the pioneer spirit of the early settlers in that area of the country.

The Shillelagh goes to the winner of the Purdue-Notre Dame game. Donated by a merchant seaman and an ardent Irish fan by the name of Joe McLaughlin, the club was actually brought from Ireland.

The Golden Egg trophy was started in 1927 in an attempt to appease Mississippi and Mississippi State fans who were intent on destroying stadiums in search of souvenirs following the playing of the "state championship" game each year.

The Beer Keg trophy got its start in a Lexington, Ky., drugstore in 1925 when Rollie Guthrie and a group of "downtown quarterbacks" decided the Kentucky-Tennessee game needed a trophy like the Old Oaken Bucket or the Little Brown Jug.

The group originally wanted to use a moonshine still, but with the preponderance of empty beer kegs around due to Prohibition, the latter seemed a more logical choice.

However, the Lexington unit of the Women's Christian Temperance Union heard of the plan and vigorously objected.

In deference to Prohibition and the good ladies of the WCTU, the beer keg was labeled "Ice Water" until years later.

Then there is the Seminole Canoe.

For years this full-sized model of a Seminole Indian war canoe was presented to the winner of the Florida-Miami game. Then, in 1970, Miami beat Florida 14–13. The Miamians took the trophy home and kept it there, even though the Gators have won the last four games in the intrastate rivalry.

But there has been no hue and cry from Florida fans for the return of the canoe, which sits gathering dust in the University of Miami athletic department offices. It just doesn't seem important enough to get all worked up about.

Like most of the other trophies awarded in college football, the canoe has lost its appeal and its importance as a symbol of football supremacy.

These trophies are relics of a time when unimportant things could be made to seem important without attendant guilt feelings, a time when college football was the biggest thing on campus.

HORSE RACING

RUFFIAN'S LAST RACE

By Pete Axthelm

From Newsweek
Copyright, ©, 1975, Newsweek, Inc.

The blow came with such sickening suddenness that it took several gasping moments to absorb its impact—and its cruel lesson in the fragility of thoroughbred racehorses and of the dreams built around them. At one point last week, the magnificent filly Ruffian was the flamelike fulfillment of generations of planning and dreaming: a huge, nearly black three-year-old with rippling muscles and those rare champion's eyes that seemed to know that she couldn't be beaten or even seriously challenged. Then, as she raced alongside the colt Foolish Pleasure in an eagerly awaited, nationally televised match race at New York's Belmont Park, Ruffian thrust her 1,125-pound body forward onto her delicate thoroughbred legs for the final graceful time.

Both jockeys heard the sound—"like when you break a stick"— as bone cracked in her right foreleg. Then Jacinto Vasquez was fighting desperately to pull her up, knowing that her marvelous competitive fires would propel her forward on three legs and further endanger the fourth. By the time she came to a reluctant halt 100 yards further on, Ruffian had pounded her ankle into a pulp of blood and tissue and shattered bone. Eight hours later she was dead.

Perhaps Ruffian was the greatest filly that ever lived. Certainly her tragically brief career was as perfect as any horse ever put together. From her first prancing step into the starting gate 13 months ago until the moment she broke down, she never allowed a rival to get in front of her for a single stride. Only one horse in the last two decades—Secretariat—excited the nonracing public as much as Ruffian did in her 10 straight victories leading up to the match race.

And she took her brilliance into her grave in the Belmont infield. As one stablehand suggested, her epitaph could have been, "She died in the lead."

The drama of Ruffian's demise can be divided into two acts, each fraught with the irony that had she been a lesser star, with just a bit less pure speed or fighting spirit, she might have saved herself.

In the tense days before the match race, hardly anyone outside the Foolish Pleasure camp doubted that Ruffian was far superior in appearance and natural ability. But to some insiders and handicappers, her speed also made her vulnerable. She was so much faster than the other fillies of her generation that her races had deteriorated into a series of leisurely gallops that did little to toughen her for all-out, head-to-head competition. Foolish Pleasure, on the other hand, had battled and jostled through victories and defeats alike in a long campaign against colts; whatever his limitations, his taste for infighting was unquestioned. The rivals could have been compared to Muhammad Ali and Joe Frazier before their first fight —one with incomparable grace but no strong recent competition, the other with a willingness to absorb punishment and wear down a foe. Frazier won that fight, and trainer LeRoy Jolley seemed determined to prepare Foolish Pleasure for a similarly gritty performance; he drilled the Kentucky Derby winner for extreme speed so he could stay close to Ruffian.

Frank Whiteley, Jr., the crafty veteran horseman who trained Ruffian, did not try to match flashy workouts with Jolley. He felt that Ruffian's natural speed would be enough to match the speed that was being drilled into Foolish Pleasure. Whiteley was right. Ruffian kept her sleek neck in front of the colt until disaster struck. But to do so, she had to sprint harder than she had done in almost a year, and some people wondered if the unaccustomed exertion contributed to her injury. "We threw a fast half at the bitch and she just unbuckled," LeRoy Jolley's father, Moody, blurted in the winner's circle. And if Moody's graceless comment was an unattractive contrast to LeRoy's tasteful tribute to the doomed Ruffian, it stood as one cold-blooded theory on the sad event.

But ultimately there could be no satisfactory answers. Speed may have been a factor, but horses have suffered similar injuries during slow gallops. The unusually hard, fast track has been blamed, but there is little evidence that it was unsafe—and it certainly wasn't "doctored" by management to produce a fast time. The hell-for-leather nature of match racing has also been cited, but from its earliest days racing has thrived on such confrontations between top horses. Finally, the claim that the mere presence of a strong male put undue pressure on a great female borders on the ridiculous. But Ruffian-lovers could be forgiven for groping at any theory as they faced the reality of the mighty filly stumbling away from the track in a clear, inflatable cast that rapidly turned red with blood.

The second phase of Ruffian's story was acted out at her Belmont barn and in Dr. William O. Reed's outstanding veterinary hospital across the street. Moods shifted violently with the hours as four veterinarians and one orthopedic surgeon fought to save her. First, the shaky filly had to be virtually lifted into her stall by the ashen-faced Whiteley and his assistants. Suffering from shock and increasing pain, Ruffian tried to lie down. Knowing that the horse would soon develop paralysis if she did, the vets worked desperately to keep her upright and deaden her pain with ice. Among themselves, the doctors gave her little more than a 10 percent chance of survival, but when they managed to tranquilize her enough to lead her to the operating room, those keeping a vigil nearby allowed their hopes to surge.

Odds: The operation took three and a half hours. Twice the vets almost lost Ruffian and barely revived her with artificial respiration and stimulants. Every minute is precious when a horse is lying down, and they had to use valuable time to wash out the badly contaminated open wound. Despite the mounting odds against them, however, the vets completed their task. Then there was nothing to do but await the moment of truth when the anesthesia wore off.

Ruffian awoke in a fatal frenzy. "Several men tried to hold her," said Dr. Alex Harthill, "and she threw us around as if we were rag dolls." Soon she kicked off a special shoe, then tore her cast to pieces. As she did so her hemorrhaging and swelling increased, and shortly after 2 A.M. the vets presented the facts to owner Stuart Janney. "I'm a realistic man," he sighed—and at 2:20, the suffering filly was injected with a fatal dose of phenobarbital. "The best filly I ever saw," mumbled the stricken Whiteley, "and the best I'll ever see."

"The same thing that made her win made her die," added Dr. Jim Prendergast. "She fought so hard."

BASKETBALL

THE ULTIMATE POL

By Murray Olderman

From Newspaper Enterprise Association
Copyright, ©, 1975, Newspaper Enterprise Association, Inc.

At 9:15 A.M. on Wednesday of the first week in June, a wavy-haired, toothy politician named Larry O'Brien was formally ratified by the board of governors as the third commissioner in the history of the National Basketball Association.

Thirty hours later, he had presided over the assessment of a whopping figure on the divestiture of a million-dollar property named George McGinnis by the New York Knicks.

This was accomplished by a group that will debate for a year on the amount of tip for room service. Its first commissioner, a rotund little man named Maurice Podoloff, used to get obfuscated by his own verbiage. Its second, the recently retired Walter Kennedy, pined for the good old days when a handshake did the job of a battery of lawyers. Neither particularly defied their bosses, the owners, which meant they were a little reluctant to make decisions.

Now the NBA has the ultimate pol, Larry O'Brien, whose most recent public exposure was presiding over the 1972 Democratic convention, the one that nominated George McGovern.

And so it is almost child's play, even though it involves millions and the futures of elongated young men, when O'Brien exercises his new power as NBA commissioner.

"I am cautious," he says, "determining facts, but I can make decisions. Miami Beach [site of the convention] two years ago was tougher than this. I didn't go to bed for two nights. I had to make rulings that effectively blocked off Hubert Humphrey and Edward Muskie from the nomination—and I was a lot closer personally to Humphrey than to McGovern."

The McGinnis ruling was really his first in office. The superb forward of the Indianapolis Pacers of the American Basketball Association had signed a contract with the New York Knicks recently, which was legal in the eyes of the law since he was a free agent. But the draft rights to him in the NBA were held by the Philadelphia 76ers, who weren't about to give them up, and the flaunting action by the Knicks threatened the constitutional foundation of the league.

Even before he officially took the commissioner's chair, O'Brien had started investigating the aspects of the McGinnis case. And at the NBA meetings, he had invited Mike Burke of the Knicks and Pat Williams of the 76ers into the chairman's suite of the St. Francis Hotel to thrash out the arguments for both sides. He had earlier requested that Burke submit the McGinnis contract to the league office for perusal. Mike could have effectively blocked an immediate ruling on the matter by not complying, since a team does not have to send in player contracts for league approval until the beginning of the season, which would have been next October. But O'Brien was persuasive.

At 2:05 P.M., on his second official day in office, O'Brien called the afternoon session in order. At 2:10 P.M., he announced the McGinnis contract with New York was void, and the Knicks would forfeit their top draft choice next year.

"Not a pin dropped," he recalls, an unusual reaction from the perennially bickering owners of the NBA, who threaten to sue each other and the league every time they stub a toe.

He had begun earning his $150,000 a year in salary.

O'Brien claims that when members of the committee to select a new commissioner, who had been dallying for more than a year, first mentioned the idea to him at a cocktail party, and then followed up with a breakfast meeting, he told them he didn't want his name presented for the job.

But Watergate, like it has many prominent American political leaders, touched him personally. He found out through the testimony of John Ehrlichman that he had been tapped and under surveillance for three years.

"Being a victim of Watergate," he says, "brought another dimension to my life. My profession was tarnished by the same guys who had tried to get me."

So he looked around for something else to do since he was bored by the life of a New York lawyer, and there was this NBA opportunity still there—he was a nut on pro basketball anyhow—so he took it.

But to paraphrase a famous quotation by his good friend, the late

John Kennedy, ask not what the NBA can do for you, but what you can do for the NBA.

"I think time will tell," he almost ducks the issue. "The fact that NBA and I entered into marriage was due to the ebb and flow of life. I did not accept it for prestige or profit.

"The great challenge in sports is what will happen to the NBA and the ABA. In 1971, when the merger talks were debated in Washington, the effort was horrendous."

So, by implication, Larry O'Brien, who is fifty-seven, can make his greatest contribution by effecting a union of the two basketball leagues whose quest for tall, agile men has resulted in the highest salary spiral in the history of sports. This was supposed to be the reason the NBA got him in the first place, because of his political clout in Washington.

Therefore, he will not stop being a politician, in the theoretical sense, though he is out of it as an organization man.

"Will I miss it?" he asks rhetorically. "Yes."

He curls up in his hotel room chair, black patent leather shoes twisted together.

"Am I going back to it? No."

Except if it concerns pro basketball.

GENERAL

CAN SPORTS SURVIVE MONEY?

By Roger Kahn

From Esquire
Copyright, ©, 1975, Roger Kahn

Briefly, during 1972, Derek Sanderson was crowned monarch of this sporting life. Sanderson, a skilled and courageous centerman, had taken splendid, but hardly infinite, hockey talents and parlayed them with the negotiating skills of Robert Woolf of Boston, an attorney who could have gotten Cain off with ninety days probation.

First, Woolf ran Sanderson's contract with the Boston Bruins from $12,000 to $50,000, an event Sanderson celebrated by remodeling a town house on Beacon Hill. Soon visitors found a two-story living room, paneled in white oak, stretching below a sleeping terrace. The terrace included a vast round bed and a beautiful roommate called Judy, who was content to live with Derek in (a) sin or (b) glory. That is multiple choice. Consider your generation and choose one.

Next, a World Hockey Association team called the Miami Screaming Eagles drafted Sanderson and asked why he was living like a pauper. Ice hockey is not precisely indigenous to Miami and the Screaming Eagles moved north and became the Philadelphia Blazers.

"I knew these people wanted Derek badly," Bob Woolf says, "but I couldn't believe the figures I was hearing." Pleasantly shaking his head, Woolf arranged a $2,750,000 long-term contract for his client. Sanderson stroked Aladdin's lamp and a Rolls-Royce Silver Ghost materialized. Subsequently, Derek Sanderson, hockey player, disappeared.

In all, Sanderson played eight games for the Philadelphia Blazers. He was a poor boy from Niagara Falls, Canada, and his early memories stir, he says, with images of knife fights in freezing alleys. Now reporters pressed him with questions, not about hockey, but about money. Abruptly he had become the highest-paid team athlete in history. The new questions and the new money disoriented him. His back went bad. Presently, Woolf had to negotiate Sanderson's release from the Philadelphia Blazers. He settled for an even five million. Derek fled to the savannas of Florida, where he worked on his short-approach game.

But he is a gritty man and pride moves him. Sanderson returned to Boston and then last season went to New York, where he signed to play one year for $100,000. Typically, the Ranger type is clean-shaven and conventional. Sanderson sports a swirling brown moustache and, after hockey and the good life, he loves irreverence. By Stanley Cup time, he had persuaded all the Rangers not to shave "until we win or get knocked off." Unfortunately the Islanders eliminated the Rangers in three games and all we ever got to see was five o'clock shadows.

"Did the big money affect me?" Sanderson says slowly, in the elegant offices of Bob Woolf Associates, Inc. "I'd say a little bit. Like, I was a good, hard-working hockey player one year and then, after I got the million, I rolled over and went to sleep."

The Blazers are gone from Philadelphia now and the Flyers preside. The Flyers, that muscular mix of teamwork, coaching, violence, and victory. When the Flyers find themselves in trouble, Kate Smith appears and sings "God Bless America." Almost invariably, the Flyers win.

What could be less commercial than good old Kate crooning to the good old Flyers? Except Ms. Smith will not warble a note for her beloved Flyers unless she is guaranteed a fee of $5,000.

A tangram is a Chinese puzzle made by cutting a square of thin material into five triangles, one square and one rhomboid. You rearrange the shapes and then recombine them, or try to recombine them, until insanity seizes the mind.

Money and sport. Is this a tangram that we see before us? The shapes appear. Someone, everyone, asks, aren't athletes earning too much money? Catfish Hunter breaks the bank in The Big Turnip. Bob Woolf wonders, just wonders, mind you, in his innocent way, if Jim Plunkett shouldn't be a million-dollar quarterback. Joe Namath strides away, gimp-legged, from a reported (or, as we shall see, unreported) $4,000,000 offer. Alan Cohen, president of the Madison Square Garden Corporation, confesses that he'd rather see the Rangers make a profit than win the Stanley Cup. (Bottom-line Cohen, sports writers call him now.) We read, or at least look at, stories announcing that major-league baseball has sold television rights for over $92,000,000.

Agents, mating with admen, proliferate. The agency people debate why Mark Spitz, who swam like a fish, metamorphosed into a commercial lox. The technocrats of television enter like boyars. At ABC, crews film automobiles in collision and after a while Roone Arledge peddles demolition derby as sport. (If that's sport, Arledge, so is lapidation, which is stoning people to unconsciousness or death.)

How did such preposterous activities start? Why is everyone talking about money all the time? Why aren't things the way they were, when we talked about the games, the scores, courage, excellence, and the time that Early Wynn stuffed a catcher's mitt with Limburger cheese one very hot day in Cleveland?

Simple as a tangram and complex as a tangram. We need not only the right answers, but the right questions. Are professional athletes, who are mostly gifted, hard-working artisans, being paid too much? I despair for an economy where Park Avenue obstetricians reap $300,000 a year, while one mile to the north in Harlem babies die for want of an intern. Our economy is irrational, but, should we decide to overhaul free enterprise, can anyone seriously suggest that the place to begin is sport? (Yes, I'm afraid Gerald Ford could suggest just that.)

Is Jim Plunkett worth a million? Did Babe Ruth deserve to earn more than Herbert Hoover? "Sure," announced the Babe circa 1929, "I had a better year than him."

Why aren't things the way they were? But in most ways things *are* the way they were. It is mostly the appearance of things that has changed. Jack Dempsey's super gates stirred people 50 years ago as much as Muhammad Ali's super gates arouse cupidity today. Contract negotiations have grabbed headlines ever since some baseball writer invented the word "holdout." Sports have always drawn hustlers, con men, as surely as home-run hitters draw groupies. I can remember being presented a Little Dizzy Dean baseball suit during the late 1930s. Dean got his royalty; the suit lasted for three games, or one washing. During the 1940s, Frank Leahy of Notre Dame dispensed football scholarships the way M-G-M issued movie contracts. Candidates were weighed, measured, examined, like so many starlets on heels. The best won four years of free college, plus fringe benefits that would have turned a teamster green. In the 1950s, when Dwight Eisenhower reigned over a placid economy and people rushed out to purchase huge, finned automobiles, 100 college basketball players confessed that they had taken bribes to lose games. Before the chain of sports explosions and the relentless onslaught of TV, then, we had amateur athletes accepting cash to play poorly. That paradigm of noncommercial sport has not been equaled in the venal Watergate 1970s, according to my notes. Emphasis shifts. The faces are new. The hustlers are slicker. But anyone who wants to weep for the carefree days, when sports and money were distinct, will have to weep alone. (And worse, pick up the tab for his own beer.)

We always resist confronting our own materialism. We bathe in bicentennial idealism on weekends, which leaves five days free for wallowing in commerce. As Herbert Marcuse points out, the American people now "recognize themselves in their commodities; they find their soul in their automobile, hi-fi set, split-level home." This is not precisely what one is taught in school or later hears from John Kennedy, so most of us live in a discomfiting duality. We would glory in the cathedrals of the human spirit, but if put to a test, frankly, we'd rather own the collection platter.

Sport became an extension of this confused American ethos. All sport was divided into two parts: the amateurs, who were glorious, pure and sensitive; and the professionals, who sweated and chewed cigars. Amateurs spouted a house poem, composed by Grantland Rice:

> When the One Great Scorer comes
> To write against your name—
> He marks not that you won or lost,
> But how you played the game.

This doggerel can be found in the same anthologies that publish Joyce Kilmer's "Trees," which is to say that it is both popular and absurd. John Lardner countered for the professionals:

> Right or wrong is all the same,
> When baby needs new shoes.
> It isn't how you play the game,
> It's whether you win or lose.

Those lines, which make a sound of truth, are remembered by five people. The professionals wanted poetry, marching bands, pom-pom girls. Coaches, sports pages, ministers, parents—in short, society—conditioned us to believe in the beauties of amateurism. Indeed, we played for nothing as children. We gloried in the growing strength of our bodies. We strove toward grace. We knew the ravishing explosion of joy that came when we made the right play at the right time. Then we proceeded to confuse children at play with the big, dirty business of putative amateurism.

College football became a monster of bribery. What, after all, is a football scholarship but a bribe? Amateur tennis players lived for years without visible employment. They survived on money pressed into their hands in cellars at midnight. Eventually, someone was driven to define an amateur athlete realistically. An amateur would not accept a check.

Consider what the sports explosion begat: 24 major-league baseball teams, where we had 16; two pro-basketball leagues (28 teams); two hockey leagues (33 teams); two football leagues; and more professional tennis players than one can count. Money is green. The cellars are empty now. We have witnessed the greening of American sport. Except in certain university communities, where football or basketball turn big profits, we are no longer afraid to call a pro a pro.

The other side is less bright. Professional sport has expanded quickly, chaotically, and when the new team in town wants to show its strength, the general manager summons the press and starts talking about his bankroll. Challenged, the established team issues releases about *its* bankroll. There are days when a man turning the sports pages wades through columns of unsubstantiated financial reports before he comes to a single final score.

Later, a general manager may complain to a favored reporter that high salaries are corrupting his athletes. This ploy runs, "Don't quote me. I don't want to get the team upset, but I'm telling you and you can use it on your own." I could take such gambits seriously only if I had ever heard a general manager complain that high front-office salaries, plus stock options, were ruining general managers.

In the old monopoly sport days, when baseball was in flower, two operating theories collided. Branch Rickey, the great thinker of the National League, had a puritan distaste for money in other people's hands. Gene Hermanski, a journeyman outfielder, negotiated briefly after a reasonably good year and came out of Rickey's office smiling in ecstasy.

"You get a raise, Gene?" someone asked.

"No. But he didn't cut me."

Rickey's teams were famous for aggressive play and, in certain instances, undertipping.

In the American League, the old Yankees were the wealthiest of players. During spring training the team was coached not only in baseball but in rudiments of style. "You are a Yankee. You are expected to behave like a Yankee. Never tip less than 25 cents for breakfast."

What happened when Rickey's hungry Dodgers played the fat-cat Yankees in the World Series? In every case but one the fat cats won.

Can it be said that money ruins athletes? The answer also applies to women. The good ones learn to survive prosperity. The old vicious amateurism confused young men, but, historically, money did not ruin Dempsey's fighting spirit, which came out of a poor boyhood in barren mountainlands. Money did not make Joe Di-Maggio lazy or Ted Williams one inch less the perfectionist. Some spirits were dulled. Some—the young Mantle and Mays—went through fat salaries as fast as banks cleared their checks. But the best have almost always been paid the most. That is one of the truths of professional sport, of true professionals. And, until time tore at their bodies, the best went right on being the best.

Nor have salaries increased as much as newspaper sports pages suggest. In his forthcoming book, *Behind Closed Doors,* Bob Woolf explains that "the Dolgoff Plan was the backbone of all the fabulous contracts signed by athletes in the boom years." The plan, named for accountant Ralph Dolgoff, works like this:

A graduating seven-foot basketball center demands a million-dollar contract. "Sure thing," says a professional general manager, "but we want you to keep some of that million, right? We don't want it all going to the government. So, we give you fifty thousand now as a bonus, plus fifty thousand a year as salary for the next four years. Then we take a hundred thousand of our money and put it in a 20-year investment program for you. We call that the Dolgoff Plan. You got to believe in America, kid. The country's growing. At the end of 20 years, the 100,000 will have grown to $750,000 through shrewd investing. Figure it out, kid. The deal's worth at least a million, and a nest egg will be waiting when you're through."

Club and player meet the press and announce another $1,000,-000 contract. Officials meet privately with veterans and say, "Don't believe what you read. We're actually giving the kid fifty thousand a year."

With taxes, vanishing mutual funds, and inflation, today's athletes are not that extravagantly paid. The exceptions, Ali, Hunter, Kareem Abdul-Jabbar, are not even that exceptional. Superstars have always drawn larger paychecks than opponents. As Jack Dempsey reached affluence in 1920, he fought a good heavyweight named Billy Miske in Michigan. "I knocked him out quick because I loved the guy," Dempsey says. "Hell of a guy, Billy Miske." Miske, a ranking contender, had begged for the fight. He was broke. Dempsey got him quickly so there would not be much pain. Miske, the broke contender, was dying of Bright's disease.

The sea change in sport is the promotion, which now sweeps almost everything before it as it rolls out of a three-block area of Manhattan. The preeminent sports promoters in the United States are ABC, NBC, and CBS. In 1974, the networks telecast a total of 1,088 hours of sport. That number floats out into abstraction like theories of sets and functions. Put differently, the networks gave sport the equivalent of 725 Johnny Carson shows last year, which is more than twice what NBC gave Johnny Carson.

Networks are as passive as the Gestapo. They do not simply buy. They dictate. They not only produce, but demand. The network people do not wander, checkbook in hand, saying, "Anything you sportin' fellers want." They have come in, calculating cost per thousand viewers and announcing, "If you want our underwriting, you'd better listen." Networks have given us the time-out for a commercial; four replays of a fly to left and analyses that are not analyses at all. You do not hear network announcers say, "That goalie is playing with a hangover. When he blinked, his eyelids stuck together. There's no other way to explain that goal." Instead, you hear, "It's tougher than it looks, stopping a hockey puck." Network announcers do not admit, "This game is the dullest mess I've seen since my date in Oakland got morning sickness at midnight." Instead they say, "Just remember, in the National Basketball Association, a 52-point lead in the third quarter is not necessarily decisive." The announcers are paid to talk about the games. They are also paid to keep you watching. This creates a hybrid—part reporter, part shill.

For some weeks, I have been ambling among promoters, prying into the business of sport. Carl Lindemann of NBC explained patiently how his network does a "black book," a study of potential viewing audiences and cost. A commercial minute on the Super Bowl sells for $214,000, as opposed to $70,000 for one minute on an average prime-time show. Don Ruck of the National Hockey League discussed "the impressive profile of the typical hockey fan and our promotions with Chrysler, Kraft, and Hertz." Bob Levinson of B.B.D.& O. described the choice or the pursuit of a sponsor.

Future sport is clear in certain outlines. The networks thrash in a frenzy, like famished sharks, to televise hot sports or to create new ones. (If demolition derby is sport, Arledge, so is defenestration, which is pushing people out of windows.) The arena is evolving into a studio. Ali fights anywhere he can find a cable. Pete Rozelle is so concerned about the football stadia being deserted that he shuttles to Washington weekly to lobby against unlimited televising. Cheers, Pete, but I have seen the future. It measures 19 inches diagonally.

But will it work? There is not yet evidence that fans are being turned off. Overall, sports ratings are secure. The most distressed, which is to say most ignored franchises, are items like the Miami Screaming Eagles, which should never have been begun. Tickets for NBA and NHL playoffs sell out in hours. I have before me a financial report, indicating that Madison Square Garden earned almost $4,-000,000 in sports and entertainment during a 10-month period, while losing about $3,000,000 on its real estate and its hotels. The Los Angeles Dodgers hope to draw three million customers this season.

We stand at the dawning of the age of network sport. It is true, as Bob Lipsyte observed in [MORE], that sport is entertainment and athletes are paid performers. But sport is a special kind of entertainment. The suspense of a great baseball game is real, not fictive. The courage of a quarterback is actual courage, not John Wayne firing blanks at collapsing extras. Sport is a scene of style and grace and skill and unpredictability. It is Bob Gibson at thirty-nine, after a bruising divorce, pitching for yet another year because he wants to, because he has to, because, even in the pain that foretells the death of his career, pitching is what he thinks he can do best. That is one touch of the mystique, and it is worth a hundred stories on Gibson's salary.

Can sport survive money? Quite simply, it always has. Can sport survive network promotion and television's babbling belief that money is, all by itself, proof of merit? The answer here leads us away from the network reporter/shills and onto the sports pages.

After *Esquire* published Randall Poe's article on sports writing last October, a ripple effect led to a low-keyed debate. Was it true, as David Shaw asserted in the *Los Angeles Times,* that the *Los Angeles Times* presented the best of all newspaper sports pages? (Was it true that Shaw had never heard the phrase self-serving?) Had *Sports Illustrated* really invented literacy? Would anyone trade Dick Young for Larry Merchant and a new journalist to be named at a later date? Would anyone trade Larry Merchant for Dick Young and a crew-cut copyreader? Fun, but a Leonard Lyons view of current history, nothing more.

In other times, when sports were actively promoted by such hustlers as Tex Rickard, the press did a weak job of reporting. Fight writers of the 1920s doubled their salaries with graft from big promoters. Ice was the euphemism; ice was graft. No less a figure than Damon Runyon not only covered fights for the Hearst chain, but owned a piece of the promotions. Any readers out there waiting for Runyon the reporter to knock a fight arranged by Runyon the promoter are still waiting.

Ethical lines are firmer now, but new journalists, old journalists, and others in between seem confused by the latest breed of hustler. They accept figures that exist only in press releases. They quiz Hunter endlessly about his insurance policies and barely touch a more mysterious mystery. The Catfish has been the most effective of pitchers in the last five years, but he doesn't throw that hard. The riddle of the Catfish is not his contract but his success.

The function of sports pages is to tell us about the games and the people who play the games, and their emotions and their humor and their bent dreams. Television offers a glossy print with fine immediacy and no depth over off-camera voices shouting, "Look at me. Look at me. (And please stay tuned for a commercial announcement.)" It is up to newspaper sports sections to take people truly into the house of sport and to let them smell the cabbage cooking in the kitchen.

Money is part of sport, as money is part of most things. It is part of writing, music, loving, living, lying. Namath walks away from $4,000,000, the newspapers tell me. Why is Namath worth $4,-000,000? Because he, plus a few others like him, are the only way the struggling World Football League can offer a package of games for which the networks might bid. Further, how do we know it was $4,000,000? How would the money be paid? Are we expected to believe that Joe Willie walked away from $4,000,000 in cash? The Joe Willie I knew wanted a fat fee to attend a luncheon where he had only to take possession of a $5,000 car. That Joe Willie? Walking away from $4,000,000? I'd have to see bank statements first.

Muhammad Ali has fought three times since promising to turn his profits back to the ghettos. Has anybody on the fight beat since investigated? How much has he contributed so far? Newspapermen view Ali with limited enthusiasm, but here is a situation that demands a follow-up. The newspaper press is deaf to that demand.

Occasionally, perhaps five times a year, good legitimate money stories appear. At those points, a valid new sports journalism would give us hard, cynical reporting. Let's see the checks. Let's see the contracts. Ah, says the gentleman from the New York Yankees. Mr. Hunter's contracts are a private matter between him and the ball club. Well, we all respect the privacy of Mr. Hunter, an amiable man, but when a figure of $3,750,000 comes out of baseball, someone is more concerned with puffery than privacy. In this heady time of sports boom, amid recession, the press has let promoters have things both ways. It accepts their figures and prints them. It does not get to see the books. That is reporting to Richard Nixon's taste.

Writing sports-money is an easy way out, a kind of trick that helps fill each day's maw of empty columns. But it is not a good way out.

It is even cheap. The old sirens of sport, Grantland Rice and his disciples, created a climate in which the word *amateur* became, all by itself, a lie. Sports pages now, with their superficial prattle about cash, are just as dangerous. I find it difficult to take seriously a new journalism that reveals that ball players drink, copulate, and speak with shaky grammar but that cannot dig for the hard stuff, the bottom line, as Alan Cohen would say.

"Sex and money," a tough editor once told me. "When you've got to get attention, begin either with money or sex." We've had multimedia sex, offered by producers who mistook the unadorned breast, which is a gland, for a form of entertainment. In time men, and even boys, yawned at the institutional boob. The producers moved onward and downward until here we are in an era when it's tough to sell a pubic hair.

So with money. Write Derek Sanderson and His Millions. Interview Kate Smith's agent. Where a good money story exists, go and get it. But please spare us these incessant money press releases disguised as news stories, before the sports pages spawn generations of auditors who never know that the grass is green and nine men are on the field at all times.

The other evening some of us sat in a New York restaurant with Jack Scott, who was talking about his friend Bill Walton. "Whatever you've read," Scott said, in his controlled, intense way, "I can tell you that Bill is living on about $20,000 a year." What everyone had read, of course, was that the Portland Trail Blazers signed Walton for more than $1,000,000.

"What's happening to the money?" someone said.

"I don't know," Scott said. "I just know how he lives." He sipped a drink. "What's interesting," Scott said, smiling to himself, "is the time he went to Notre Dame with a UCLA basketball team that hadn't lost in years. Notre Dame beat them, but Bill's got sensible values. He didn't slit his throat. He just walked off the court, whistling the Notre Dame fight song."

Let the bookkeepers spend their lives with ledgers. Myself, I'd rather listen to a seven-foot whistler, cheerful in defeat, as he chirps away half a note flat, high above the tumult of the crowd.

BASKETBALL

A GRAND FINALE

By Joe Gergen

From Newsday
Copyright, ©, 1975, Newsday, Inc.

There is more to the man than the record and there is more to the record than the man. But, in the final analysis, the record is his and his is the record that will be the standard of measurement in college basketball for the foreseeable future. John Wooden won a tenth national championship in his last attempt, and that's something worth remembering.

In the concrete cavern that is the San Diego Sports Arena, John Wooden walked off the basketball court last night and into the uncertainty of retirement. He walked off with a basketball in his hands while his players, the ones who wore the blue and gold of UCLA, bounced along excitedly in front of him, pausing to thrust their fists into the air in acknowledgment of their conquest. He walked off a winner.

And if that fact appeared to find greater expression in his players, it's only the way the man intended it. John Wooden is a proud man, a man as proud of his self-control as he is of his team. He smiled, he accepted congratulations, and he stepped aside to watch his players do the celebrating after the 92–85 victory over Kentucky in the NCAA tournament's title game.

"I played my heart out for Coach Wooden," said Dave Meyers, the captain and intense leader of the Bruins. "It meant that much to me. He deserves to go out a winner."

And, meanwhile, the man said yes, thank you, it was nice, and wasn't it really quite a game. "I suppose anyone would like to go out with a victory," he finally revealed. "The fact that the victory was for the national championship doesn't lessen the pleasure."

As ever, there was the understated touch, the kind he had displayed before the game in the briefest of talks to his players. "He just said, 'Good luck, fellows,'" recalled junior guard Andre McCarter. "It was like he was stepping out of it and just leaving it up to us. But he had us prepared. And I feel his retirement was a great motivation factor even though he stressed winning it for ourselves."

What the Bruins did win for themselves was the recognition that they had done as much as any UCLA team of the past, as much as any team can be expected to do. They had won the national title, and in so doing they had surpassed the performance of the 1974 UCLA team, a team with superior talent.

"I know it means a lot to me," said Meyers, the only returning full-time starter from that team, "because we lost Bill [Walton] and Keith [Wilkes]. We lost more than any other team in the country. You didn't see any other team from the final four back here this time except us. That says a lot for our players and it says a lot about our coach. He's the best coach in the country."

Or, at least, he was. It's time to consign the "Win with Wooden" buttons to the attic treasure chests where the "Win with Wilkies" buttons are stored. Suddenly, John Wooden belongs to the past. "The sadness is in leaving the youngsters," Wooden said. "That and the association with people I've been with for many years. Oh, I'll still be there for a spell. I'll have to clean up some things. I don't want to leave all that work for the next man."

The next man will have quite an act to follow. In 27 seasons at UCLA, Wooden's teams won 620 games. They won the NCAA championship in 10 of the last 12 years. They won the grudging respect and admiration of every basketball man and fan in the country.

It was in recognition of those achievements that the 15,151 spectators accorded him a standing ovation as he walked to his seat on the UCLA bench before the game. As ever, he sat in the second seat from the end nearest the scorer's table. He rolled up his program, crossed his legs, and sent a UCLA team onto the court for the seven hundred and sixty-seventh and last time.

Kentucky didn't concede easily. The Wildcats went right to their muscle game at the start of play. Within nine seconds, Meyers was on the floor, courtesy of 240-pound Bob Guyette. Kevin Grevey, who had shot poorly in all four previous tournament games, was on target at the outset and Kentucky raced to a 17–12 lead. Then Meyers blanked a jump shot for UCLA and Guyette pounded him for his third personal foul, earning a seat on the Kentucky bench.

Rick Robey, the 240-pound freshman center, also encountered

foul trouble and soon gave way to 245-pound freshman Mike Phillips. But the Wildcats were forced to play with two small forwards, Grevey and Jack Givens, and Wooden took the opportunity to insert 7-1 center Ralph Drollinger into the lineup. Between Drollinger, the 6-8 Meyers, and 6-9 Richard Washington, the tournament's outstanding player, the Bruins began to dominate the boards and get two and sometimes three shots. "They had us outheighted," Grevey said.

The Bruins pushed a three-point half-time margin (43–40) to 10 (66–56) after eight minutes of the second half. It appeared the Wildcats were about to be inundated when Grevey, who had 18 points in the first half, rediscovered his touch.

Grevey, who finished as the game's high scorer with 34 points, connected on one three-point play and then produced another two minutes later. The lead melted away point by point until, with 6:49 remaining, it was down to one. The critical moment was at hand.

UCLA worked to set up Meyers from the top of the key but, as the Bruin forward went up to shoot, Grevey appeared in his path. Both men went sprawling, and Meyers was whistled for the foul, his fourth of the game. "I was very upset," Meyers said, "because I felt he went underneath me as I went up. It was that good old Midwestern play, he fell down."

What he said to the official, Hank Nichols, was more pointed and drew a technical. Now Grevey, Kentucky's best shooter, had the opportunity to shoot a one-and-one from the free-throw line and then a technical, and the Wildcats also would gain possession. If everything went perfectly, Kentucky would have five points and a four-point lead. The Wildcats got none. Grevey missed the front end of the one-and-one and then he missed the technical and Kentucky committed a turnover. The game was lost then and there. "I guess I kept thinking about that too much," Grevey said later, "and I hate thinking about it now."

The Wildcats never climbed closer to three points after that and McCarter clinched the victory by driving the open lane and scoring a lay-up for a 90–85 lead with 40 seconds left. UCLA had used only six men to combat perhaps the strongest team in the country, but those six were magnificent last night.

"Kentucky kind of wore down in the second half," said Washington, who had 28 points and 12 rebounds. "They weren't as physical." Pete Trgovich, the senior guard, was more direct in his evaluation. "I think Louisville had a better team and played a better style," he said.

And it really didn't matter that one fan in the crowd raised a banner that said, "In Your Hearts You Know Indiana Is No. 1." Indiana, like every other team in the nation, had fallen along the route to the national championship. Only UCLA was standing at the end, which is the way it has been for the better part of two decades in the era known as the Wooden Years.

"There'll be a whole new coaching staff here next year," Trgovich said. "With the system they have, they'll get a fine man. The school has too much of a reputation as a basketball power to go down drastically. But it won't be quite the same without John Wooden."

No, it won't. Even the man himself seemed finally to realize it some 45 minutes after the game, after he had spoken to his players and to newsmen and to well-wishers. In the corridor leading to the UCLA dressing room he encountered Nell Wooden, his wife of 42 years. And John Wooden, who had stared clear-eyed through those spectacles that gave him the appearance of a midwestern school-master, silently cried. The two of them stood there, locked in each other's arms, for what seemed like an eternity.

The work of a lifetime was over. Now just the record remains.

GENERAL

NAMATH'S MOTHER ALSO SCORES

By Gerald Eskenazi

From The New York Times
Copyright, ©, 1975, The New York Times Company
Reprinted by permission

Joe Namath was always collecting things in his bedroom.

"You couldn't walk through there," his mother, Rose Namath Szolnoki, recalled yesterday. "The bats were here, the football there, the basketball. Oh, it was a mess."

Young Joe just wasn't the way people think of him, she explained at her first news conference to discuss her book, *Namath: My Son Joe.* The writing was done by a former hopeful at quarterback for the Jets, William Kushner, who flunked a 1970 tryout with the team.

Mrs. Szolnoki, who still lives in Beaver Falls, Pa., proved to be a charming woman who knows how to sell a book ("You want to learn more? Buy the book.") It is published by Oxmoor House and will be out in September.

She worries about him just like any other mother would, she said about her bachelor-son, who will be thirty-two years old next Saturday.

"He always had that slouch," she said. "His brothers had it too. 'Straighten up,' I'd say. We must have inherited it from somebody."

Mrs. Szolnoki sees a change in Joe. "As the years go by," she said, "Joe is starting to like peace and quiet. He likes to stay home in the evenings, now."

But there was the time when the young quarterback got in trouble with Coach Bear Bryant at Alabama.

Mrs. Szolnoki called a mutual friend in Alabama and asked, "Should I talk to Bear? Is he angry?"

"I think so," the friend replied. "He just threw Joe's locker out of a second-story window."

There are other little-known stories that only a mother could tell. There was that incident in Joe's first year of high school when he had a knee problem.

"We thought it was polio," said his mother. "It turned out it wasn't." But she believes his knee problems stemmed from that time.

Before she went on stage at the American Booksellers Association convention at the Hilton, she met another author, Muhammad Ali, whose book is called, of course, *The Greatest: My Own Story.*

"I'm number one," Ali told Namath's mother.

"No. I'm number one," she replied.

Ali also disclosed that he had invented a new tactic called The Russian Tank. It replaces the Rope-A-Dope. The Russian Tank will be employed against Joe Bugner on June 30. It is, simply, a cover-up technique with arms, parallel to the ground, crossed in front of his face.

Mrs. Szolnoki covered up only once, when she was asked what effect her divorce from Joe's father had. At first she refused to discuss it, then relented.

"We had a nice life while it lasted," she said. "Joe was thirteen at the time. Joe was close to his father. He still is—and I've never stood in the way."

The divorce also broke up young Namath's relationship with his closest friend, a black youngster named Linny. In fact, most of Joe Namath's early friends were black—his family was one of the few white ones in a black neighborhood.

Until Joe was thirteen, he often would spend the night at Linny's house. He also started on an otherwise all-black football team.

"The man," a teammate once said, "really can throw the ball."

Indeed he could. His mother recalls that Joe "was always throwing a football higher than the telephone wires."

Mrs. Namath refused to be brought into the current question of whether Joe would sign again with the Jets. But her publisher, John Logue, said that when she was asked whether she should hold off from writing the final pages, she told him, "No, I think we can end it here. With Joe still playing for the Jets."

GENERAL

NAME THE U.S. CONGRESSMAN WHO HOLDS THE NFL
RECORD FOR THE MOST FUMBLES RECOVERED, LIFETIME

By Stanley Frank

From TV Guide
Copyright, ©, 1975, Triangle Publications, Inc., Radnor, Pennsylvania
Reprinted with permission

You probably never have heard of Seymour Siwoff, but you posi-
tively have heard the product of his labors. Siwoff is the official
statistician for the National Football League, the National League
in baseball, and the National Basketball Association. Without his
stupefying masses of figures, many sportscasters would be speech-
less for minutes on end.

"Overemphasis on statistics is the abomination of sportscasting,"
Howard Cosell says with characteristic restraint. "The principal job
of announcers should be to relate the audience to the athletes.
Harping on picayune percentages has made the reporting of events
as dull as recitals of insurance tables."

It may seem odd, but Siwoff agrees. "It's nonsense to spout numbers that have no significance," he says. "Used properly, statistics
describe performances in a comparative frame of reference. A .300
batting average means nothing unless you know that only about 20
players achieve it in a season. Conversely, a .300 passing average is
lousy in football and a .300 shooting average is mediocre in basketball.

"The real value of statistics lies in analyzing data in depth on a
team-vs.-team basis. We've done that for all the networks, which pay
us a fee for a special service we call color cards. We can make
commentators instant experts by helping them to anticipate the
turning points in a game or a series."

Asked to cite an example of such astute diagnosis, Siwoff said,
"Sure—the NBA championship playoff between the Golden State

Warriors and the Washington Bullets. Before it started we alerted Brent Musberger, who did the play-by-play for CBS, that the Bullets were strictly a six-man team and the Warriors were much stronger in reserves. You know what happened—the Warrior bench was the payoff."

Indeed it was. The Warriors' reserves outscored the Bullets', 147–61, accounting for more than one-third of their team's points.

"Siwoff made me look like a ruddy genius when I began stressing his dope on the reserves in the first game," Musberger admits. "I wouldn't have dug up that key to the series in a month of research. You've got to be careful with Seymour, though. He'll turn you into a talking computer if you repeat all the stuff he feeds you. I suppose too many of us use statistics as a crutch, a substitute for homework and imagination. In a good game the announcer can shut up and just throw in an occasional comment. In bad games there's a tendency to run off at the mouth to distract the audience. That's when you get rehashes of averages and overdoses of phony team records that drive fans up the walls."

Siwoff's statistical summaries are commissioned and paid for by the respective league offices. His New York office is open seven days a week throughout the year to process box scores immediately after the completion of games. In football and basketball, the tabulations are phoned in by the official scorers of the home teams; the baseball box scores are received by Teletype from newspaper wire services.

Another reason the office is open so late is to answer reporters' questions—although sometimes Siwoff doesn't wait for the queries. When a record is in the making, he watches TV to stay on top of the ball. In 1973, when O. J. Simpson ran wild in the first half against the New England Patriots, Siwoff phoned the broadcasting booth, checked Simpson's yardage on every attempt, and maintained direct contact until Simpson set a new single-game rushing record of 250 yards. Three months later, in Buffalo's final game, Siwoff helped Simpson become the first player in NFL history to gain 2,000 yards rushing in one season. Simpson went into the game needing 197 yards, and Siwoff informed the Buffalo coaches, via the press-box phone, of O. J.'s progress. Although Buffalo clobbered the Jets, 34–14, Simpson remained in action until he reached 2,001 yards on his thirty-fourth carry of the day.

Later that night Siwoff audited the official scorer's work sheets. "We verified the line of scrimmage before every Buffalo running play," he says. "There were two errors because the mud had obscured the markings on the field. O. J. actually gained two more yards for a total of 2,003. We sent out a flash to all the wire services to set the record straight."

On July 25, there was a sudden flurry of activity in Siwoff's office. The radio was tuned to the Mets-Cubs game in Chicago, and the announcer reported that Paul Reuschel was the new pitcher for the Cubs. His brother Rick had started the game.

"Oh-oh, get ready," someone said. "They'll be calling from Chicago to find out the last time brothers pitched in the same game."

"Look up the Atlanta box scores toward the end of last season," Siwoff snapped. "I think Phil and Joe Niekro worked in a game, but check it."

Five minutes later, when the call came from the press box in Wrigley Field, Siwoff was ready to report: the Niekro brothers appeared in the same game on September 7, 1974.

"Oddities and trick records intrigue the fans, but the chief charm of statistics for me is the bridge they build for establishing the marvelous skills of former stars," Siwoff says. "There's no way to compare the interpretations of Hamlet by Laurence Olivier and John Barrymore. Even if a film with Barrymore's version were available, it would be one-dimensional. But sports statistics is a method —even a language—for making performances come alive. The fans always identify old favorites by their averages. Statistics are the final authority in settling saloon debates. They're the fuel that keeps the hot-stove league going full blast during the off-season.

"It's depressing to realize that few football fans today have heard of Sammy Baugh, maybe the best quarterback ever seen," he says. "Baugh completed 56.5 percent of his passes, less than one point behind Bart Starr, the all-time leader. Baugh still holds the career and season records for best punting averages. In his day everybody played the offense *and* defense, and he was the first man to intercept four passes in a game. The statistics prove his class."

The most publicized record in sports history, Henry Aaron's seven hundred fifteenth home run last year, prompted Siwoff to add a statistical category to affirm Babe Ruth's preeminence as a slugger. He compiled a table relating homers to times at bat. The Babe was far in front with a home run every 11.76 trips to the plate. Aaron, with 15.86, was ninth on the list, behind Harmon Killebrew (14.02), Ralph Kiner (14.11), Willie McCovey (14.40), Ted Williams (14.79), Mickey Mantle (15.12), Jimmy Foxx (15.23), and Hank Greenberg (15.69).

NBC's Curt Gowdy supports Siwoff's argument for statistics. "Statistics dramatize the feats of former stars and draw attention to promising rookies. Fans always associate players with their statistics.

They refer to Ted Williams as the last .400 hitter in baseball; they remember the 26 passes Johnny Unitas completed in the sudden-death playoff with the Giants in 1958, and the 100 points Wilt Chamberlain scored in a game 13 years ago. The numbers give sports the continuity that sustains interest through the years."

Now fifty-four, Siwoff went to work as a $12-a-week office boy for the Elias Baseball Bureau in 1939, and the thrill of meeting the heroes of that era sustained him through 13 consecutive weeks without a payday.

In 1952 Siwoff took over the moribund Elias Bureau, which compiled only baseball averages, and since then he has expanded his service by introducing more than 50 categories in three sports. He has added such items as saves by relief pitchers, yards lost attempting to pass, and blocked shots in basketball. It was just a warm-up for a broader concept of his work.

"Statistics is a science that should have more important applications than turning out mere numbers," he says earnestly. "I've always wanted to develop a method for measuring the effectiveness of athletes. It involved feeding a lot of data into computers, an expense I couldn't afford until Bowie Kuhn's office commissioned me to set up criteria for evaluating a player's contribution to the success of his team.

"This opens up a revolutionary approach to contract negotiations," Siwoff points out. "For instance, what's the relative importance to a team of a slick shortstop who hits .260? An outfielder who drives in 100 runs? A pitcher who wins 15 games?

"There will be loud screams on both sides of the bargaining table when this system is used by management. I'll catch a lot of flak, but at least people will no longer say statistics are Mickey Mouse stuff."

And now for a few loud screams from those who failed to answer the question at the beginning of this article. The holder of the NFL record for most fumbles recovered, lifetime, is Jack Kemp (Pittsburgh Steelers, 1957; Los Angeles Chargers, 1960; San Diego Chargers, 1960–62; Buffalo Bills, 1962–69; House of Representatives, 1971 to present).

"Actually," says Siwoff, "Kemp recovered mostly his own fumbles."

BASKETBALL

THE CARDIAC KIDS END AN INCREDIBLE SEASON

By John Simmonds

From The Oakland Tribune
Copyright, ©, 1975, The Tribune Publishing Co.

As the buzzer sounded Rick Barry tossed the basketball high in the air and a moment later the Warrior dressing room was a scene of total bedlam.

Corks popped out of champagne bottles and the bubbly stuff flowed over everyone. Players hugged and cheered and a flood of reporters and cameramen turned the cramped dressing quarters into a room of wall-to-wall people.

An incredible season had ended on an incredible note for the Golden State Warriors, CHAMPIONS of the National Basketball Association.

With less than four minutes gone in the first quarter yesterday at Capital Centre the Warriors had lost their coach. They were down by 14 points in the second quarter and by eight with four minutes remaining in the game.

Yet the Cardiac Kids came roaring down the stretch to hand the Washington Bullets the killing blow in the championship series with a 96–95 victory and become only the third team in NBA history to win the title with a four-game sweep.

"I've never been associated with a greater bunch of guys," bubbled Barry, who scored 20 points and won *Sport* magazine's Most Valuable Player Award for the series.

"It's utopia to be out there with them," Rick continued. "They're incredible and this is something I'll never forget the rest of my life."

Meanwhile, guard Charles Johnson stood on a bench and sipped a beer instead of champagne.

"It hasn't really hit me yet that we're number one," he said. "But I hope I'm alone somewhere when it does because I'm going to explode."

Keith Wilkes, the rookie sensation whose big rebound near the end helped the Warriors get the final victory, was asked to compare this championship with the NCAA titles scored by his UCLA teams.

"Right now this is my top thrill," Wilkes answered. "It's a lot like my sophomore season at UCLA. We weren't supposed to be that good but went on to go 30–0 and win the NCAA championship.

"This team wasn't supposed to go anywhere either. We lost a lot of people from last season and made a lot of changes. But we won our division title, the conference title, and then beat Seattle, Chicago, and Washington in the playoffs."

"This year we proved we deserve to be where we are," added coach Al Attles. "If this is not the best team this year, I don't know who is."

Center Clifford Ray called the championship win the "greatest feeling I've ever had."

"These guys busted their rears all season long," he beamed.

"I don't know what to say, it's an unbelievable feeling. We had the desire and came from last to the top. This should help younger teams. It shows you can accomplish a lot when you stick together and have a lot of harmony."

General Manager Dick Vertlieb called it a season where everything worked.

"We had good coaching, good athletes, and no injury of any consequence," he said. "Everything worked and when it does you win a championship."

"This is the highlight of my pro career," said veteran guard Jeff Mullins as he wiped champagne from his eye, and forward Bill Bridges, who is making this thirteenth season his last, echoed that thought.

"It's my top thrill, definitely so," he said.

The game almost turned into a riot in the first quarter.

Mike Riordan, using everything but a blackjack on Barry in the early going, picked up his third foul when he grabbed and slugged Rick from behind and Attles had seen enough.

Al charged off the bench toward the Bullet forward but was intercepted by several players and Assistant Coach Joe Roberts before he could reach his target.

Al left with the score 10–4 for the Bullets and turned the coaching reins over to Roberts. Things got much worse before they got better as the Bullets' quick guard Kevin Porter burned the Warriors time after time by slipping behind the defense for baskets.

But the Warriors shot 67 percent in clawing their way back in a sloppy second quarter, closing to within two points just before the half after trailing 36–22 earlier in the period.

The Warriors didn't get a lead, though, until late in the third quarter when Phil Smith notched a jumper to push them in front, 66–65.

Washington immediately regained control and seemingly had its first series win locked up when Elvin Hayes hit a jumper to put the Warriors down, 92–84, with 4:44 left in the game.

But the pressure got to the Bullets—the team that was supposed to replace the Boston Celtics as NBA champions—instead of the Warriors in the dying moments.

Wilkes hit a jumper and then Porter missed two straight free throws that would have put the Bullets back up by eight. The Warriors got four quick points and then Porter failed on a short jumper when Ray stepped out on him.

Then Wilkes reached over bulky center Wes Unseld for an offensive rebound and put the ball back up to tie the score at 92 with 2:12 remaining.

"The ball went up and I went to it and got it in good position," Wilkes said. "When I went back up I figured I would at least get fouled."

Butch Beard then fouled Hayes, but the Big E made only one free throw and the Bullets led by a point. Butch put the Warriors ahead for good when he drove around Porter and down the side of the key past Unseld for a lay-up.

The Bullets blew an opportunity when Unseld passed poorly to Phil Chenier and out of bounds. Moments later, Dick Gibbs blew an easy lay-up after taking an Unseld pass.

Washington had the ball again with 30 seconds to go but Unseld bounced the ball off his knee and into the backcourt and the Warriors regained possession.

Porter fouled Beard, who hit one free throw with 19 seconds left for a 95–93 Warrior lead. Chenier missed a jumper against Ray with nine seconds left. Beard got the rebound and was fouled by Hayes.

With three chances to make two, Butch missed the first two shots. But the third one went in and the Warriors had an insurmountable three-point lead.

"After I missed the first two I told myself to relax," Butch said. "But I thought the second one was in the basket."

Attles watched the last three and a half quarters on television in the Warrior dressing room but insisted it didn't bother him that much.

"I thought I did the right thing in going out on the floor and I had all the confidence in the world in Joe and the players," Al said.

"The only thing that concerned me was that we might get the

feeling that if we don't get it today we'll get it next time."

Roberts accepted his temporary head coaching duties calmly.

"I just used the guys who were producing," he said before taking a swig of champagne. "I knew the Bullets were tired and I felt if we could run them we could beat them."

It was another big day for backup center George Johnson, who swatted away four Bullet shots, took 11 rebounds, and once drove around Unseld for an easy basket.

Wilkes, Bridges, and Derrek Dickey did another fine job on Hayes, limiting him to 15 points, only five in the second half. Elvin fouled out in the waning seconds.

Lost in defeat was a super effort by Chenier, the Berkeley High product, who scored 26 points, passed for 11 assists, and had five steals.

GENERAL

HOW IVAN DOES IT

By Wally Provost

From the Omaha World-Herald
Copyright, ©, 1975, Omaha World-Herald Company

Late in June a friend passed along a brittle issue of a sporting tabloid published in Caliente in 1944. Adm. William Standley, recent ambassador to the Soviet Union, had visited the Mexican racetrack and relayed this report on hoofing in wartime Moscow:

"They had all the daily doubles, quinielas, and mutuel betting. Tremendous crowds attended. One-hundred-ruble bets were common. The track is government controlled. They race seven days a week."

That was a tantalizer.

In Moscow two weeks ago, I learned that races were being held each Sunday, Wednesday, and Friday with first post at 6 P.M. on the weekdays.

"Let's see how Ivan does it," Mrs. Ogle said on a Friday. We found a cooperative taxi driver near Red Square and went bouncing toward a new racing adventure.

Several miles from downtown Moscow, but still well within the city, we arrived at the track. Or so the cabbie said. We were reluctant to release him. Nothing in sight resembled a racetrack grandstand.

We had stopped at a cul-de-sac in what looked like a typical old Moscow neighborhood—solid façades of shops, apartment buildings, and offices.

The structure immediately before us had the appearance of one of the city's countless vintage institutes: exterior of yellow stucco with white trim, a columned portico, granite steps.

Are you certain this is the Hippodrome (and not the Lenin Moustache Cup Museum)? The driver nodded affirmatively and gestured that we should go on in.

Sparing readers the various means of discovery, there were three entrances to three wholly segregated grandstand sections, the price depending on proximity to the finish line. Most expensive was 80 Russian pennies, 100 of which are worth about $1.40.

If Russian society is classless, horseplayers don't know about it.

When you have a ticket in Russia, you next look for a doorway with an elderly woman sitting on a chair. She'll be the ticket-taker.

Past the seated woman was a dingy hall, an untidy room for refreshments and snacks, more hallway, a pari-mutuel room about 40 by 40 and through the far doorway in this room the actual entrance to the grandstand.

Excelsior! Or whatever they say in the Land of Skavinsky-Skivar.

Let slide the fact that it turned out to be sulky racing instead of thoroughbreds. We were interested in atmosphere and procedures.

The track still has exactas and quinielas. That could be determined by prolonged study of signs over the mutuel windows. There also apparently was straight betting on win and place.

All the clerks were women and they seemingly doubled as sellers and cashiers. Mutuel tickets were in small stacks according to number, each stack secured by a rubber band.

The basic wager is one ruble ($1.40). Each bet is recorded by hand on a large tally sheet. Just before each race, the clerk adds up the amount bet on each horse or combination.

Presumably some mathematical sharpy in an inner office calculates the eventual payoffs. A huge electric message board in the infield shows the winning numbers but we never did see prices posted. In fact, the board broke down after the third race.

Finally despairing of making accurate window identification, the country boy picked out a handicapper of crafty mien and got behind him in line.

After that dude made his bet, I thrust the identical number of rubles through the wicket, nodded toward the departing player, and said, "Same."

The clerk thought I was mispronouncing "siem," which is Russian for the number seven. Worse yet, it was an exacta window. I gave her three more numbers and walked away with three combinations based on number seven winning the next race.

Number seven came in fifth. I felt right at home.

There were two tiers of high-walled "boxes" in the high-priced upper section of the Hippodrome. No seats. The players stood—or mostly leaned on the parapets. Above was a balcony with bench-type seats.

Few women in attendance. Most of the men were dressed like a U.S. hard-times party, circa 1935.

Strangest of all, there was no cheering, no roaring of the crowd. Some muttering, of course.

The start and finish of each race was signaled by one clang of what sounded like a giant dinner bell.

The sulkies would take off at a brisk pace, but position changes were few after drivers reached midpoint of the backstretch. Maybe there really wasn't much to cheer about.

Mrs. Ogle and her escort sat next to a quiet young couple in the balcony for several races, bemoaning their failure earlier in the day to find a race-going interpreter who could have explained all the fine points.

Then the young couple departed. As they squeezed past, the man said, "Excuse us, please" in flawless English. We were too stunned to chase after them.

FOOTBALL

A THROWBACK TO FOOTBALL'S STONE AGE

By Glenn Dickey

From the San Francisco Chronicle
Copyright, ©, 1975, Chronicle Publishing Co.

Pittsburgh dropped its Steel Curtain on Minnesota with a thud yesterday in Super Bowl IX, whipping the Vikings decisively, 16–6, in a game that lived down to everybody's expectations.

It was a game only a winning football coach could like. It was a throwback to football's Stone Age, muscle against muscle, and the Steelers had more muscle.

The flying wedge would not have looked out of place in this one. It was a game that made all those beautiful football clichés come alive, being won in the pit or the trenches, take your pick. If you liked The Flintstones, you would have loved this one.

At that, it could have been worse. At half time it was 2–0 Steelers, and only the tension and the weather kept the fans awake. It was 46 degrees at game time, declining to 43 at half time, and a sadistic public address announcer told everybody that the wind made a chill factor of 22. It didn't seem that warm.

Clearly, NFL commissioner Pete Rozelle blew it. The day before the weather had been warm, almost balmy, and the game obviously should have been scheduled for that day. For the money Rozelle is paid, he should be able to pick the right day.

Yesterday was a day of firsts for the Steelers, their first time in the Super Bowl and the first time a newcomer has beaten a repeater. The credit is not all theirs, however, since they were playing the Vikings, a team that has now been to the game three times and lost each time. They strive for consistency, and by God they achieve it.

The Pittsburgh win further established the dominance of the American Conference in the interconference rivalry. The AFC or AFL has now won six of the past seven Super Bowls, and this win comes on top of a decisive AFC lead in interconference season games. Indeed, it could be argued that the top three teams in football are AFC teams—Pittsburgh, Oakland, and Miami.

All week, Pittsburgh's physical superiority had been conceded by all but the most rabid of Minnesota fans, but the question remained whether the Steelers would feel the pressure of their first visit to the Super Bowl.

That question was quickly answered, in the negative. The Steelers played their game from the beginning, and forced Minnesota to do the same. Even when it was 0–0 in the first half, the Steelers were dominating the game, and their dominance became more pronounced as the game went on.

As they had against Oakland in the AFC championship, the Steelers took away the run, allowing the Vikings only 21 yards in 20 carries, an even poorer showing than the Raiders made.

But unlike their game with the Raiders, the Steelers also took away the pass yesterday. The beleagured Fran Tarkenton completed only 11 of 27, with three interceptions, for 102 yards. Possibly even more telling was the fact that only one of those completions went to an outside receiver.

Tarkenton, playing more aggressively than Ken Stabler did in the AFC championship, completed a pass on the first Minnesota offensive play of the game, and he often went to a pass on first down to try to loosen up the Pittsburgh defense, but it did no good.

The Steeler defense was simply overwhelming. There was no great mystery to it: The front four (with Dwight White making an amazing recovery after his week in the hospital) forced Tarkenton to throw under pressure almost always, and the linebackers and defensive backs covered his receivers completely.

The nimble Tarkenton was never sacked, but only because he dumped the ball off time after time to running backs for short gains at best. Even when the Vikings got a break, they couldn't take advantage of it.

The most notable instance came with Pittsburgh ahead, 9–0, early in the fourth quarter and the Vikings, despite their ineptness, only a break or two back. They got a break, with pass interference being called on a long pass play at the Pittsburgh five, but on the next play, Chuck Foreman fumbled and Pittsburgh recovered.

Indeed, had it been up to the Viking offense, the NFC champions would have been shut out. The only Minnesota score came on a blocked punt, and the Vikings got inside the Pittsburgh 20 only on the pass interference call.

For a time yesterday, it appeared the game might go four scoreless quarters into an overtime that nobody wanted, because Minnesota was obviously incapable of scoring and Pittsburgh didn't seem to want to.

Twice in the first quarter, the Steelers had a chance to score but let it go by. The first time, Roy Gerela missed a 38-yard field goal, the ball sailing wide to the left, and the second time the Steelers missed first a touchdown and then a field goal.

Moving from their own 47, the Steelers had a first down on the Minnesota 29 when quarterback Terry Bradshaw pulled a beautiful play, faking a handoff to the left side and then rolling to the right. He made 11 yards and probably would have scored if wide receiver Rob Shanklin could have blocked cornerback Nate Wright, but Shanklin merely waved at Wright going by and the Viking made an open-field tackle at the 18.

Three plays later, the Steelers, having advanced only two yards closer to the goal, tried another field goal. This time, holder Bobby Walden fumbled the snap and tried to run with it, being downed on the 23, with the Vikings taking over on downs.

Minnesota got its chance to miss a field goal early in the second quarter, Fred Cox kicking wide to the right on his only attempt of the day, and then Pittsburgh finally got on the scoreboard, fittingly enough with a defensive effort.

After a punt had pinned Minnesota down on its seven, Tarkenton tried to hand off to Dave Osborne, who ran a little wider than he should have. The ball was fumbled, Pittsburgh and L.C. Greenwood kicked it, and Tarkenton finally fell on the ball as he slid into the end zone for a safety.

"You can't afford to let this Pittsburgh defense have a 2-0 lead," remarked sage Dan Jenkins.

That insurmountable lead went to 9-0 early in the third quarter after Pittsburgh benefited from an error of its own. Gerela slipped as he kicked off to start the second half, the ball bouncing crazily from about the Minnesota 40 to the 30. Bill Brown bobbled it there and Jon Kolb recovered for the Steelers.

Franco Harris then took over. First he ran for 24 yards to the six and then, after being thrown back three on the next play, sprinted around the left side for the touchdown, getting a block from tackle Gerry Mullins at the line of scrimmage and going in untouched.

The game then reverted to its earlier pattern, which was Pittsburgh making errors and the Vikings unable to do anything about it. One time, a Bradshaw pass went directly to Minnesota linebacker Jeff Siemon, but the Vikings were offside. Another time, Harris fumbled and the Vikings immediately followed with the long pass that resulted in the interference call mentioned earlier. Then Minnesota fumbled the ball back.

Finally, the Viking defense, realizing that just getting the ball for the offense wasn't enough, took over completely and blocked a punt for the touchdown. The PAT was wide, and the score was 9–6, Pittsburgh.

Only a field goal back, Minnesota was still in the game, in theory, but Pittsburgh's superiority was so obvious at that point, it would have taken another big break for the Vikings to tie or take the lead.

That break was not forthcoming. Instead, the Steelers followed with the only sustained drive of the game, going 66 yards for a touchdown in 11 plays that took slightly more than seven minutes, leaving the Vikings with only three and one-quarter minutes to effect a miracle after the Steelers' PAT made it 16–6.

The big play came on third-and-two from the Pittsburgh 42. Bradshaw hit tight end Larry Brown at the Minnesota 40 and he ran to the 28. Just before he hit the turf, Brown fumbled and the Vikings seemed to recover—but the play was, correctly, ruled dead.

Seven plays later, the Steelers faced a third down on the four and obviously wanted the touchdown, because a field goal would still have given the Vikings a chance to overcome them with a touchdown.

Bradshaw rolled to the right and it appeared for an instant that he might run in. Linebacker Siemon came up to prevent that, leaving Brown one-on-one with safety Paul Krause and a step behind him, and Bradshaw threw a bullet strike to the tight end for the touchdown.

For practical purposes, that was it. On Minnesota's next play, Tarkenton threw his third interception and Pittsburgh then ran the ball and the clock down, finally yielding the ball on downs at the Minnesota 23, just in time for two meaningless Viking plays before the end.

GENERAL

CURE FOR THE BLUES

By Regis McAuley

From the Tucson Daily Citizen
Copyright, ©, 1975, Tucson Daily Citizen

Once upon a time, before lawsuits, drug abuse, armed robberies, and traffic violations were all part of the sports scene, it was fun to be a writer.

One of the fringe benefits of rounding third base in your career is that when the news gets too depressing you can just lean back in your chair, close your eyes, and think of all the hearty laughs you've had as you traveled the road when sports was still a game.

Like the night Bob Lemon had a two-strike count on Ted Williams and the next pitch cut the corner of the plate, but the umpire called it a ball. Lemon, in one of his few squawks at an umpire, came charging off the mound and ran all the way across home plate where he shook his red face violently back and forth as he told off the umpire. Then on his way back to the mound he said something to Williams and the Splendid Splinter doubled over with laughter.

After the game we asked Lemon what he had said to the greatest hitter in baseball. "I said, 'and as for you, you big idiot, why didn't you swing at it?' "

Lemon was involved in another situation, which shows how cool this star Cleveland Indian pitcher was. It was the night he pitched his no-hitter against Detroit in old Briggs Stadium. Johnny Berardino, who is seen daily now in the television soap opera, "General Hospital," was a utility infielder for the Indians at that time and was being used at first base, an unfamiliar spot for him. George Kell, the hard-hitting third baseman for the Tigers, was up with two outs in the ninth. Berardino was trembling at first base, lest the ball be hit at him. Kell hit a one-hop smash right back at Lemon, but at the crack of the bat, Berardino fell down on all fours. Lemon trotted over toward first to give Berardino time to scramble over to the bag and then he said, as he tossed the ball underhanded for the final out of his famous no-hitter, "Now don't drop it, stupid."

And there was the day here in Tucson when we were leaving Del Webb's Hiway House to go to Phoenix for a game with the Giants. I left my sports jacket neatly folded on the bed and forgot to take it with me. That night, manager Jimmy Dykes invited us to dinner at the famous Camelback Inn.

When Harry Chiti, the big second-string catcher, heard that I wasn't going because I had forgotten my jacket, he came to my room and offered me his. I put it on and could feel it hitting somewhere near my knees. "How does it look?" I asked him and he said, "Well, where are you going?" I went to the dinner anyhow.

I tried to sneak into the Camelback inconspicuously and on our way out after dinner, a well-dressed, executive-type gentleman sitting at a table with his wife and another couple tugged me by the coattail and whispered, "Sir, would you mind giving me the name of your tailor?" I could have strangled Dykes, who had gone on ahead, puffing his cigar and chuckling.

When Early Wynn finally won his coveted three hundredth game, it was in Kansas City and the team had to dash to catch a plane for Minneapolis right after the game. The late Charley Morris, Indians' traveling secretary, called ahead and ordered the proper refreshments sent to a hotel parlor because the bars close at 1 A.M. in Minneapolis.

In the midst of our toasting Wynn, somebody remembered that we didn't buy him a present. So George Strickland, the coach, stepped up on a velvet-covered sofa, took an oil painting down from the wall, and presented it to Wynn in one of the most flowery speeches ever heard.

Wynn gave a speech that night, too. He told of how he had unlaced catcher Clint Courtney's glove one day in Chicago and smeared Limburger cheese in the padding, then laced it up again.

"I didn't like the umpire who was working the plate that night," Wynn said, "and every time the ball popped into Courtney's glove, that umpire would wince and turn his back. But Courtney didn't even notice it."

And that wonderful day the Indians won the 1948 pennant and owner Bill Veeck, who had been criticized editorially by *The Sporting News* for signing an old clown like Satchel Paige to a contract (Paige won 12 games to help the Indians win the flag), sent this telegram to publisher Taylor Spink:

"May I please nominate Satchel Paige for your paper's 'Rookie of the Year' award?"

Those were the days, my friend.

GOLF

WOMEN'S GOLF: THE REWARDS ARE ELUSIVE

By Joan Libman

From The Wall Street Journal
Copyright, ©, 1975, The Wall Street Journal

A crowd of close to 200 watches silently at the tenth green of the Pasadena Golf Club in St. Petersburg, Fla., as the perfectly coiffed woman leans over a putt. Kathy Whitworth, who has earned more than a half-million dollars as a professional golfer, taps the ball 25 feet downhill and into the cup for a birdie. The crowd cheers.

Across the fairway, only four spectators gather at a tee as Jane Ferraris, a pro from San Francisco, blasts a drive 260 yards. Two of the onlookers are so engrossed in a conversation about a roast-beef dinner that they ignore the shot. "Imagine that," says a man in pastel Bermuda shorts, "for only $3.75 they let you go back for seconds at no extra charge."

The lack of attention from her tiny gallery doesn't bother Miss Ferraris. At the Orange Blossom Classic here, as at most big tournaments, the crowds gravitate toward stars and big money-makers such as Kathy Whitworth, Jane Blalock, and Laura Baugh.

Jane Ferraris is neither a star nor a big winner on the Ladies Professional Golf Association (LPGA) tour. Last year the twenty-eight-year-old pro's U.S. winnings totaled only $10,000 (she finished fortieth on the official money list). In nine years on the circuit, she has never wound up higher than sixteenth. She has won only three tournaments and faces the prospect that, after hundreds of rounds of tournament golf, she may never be rich or famous.

But for Miss Ferraris, as for many others on the LPGA tour, being a woman professional athlete is bringing increasing satisfaction. Golf is starting to benefit from the public's interest in women's sports, and many women who couldn't have survived playing golf in the past now are making a modest but adequate living.

Although golf hasn't made the dramatic advances of women's tennis, it has come a long way. Betsy Rawls, a top pro, recalls how 25 years ago 15 women traveled from tournament to tournament by car caravan, competing for a total season's purse of about $25,000. Last year, the LPGA tour swelled to 112 members who jetted around the country to split a $1.8 million total purse.

"In those days, you didn't do it for the money," Miss Rawls recalls. "You had to love it." Today, it's hard to imagine anyone loving the life—a constant grind of tournaments and practice—but the rewards are far more tangible.

Miss Ferraris, for example, grossed $25,000 last year. That included her $10,000 LPGA money, $10,000 from a Japanese tournament, and $5,000 from a television dishwashing-liquid commercial. Her expenses, including caddies, motels, car rentals, air fare, and food, came to about $12,000. While on tour, she cuts expenses by sharing a room with a young Australian golfer, Penny Pulz.

Her income has enabled her to build up some savings, to a point that she complains about the problems of investing. "Wherever you go, people have a hot deal for you. It's hard to know who to trust with your money," she says. She keeps $10,000 cash readily available "to grab hold of whenever I want to." Recently, she doubled her money on a land investment near a Cape Cod golf course. She also owns part of a Palm Springs, Calif., condominium and is pondering how to invest some funds tied up in bankers' acceptances.

Sometimes Miss Ferraris, a solidly built woman with a pixieish manner, thinks about quitting the tour and teaching golf. (She dropped out of college after her freshman year so her career choices are somewhat limited.) But the lure of the pro circuit is strong. "How many other ways are there for a woman to clear $13,000 by actually working 30 weeks a year?" she asks.

Actually, the 30 weeks of tournament play are spread over about 10 months, and Miss Ferraris is on the road most of that time. She also makes several trips to Japan and Australia each year to compete in tournaments. "The traveling is getting to me," she admits. "I don't enjoy packing and unpacking. I don't enjoy going to the laundry to wash clothes. And I don't enjoy eating hotel food. Being Italian, I like eggs fried in olive oil. I can't get that, so I've given up eating breakfast, even before a tournament."

The tedium of traveling between one golf course and another is apparent as Miss Ferraris talks to a reporter in her motel here. Reaching for another beer and lighting a cigarette, she says, "When you first start on the tour, you do a lot of sightseeing. But after you've seen the Alamo five times, what do you do?" Most often, she says, she collapses in front of the television set in her motel room at night and watches "cop things" like "Kojak" or "Columbo."

Following the sun on the pro tour does little for one's social life, she adds. She avoids casual dates. "One-time-going-out-to-dinner really gets boring, and I would just as soon watch TV as tell my whole life story all over again," she says.

She prefers to date men who are athletes. "When he [her athlete-date] is talking about mental pressures before a game and the let-downs after one, I know what he's talking about," she says.

To break the routine, Miss Ferraris occasionally skis. "It's really good to look down and see white," she says. "You get tired of seeing grass all the time." But the diversion isn't entirely relaxing, "be-cause you have to worry about hurting yourself," she adds. "One cut on the hand can mean having to change your whole [golf] grip."

Although Miss Ferraris is glad to be earning a living at pro golf, she criticizes the LPGA for not trying harder to promote players. And she chides her sister golfers for failing to demand more promo-tion.

"Look at the St. Petersburg tournament," she says. "Men wouldn't play for $35,000 total prize money. We don't have anyone to market the LPGA. Publicity is how you get the purses up, which increases outside interest and creates more ways [such as product endorsements] to earn money."

Betsy Rawls disagrees. "There's no God-given right to make a living at golf," she says. "I don't think we should be playing for $100,000 a week like men do, because they are more spectacular and that's a different kind of show. You can't create publicity out of thin air."

Despite her frustrations, Miss Ferraris enjoys the competitive life. She took up golf at age ten when her father, an orchestra leader at a well-known San Francisco hotel, would take her to the golf course to keep him company. At thirteen, she entered her first tournament.

Those who watched her compete in those days say Mr. Ferraris pushed his daughter hard. "I remember one tournament when she was doing badly," one observer recalls. "Instead of playing through, he pulled her out so they could rush over to enter another tournament."

The pressure continued in high school, when Miss Ferraris remembers having to juggle activities around to please her father. She ran through nine holes after school in order to get back to campus in time to watch a basketball game or play on the volleyball team. "Back then," she recalls, "women athletes were regarded as weirdos. You had to go overboard to show everyone you weren't."

These days, she and her father don't discuss golf at all.

As an adult, she finds that winning is a constant preoccupation. "You really have to be blood and guts to succeed out here," Miss Ferraris says. "You can't let too many things interfere with what you have to do. The biggest challenge is to play better. I feel my potential lies in the top 10 and that's frustrating. You play with people and you know in your heart you're better than they are, yet they beat you every week."

Blood and guts notwithstanding, friends praise her for being a helpful critic. On the practice day before the tournament here, she looks across the green at roommate Penny Pulz, a twenty-three-year-old newcomer to the tour, and yells, "You're getting the idea, but you're not driving enough with your legs. Not so much body."

On the second hole of the practice round, it starts to rain, and Miss Ferraris, who has a cold, tries to continue. Drenched by the time she reaches the third hole, she gives up, heading for the clubhouse. The rain lets up and her threesome starts to play again, but one hole later, the practice day is rained out for good.

Her cold isn't much better at the start of the tournament the next day, but Miss Ferraris shows up at the practice tee; she is wearing blue-checkered pants and a blue shirt. A local photographer asks for a picture. She complains, "I don't know why they have to do this today when they could have done it yesterday." But when the photographer gives the cue, she leans on the golf bag and smiles for the camera.

Her nerves begin to show almost immediately. On the first tee, she hits what looks like a beautiful shot, but the wind takes over, sending the ball into a water hazard. She also has trouble putting. By the sixth hole, three putts have circled the cup but missed.

Difficulty with putting is a common malady at the tournament. On another green, Hollis Stacy of Savannah, Ga., is in trouble too. At one point, her exasperated thirteen-year-old sister, Martha, a golf enthusiast, pulls Miss Stacy aside. "Look," Martha is overheard demanding, "would you just relax on the putts?"

On the last hole, Miss Ferraris hits the ball into the water again, taking a two-stroke penalty and winding up three over par. The rest of the tournament goes much the same way, but there are bright spots. "Wow," says a man shaking his head at her 5-foot-4 frame, "that little body, and she hit that ball 250 yards. I wish I could do that."

But Miss Ferraris fails to pick up momentum. By the third and final day, thousands of spectators have gathered, most watching two separate rounds featuring Amy Alcott, a freckle-faced eighteen-year-old from Santa Monica, Calif., who has a one-stroke lead over veteran Sandra Post going into the final hole. It is Miss Alcott's first tournament as a pro.

Sandra Post arrives at the final hole first, sinking a long putt to finish one under par and tie the tournament. Miss Ferraris sits on the grass drinking a beer, watching as Miss Alcott, wearing a red ribbon in her hair, sinks a spectacular 15-foot putt to win the tournament by one stroke. The crowd goes wild.

A poised Amy Alcott accepts the $5,000 prize and is bombarded by reporters and photographers. No one gathers around Jane Ferraris, a former rookie of the year, who in 1972 won this very tournament. This time, she wins $140 for finishing eight over par.

"Well," she says philosophically, heading for her car, "$140 is better than a kick in the fanny."

GENERAL

THEY DO IT TO HEAR BUBBLES

By Phil Hersh

From the Baltimore Evening Sun
Copyright, ©, 1975, Baltimore Evening Sun

This time it was for fun, the girls out on the river to accommodate a photographer, a few sprints and some paddling around.

But the wind was serious and the chill dipped the temperature below 50 degrees and the Washington College women's crew was wearing shorts and short-sleeve shirts to look prettier for the pictures.

This was a day for bulky sweat suits like the ones they wore in mid-March, when the cold made their hair freeze and the blisters on their hands oozed blood.

"It is an excruciating sport," says their coach, Barry McArdle, "and they do it."

They do it to hear bubbles, the curious reward when natural forces combine if the boat is balanced and moving quickly and everything is set up perfectly. Then the eight-oared shell fairly planes along, the rush of the water bubbling under its midsection.

"Did we have bubbles at Barnard?" asks Debbie Gitt, who pulls the number-four oar. "Damn, I wish I'd heard them."

She is a freshman who never played anything at Mount Hebron High School and she started rowing only two months ago. Suddenly this strange sport where you go backward sitting down has become a dominant force in her life.

The day the crew voted not to enter next weekend's Eastern Sprints—the vote had to be unanimous, and the seniors had term papers to do—Debbie took a 10-mile bike ride to calm down.

"I couldn't believe how upset I was," she says. "I was noncompetitive when I came here and about the least competitive on the team, and I wasn't ready to quit."

The end seemed so abrupt for a bunch that had gone any lengths to race in its second season of varsity competition.

They opened the season with a crushing loss to Vesper in Philadelphia, then came back the next day to beat George Washington on the Chester. That was the race when the number seven, Cindy Morton, rowed 600 of the 1,000 meters on the bottom of the shell after her seat slide went off its track.

Three more races and three victories and they were ready for the President's Cup at Poughkeepsie, N.Y. They woke up at 6 A.M. for a 9:15 race but the winds were too high so they took off for New York City, beat Barnard, and went back 60 miles to Poughkeepsie because the races were supposed to be on again for 6 P.M. They didn't want some other crew to think it was better.

"Did you ever coach girls?" asks McArdle, also Washington's dean of men. "They're very grouchy and sometimes hard to get along with, and they're much more competitive with themselves than outsiders. They're pretty hard on themselves and each other."

Most of the time they are linked in a sorority of pain, running five miles a day and doing weight training to strengthen the legs that drive the boat. Coxswain Michele Williams is the boss in the shell and the stroke, Mary Ann McArdle, is the coach's sister, but on the water the only identity is eight oars and a voice blending together.

They have the group distinction of being the only women's crew in Maryland, which sounds impressive until you realize that only Washington and Navy have any crews at all. The girls feel a kinship to the Middies, using one of their old shells until an angel financed a new one this year. On the road they still row in borrowed boats because the school has only one shell trailer and the men need it, too.

"It isn't discrimination against women," says Penny Fall, director of women's athletics. "From what I've seen at other schools I think our girls are probably in the best position of any of them."

Fall is nominally the women's crew coach, but the teaching is all done by McArdle. He had never rowed but volunteered to coach when the school found itself with shells and interested students but no money to hire a full-time, experienced coach.

"The girls would be a lot better off now with a coach who knew what he was doing," says McArdle, who learned the sport from books. "But we were stuck with each other and made the best of it."

Only three of the eight girls, seniors Morton, McArdle, and Bowie Johnson, had rowed before March. The boat was filled out by sophomore Kathy Campbell and freshmen Williams, Gitt, Shari Moore, Jerae Lowman, and Robin Brown.

It took them seven and a half minutes to cover 1,000 meters then, which was more paddling than rowing. By the end of the season it was down to three minutes and nine seconds.

And bubbles.

BASKETBALL

MILLION-DOLLAR QUESTION: BUCKS OR BOOKS?

By Dave Hirshey

From the New York Daily News
Copyright, ©, 1975, New York News, Inc.

Any minute now, the word will filter down from the tundra that there's this 6-foot-10 kid by the name of Stan Dout in Phee Nom who is averaging 300 points a game and the pro scouts will fall over each other trying to sign him up.

Oh yea, Stan Dout is six years old.

But that probably wouldn't deter anybody now that Moses Malone has shown you can do quite nicely by skipping college and going right into the pros. "I never really thought about going pro until I read about Moses Malone," Darryl Dawkins was saying yesterday. "I still think I want to get a college education but if a super offer comes along. . . ."

Darryl Dawkins is this year's leading candidate for "High School Millionaire of the Year." He has all the right credentials: He has a height (6-feet-10), a nickname (Dr. D), a mother on welfare, and a phone number that's been changed four times. He averaged 26 points and 15 rebounds in leading Maynard Evans High School of Orlando to the Florida Class AAAA championship.

"He can play with anybody," his coach, Fred Pennington, said last week after Dawkins applied as a hardship case, making him eligible for next month's NBA draft. The line forms on the right, fellas, and only those with large checkbooks need apply.

Already, scouts from Philadelphia, Chicago, Utah, and San Diego have descended on Orlando and none of them were there to visit Disney World. Of course, this has caused a great deal of outrage among the guardians of the nation's morals, who view the possibility of a callow eighteen-year-old seduced into the worldly temptations of the NBA as tantamount to child abuse.

I can't understand what all the fuss is about. After all, Alexander the Great conquered half the world by the time he was twenty-one and he didn't even have a jump shot. Did anybody tell Howard Hughes he had to wait till he was twenty-two to pursue his fortune?

Lest we forget, this is the same nation that gave us Horatio Alger, Mason Reese, and Shirley Temple. So why should Darryl Dawkins waste his time becoming a brain surgeon?

Because. . . .

1. A college education is a very valuable thing to have and a man should always prepare himself for when he can no longer fast-break downcourt.

There are dozens of millionaires out there who are muddling through without that sheepskin. And besides if Darryl Dawkins really wants an education, he can go out and buy a college with his first paycheck.

Let us take a pearl of wisdom from the Bible according to Moses. "College would have been a complete waste of time for Moses," says his coach, Tom Nissalke, of the Utah Stars. "He has no interest whatsoever in academics. He's a basketball player. Period."

2. Any educated pro is a better pro, more able to cope with the pressures and demands of big-time sports.

What college did Bobby Orr go to?

3. Signing kids out of high school will establish a trend that could destroy college basketball.

The only kids the pros will go after are the ones who will be the objects of ugly recruiting wars anyway and there will always be plenty of Bill Bradleys who will go to college no matter how many bucks are dangled in front of them.

4. Is it ethical to throw a mere child in with a bunch of hardened elbow-swinging, eye-gouging, referee-baiting over-thirty types?

Any NBA team signing an eighteen-year-old is perfectly aware he's likely to be a piece of china in a bull shop. Moses Malone was the test case and he hasn't cracked yet. "You can't use Malone as the barometer," believes 76er general manager Pat Williams. "He's an exception. The thing is, you have to be sure the kid is worth the gamble. If he fails to make it, he loses the money, the education. It could ruin his life."

Jama-Keith Wilkes played four years for John Wooden at UCLA, then became an outstanding rookie with the Golden State Warriors. He worries about the wrenching emotional adjustment a youngster has to make stepping directly out of high school and into the pros.

"There are so many hassles—the travel, the press, the women," Wilkes knows. "I had four years of college and I still find it difficult.

Throw an eighteen-year-old kid into that situation and it could have a traumatic effect."

For that matter, throw Bill Walton into the same situation . . . and it DID have a traumatic effect. Maturity doesn't automatically arrive at age twenty-one along with the right to act in a porno movie without your parents' consent.

Some like Orr, a shooting star at eighteen, and Pelé, playing brilliantly in a World Cup final at seventeen, can handle the transition gracefully, others have to be fed Pablum at half time. There's only one way for a kid to find out whether the waters are troubled or calm and for a million dollars who can blame a guy for closing his eyes and diving in?

It would be nice to report that Darryl Dawkins doesn't need the money. Nice, but not true. He and his three brothers chop wood every afternoon to heat their home. For three days in December, he is excused from school to pick oranges so that his family will have Christmas presents. Darryl Dawkins is eighteen, black, and indigent. For him, college would be a rare and exceptional opportunity. But not quite as rare as a chance to become an instant millionaire.

BOXING

SHELBY'S MOMENT OF GLORY

By Royal Brougham

From The Seattle Post-Intelligencer
Copyright, ©, 1975, The Seattle Post-Intelligencer

Scene: the cowboy town of Shelby, Mont.
  Date: Midsummer, 1923.
  Place: backroom of the Red Dog Saloon on Main Street.
  Jim Johnson, leading spirit of the community, had the floor. When Jim spoke, everybody else listened. He was mayor of the town and president of the bank.
  The mayor dropped a bombshell.
  "Those New York fellows say they will award the championship Jack Dempsey-Tom Gibbons fight to the highest bidder. What a great chance to put little ol' Shelby on the map! Let's stage the fight right here. What are we waiting for?"
  The vote was unanimous.
  What more spectacular way to get the jump on rival cities like Cut Bank, Great Falls, and the others, establishing Shelby as the commerce capital of the region?
  The telegram to manager Jack Kearns read:
  "Shelby bids a quarter million for the fight."
  They were dead game sports in Montana, imbued with the spirit of the Wild West. And good gamblers, from the mayor down to the last barkeep, sheepherder, and cattle rustler.
  Kearns, envisaging a bonanza gate with Californians and Alaskans paying for ringside seats with gold nuggets, accepted.
  The stage was set for the most incredible, inconceivable, weird and whacky prize fight promotion in the long history of the cauliflower-ear pastime.
  The shrewd Kearns, a shifty fast-talker who could sell a pile of sand to an Arab, was a little shaken when he checked into Shelby

—one street, a leaky-roof hotel, a couple of noisy dance halls, and 12 saloons. (Check your guns with the manager!)

But Kearns was impressed when the townsfolk passed the hat, twisted a few arms, and raised the first installment.

As a wide-eyed, bushy-tailed young reporter, I arrived a couple of weeks before the fight, joining such veterans as Westbrook Pegler, Heywood Broun, Damon Runyon, Hugh Fullerton, Dick Little, and others. Of necessity, most of us were bedded down in our Pullman cars.

Dempsey and his entourage established training quarters near Great Falls among the cottonwoods on the banks of the muddy Missouri River. They were a bizarre assortment—the champ, his trainer Jerry "The Greek" Luvadis, camp jester Joe Benjamin, and three or four beat-up sparring partners who were cannon fodder for Dempsey's punches.

The challenger's more modest bivouac was a bungalow just outside town.

Overnight the community of 2,000 inhabitants mushroomed into a seething mob of drifters, hoods, gamblers, pickpockets, and their paramours.

It was a 24 hour-a-day rat race. There was a bulge on every hip, either a gun or a pint. It was reported that a frustrated deputy sheriff accidentally shot himself in the foot. A rodeo put in an appearance, featuring a five-legged calf.

A little old lady in a red and green kimono, Madame Labelle, would tell your fortune for four bits, giving you the winner of the forthcoming fight. For another half dollar she'd name the round.

In short, the joint was jumping. Shelby was on the map.

But trouble was looming. Kearns demanded to see the color of the second $100,000 installment. The expected rush to buy ringside seats, which was to bail out the promoters, wasn't forthcoming.

A monumental fiasco was evident when the hard-dealing Dempsey manager issued the ultimatum:

"No dough, no fight."

That killed whatever chance there was to draw a crowd. Because of the uncertainty, special trains from New York, Chicago, and California were canceled.

At the last minute, Kearns agreed to go through with the match, but insisted on taking all the gate receipts. Shelby and poor Tommy Gibbons were left holding the sack.

To add to the confusion, the first rainstorm of the season inundated the town. Hardly pennies from heaven, it turned the streets into a quagmire.

This was a most unusual happening. Toole County is an arid area. Natives say they have seen bullfrogs that were eight years old before they learned to swim.

Verily, the golden dream in the Red Dog Saloon had turned into a migraine headache.

Fight day came, boiling hot, the temperature matching the tempers of the fans. Kearns and Dempsey were the hated villains. A bare 7,000 paying customers were in the stands. Another 8,000 crashed the poorly policed gates.

The crowd banked around the ring had to be the most incredible, heterogeneous collection of oddballs in prize-fight history.

Massed in ringside seats on one side was a score of Blackfeet Indians, resplendent in full war regalia. Cattle barons in wide Stetsons, cow and sheep hands in Levis, New York dudes in Abercrombie and Fitch cowboy suits, well-known mobsters from Chicago, and painted ladies in all their finery, some wearing wide-brim hats with white plumes, several bearing gay parasols, which drew the voiced complaints of grumbling fans in the seats behind.

A part of the scene was Wild Bill Lyons, Dempsey's bodyguard, sporting leather chaps, a six-shooter on each hip. Also, the famous gate-crasher, One-Eyed Connolly, peddling lukewarm "ice water" out of a rusty bucket to parched customers at one dollar a cup.

A Gibbons camp follower tipped us off that the Blackfeet braves were in an ugly mood. They had inducted the popular Gibbons into their tribe with the title Chief Thunderbird.

Remembering Chief Crazy Horse and Custer's Last Stand, Dempsey was apprehensive when he heard the rumor.

"Some of those Injuns had long hunting knives and tomahawks," the champ told me afterward. "You notice I did most of my fighting on the other side of the ring."

There were but a few scattered cheers for the champ when he took his place on his corner stool, a scowling, menacing figure with a three-day growth of beard and saddle-brown tanned torso.

The challenger drew resounding applause, including war whoops from his Indian rooting section.

Because of the tension the fight was exciting but not sensational. Dempsey was in full command from the start. Gibbons had courage, desire, and a good left hook. That was all. He fought flat-footed, his short arms being no match for the titleholder's long-range punches. Jack was satisfied to maintain his lead. What did he have to worry about?

Jim Dougherty, the Baron of Leipperville, was the hand-picked referee and a Kearns buddy. You had the feeling the champion couldn't lose, barring a knockout.

Dempsey won the clean-cut decision. The fastest action of the night was the champion's sudden departure from the ring after the ref raised his arm. It was an all-time record for exits.

Following a prearranged plan, Dempsey leaped through the ropes, raced down the aisle to the arena entrance where he was joined by Kearns, carrying all the gate receipts in two bargain-basement straw suitcases.

Nobody before or since ever got out of town faster than the two Jacks. Sprinting to the nearby railway station, they hopped on a waiting engine with steam up, leased for the getaway, and said good-bye forever to Shelby.

An amusing aftermath was the fate of many spectators who sat through the 95-degree heat on the raw pine boards, hastily converted from trees to seats.

As the mercury soared, sap came oozing to the surface. It was reliably reported that dozens of fans left the seats of their pants in the arena when they arose from sticky perches.

Maybe that's where the term "hot pants" originated. So it went with the Rape of Shelby.

BASKETBALL

THE MYSTERY MAN OF THE BLAZERS

By John Schulian

From The Washington Post
Copyright, ©, 1975, The Washington Post

William Theodore Walton III was born November 11, 1952, which makes him a Scorpio, but the sign he really lives under is a question mark.

He created it himself with an outspoken style that stopped short of full confession, and, as a result, turned him into an enigma.

The sporting public, ill prepared for a 6-foot-11 basketball player who protests wars and has his name bandied about with that of Patty Hearst, cannot figure out Bill Walton—if, indeed, exasperation has not stilled all desire to do so.

"I don't worry about what other people worry about," he said.

But even Walton's teammates on the Portland Trail Blazers would like to know some things about him occasionally, although their questions are seldom of national consequence. The other day, for instance, they simply wanted to know if he was going to show up for practice.

It was scheduled to begin at 3 P.M. in the University of Portland's purple-and-white gymnasium that looks not unlike a nightmare left over from the psychedelic era. Fifteen minutes later, Coach Lenny Wilkens was telling jokes, forward Sidney Wicks was trying to dunk two balls on the same jump, and Walton was nowhere to be seen.

When he shambled onto the floor at last, the rest of the Blazers were sweat-soaked. "What time is it?" boomed Wicks. It was 3:40 P.M.

Although it is the twists and turns of Walton's mind that many say cause the most difficulty, this time it was his body that had led to the delay.

"I need 40 minutes just to get him ready," said Ron Culp, the team's trainer, plopping down on the gym's foldout bleachers. "He'll be the first man in the history of the National Basketball Association to play without any exposed skin."

The latest part of Walton to be taped is his left wrist, which he sprained severely in the Blazers' game Friday against the Chicago Bulls. Before that, it was a sprained ankle and a broken toe and, courtesy of an auto accident, a matched set of bruised knees.

Yet, Wilkens insists on describing his fragile center as healthy.

"Compared to last season, he is," Wilkens said. "Last season, he had a broken finger. Then there was something wrong with his foot. Then his left knee got so bad we had to sit him out of our final game.

"He had the knee operated on in the off-season so there's one problem taken care of. Then we got him to put on some weight (41 pounds, from 212 to 253). No, we didn't ask him to stop being a vegetarian. I'm not going to follow him around to find out what he eats. We just had him start working with weights, and it's paid off."

Already, Walton has played half as many games as he did in all of the 1974–75 season, his scoring has climbed three points to 15.2 a game, and Wilkens is calling him "the best defensive rebounder in the league."

"I still don't feel right, you know," Walton said.

He was traversing the university campus with strides as wide as the Willamette River, responding to shouts from the dorms with a wave of an arm, but never looking up.

"I mean, I really like playing basketball a whole lot," he said. "It's one thing that really makes me happy. But it's not all that much fun when parts of your body aren't working at it."

Some skeptics, of course, think his ailments are the products of an overactive imagination. Walton, however, gets no more excited about them than he did about the discovery that the doorlocks of his Toyota Land Cruiser, just out of the body shop, had been painted over.

"I guess," he said after hauling his $250,000-a-year body through an open back window, "it's all just part of life."

An unwritten personal rule—perhaps Walton could have no written rules—does not allow him to get upset outwardly about anything.

Not the way his name was dragged into the Patty Hearst mess: "I couldn't do anything about that."

Not criticism that he had become a puppet for sports activist Jack Scott: "We're just friends. I've got a lot of friends."

Everything seems so free and easy, just the way you expect it should be for a golden boy from southern California.

But as Walton gunned the Land Cruiser downtown to the Coliseum, where the Blazers play their home games and where his sprained wrist would be treated, the tight spots in his makeup showed through.

He doesn't know whether Johnny Wooden's protective shield at UCLA hurt him more than it helped him. He doesn't know how—or if—he is ever going to get people to understand his liberal politics.

He doesn't know why a sad song, something moody and poetic by Dylan, can make him feel good.

"You're asking me a lot of questions that I don't have any answers for," he said.

So Walton, with a red beard bushing from his jaws and only the lightest fuzz on his upper lip, turns out to be not quite Dobie Gillis, not quite Franz Fanon.

Concern still clouded his face as he pulled into the Coliseum's special parking lot. The guard had to look twice at Walton before letting him in.

"I get my car back," said Walton, "and he doesn't even know who I am."

Maybe nobody does, not even Bill Walton.

GENERAL

MAMA CLEARS THE SMOKE

By John Soucheray

From the Minneapolis Tribune
Copyright, ©, 1975, Minneapolis Tribune

The face of his mother, Mrs. Gloria Connors, is heavily lined and caked and perfumed, the skin drawn tight up to the temples, pulled there and secured by a bun of strawberry hair. She is worried, worried that Jimmy will catch cold, worried that Jimmy's bronchial condition will worsen because of cigar-smoking tourists packing Caesars Tennis Pavilion to watch Jimmy practice, worried because her Jimmy appears to be enjoying himself.

"Behave yourself, Jimmy," she told him before practice began Thursday morning. "You're only twenty-two, Jimmy."

"I feel good," Jimmy told her. "Look." He did a little shuffle, like a boxer.

"Practice hard," she said.

Outside the desert sun was cracking the white ground where they cleared away the mesquite to build Caesars Tennis Pavilion, a green steel-pole building that holds 3,500 high rollers for a good match. On Saturday Jimmy will challenge Australian John Newcombe for $250,000 plus TV money. Caesars Palace put up the money, to get the high rollers.

Jimmy and his mother wanted to buy the 500 or so courtside seats to keep out the celebrities who heckled Jimmy ceaselessly during his February challenge match victory over Rod Laver on the same court. The Palace refused. Jimmy shrugged it off. Jimmy also wanted a new court surface installed for this match, a slower one. Newcombe refused and they settled the matter with a coin toss, which Newcombe won.

Jimmy began working out with John Feaver, an Englishman, and Vitas Gerulatis, a New Yorker of Lithuanian ancestry. Both have cannon serves like Newcombe's. Jimmy's coach, Pancho Segura, walked around the court, glancing at Mrs. Connors to meet her needs. Jimmy would hit and grunt. Vitas would return. Jimmy would make a face.

"This smoke," said Mrs. Connors, waving her hand. "There can't be any smoke in here Saturday. Jimmy won't be able to breathe. Bill, Bill."

Bill Riordan, the manager, stopped talking to a fat man with a cigar and came to her side. "No smoking in here," she said.

"Good point, good point," he said. "Gets cloudy with smoke in here." Riordan went to the fat man and told him the problem. The fat man puffed and puffed on his cigar and said he would see to it.

"You're absolutely right, Gloria," Riordan said. "Bothers him."

Her eyes shifted back to the court, to Jimmy sweating hard now. He missed a shot and her face cracked for an instant, a frown. She made Jimmy what he is today. She and her mother, Two-Mom, took Jimmy to the courts in St. Louis when he was three years old. It's all Jimmy has known, tennis. He beat every kid in St. Louis, played through the winter on armory floors and by the time he was sixteen he won the national junior title. Mrs. Connors moved him to Los Angeles and there he met Segura.

Their work has brought them back again to Las Vegas, the perfect place for Jimmy to prove once again that he is the master of the pressure game. He sees his name in lights, he sees his face at every turn in the mirrored halls of Caesars Palace. He feels himself getting older.

After practice Riordan ushered Jimmy into a small room to answer questions.

"I want to announce my retirement," Jimmy said. There was much laughter at this, the loudest from Riordan, who almost choked at the joke. Riordan first met Jimmy in Chattanooga, Tenn., when Jimmy and his mother and Two-Mom were there for a junior tournament. Riordan was a rookie tennis promoter, having graduated from department-store public relations. "Before Two-Mom died," said Riordan, "she told Gloria to put Jimmy's affairs in my hands. She said I had class."

A door was open from the press room to the outside. Mrs. Connors, who waits nearby during such conferences, stuck her head in the door and made a covering motion with her arms. "Keep warm," she said to Jimmy.

"Gentlemen," said Riordan, "that will have to be enough. Jimmy is cooling down too fast in here and he has another workout later, thank you."

Jimmy shrugged, got up, and was gone, followed back to his suite of rooms by his mother and a swarm of middle-aged tourists with bulging thighs and instant desert tans. "Keep warm, Jimmy," said his mother.

Riordan's hand reached through the swarm and adjusted the towel around Jimmy's neck.

FOR THE RECORD

CHAMPIONS OF 1975

ARCHERY

World Champions

Men—Darrell Pace, Reading, Ohio
Women—Zebiniso Rustamova, USSR
Men's Team—United States.
Women's Team—USSR.

National Archery Assn. Champions

Men—Darrell Pace, Reading, Ohio
Women—Irene Lorensen, Phoenix, Ariz.
Professional—John Williams, Rialto, Calif.

National Field Archery Assn. Champions

FREESTYLE

Open—Terry Ragsdale, White Oak, Tex.
Women's Open—Barbara Morris, Frankfort, Ky.
Amateur—John Ashburn, Jr., Barrington, Ill.
Women's Amateur—Michelle Sanderson, Hastings, Minn.

BAREBOW

Open—Al Tuller, Platte City, Mo.
Women's Open—Gloria Shelley, Waterbury, Conn.
Amateur—Don Morehead, Wheaton, Ill.
Women's Amateur—Eunice Schewe, Roscoe, Ill.

AUTO RACING

World—Niki Lauda, Austria.
USAC—A.J. Foyt, Houston, Tex.
NASCAR—Richard Petty, Randleman, N.C.
Formula 5000—Brian Redman, England.
IMSA Camel GT—Peter Gregg, Jacksonville, Fla.
IMSA Goodrich—Nick Craw, Washington.
Indy 500—Bobby Unser, Albuquerque, N.M.
U.S. Grand Prix—Niki Lauda.
24 Hours of Daytona—Peter Gregg–Haywood Hurley, Jacksonville, Fla. (Porsche).
24 Hours of Le Mans—Jacky Ickx, Belgium–Derek Bell, England (Ford).

BADMINTON

United States Championships

Singles—Mike Adams, Flint, Mich.
Women's Singles—Judianne Kelly, Norwalk, Calif.
Doubles—Don Paup, Washington–Jim Poole, Westminster, Calif.
Women's Doubles—Diane Hales, Claremont, Calif.–Carlene Starkey, LaMesa, Calif.
Mixed Doubles—Judianne Kelly–Mike Walker, Manhattan Beach, Calif.
Senior Singles—Jim Poole.
Senior Doubles—Bob Carpenter, New York–Bill Goodman, Wellesley Hills, Mass.

Senior Women's Doubles—Ethel Marshall–Bea Massman, Buffalo.

All-England Championships

Singles—Svend Pri, Denmark.
Women's Singles—Hiroe Yuki, Japan.
Doubles—Tjun Tjun–J. Ahjudi, Indonesia.
Women's Doubles—M. Aizawa–E. Takenaka, Japan.
Mixed Doubles—Elliott Stuart–Nora Gardner, England.

BASEBALL

World Series—Cincinnati Reds.
National League—East: Pittsburgh; West: Cincinnati; playoffs: Cincinnati.
American League—East: Boston; West: Oakland; playoffs: Boston.
All-Star Game—National League.
Leading Batter (AL)—Rod Carew, Minnesota.
Leading Batter (NL)—Bill Madlock, Chicago.
Cy Young Pitching Award (AL)—Jim Palmer, Baltimore.
Cy Young Pitching Award (NL)—Tom Seaver, New York.
American Association—Evansville.
International League—Tidewater.
Little World Series—Evansville.
Pacific Coast League—Hawaii.
Mexican League—Tampico.
Eastern League—Bristol.
Southern League—Montgomery.
Texas League—Lafayette and Midland.
National Collegiate—University of Texas.

BASKETBALL

National Association—Golden State Warriors.
American Association—Kentucky Colonels.
National Collegiate—University of California, Los Angeles.

NCAA Division II—Old Dominion.
NCAA Division III—LeMoyne-Owen.
NAIA—Grand Canyon.
Women's Collegiate (AIAW)—Delta State.
National Invitation—Princeton.
Atlantic Coast—North Carolina.
Big Eight—Kansas.
Big Sky—Montana.
Big Ten—Indiana.
East Coast—East: American University and LaSalle; West: Lafayette.
Ivy League—Pennsylvania.
Mid-American—Central Michigan.
Middle Atlantic—North: Philadelphia Textile; South: Widener.
Missouri Valley—Louisville.
Ohio Valley—Middle Tennessee.
Pacific-8—UCLA.
Southeastern—Alabama and Kentucky.
Southern—Furman.
Southwest—Texas A&M.
Pacific Coast Athletic—Long Beach State.
West Coast Athletic—Nevada-Las Vegas.
Western Athletic—Arizona State.
Yankee Conference—Massachusetts.
AAU—Capitol Insulation, Los Angeles.
Women's AAU—Wayland Baptist.

BILLIARDS

U.S.Pocket—Dallas West, Rockford, Ill.
U.S. Women's Pocket—Jean Balukas, Brooklyn.

BOBSLEDDING

World Two-Man—Italy.
World Four-Man—Switzerland.
AAU Two-Man—Jim Morgan–Jeff Beamish, Saranac Lake, N.Y.
AAU Four-Man—Lake Placid (N.Y.) Club.

BOWLING

American Bowling Congress Champions

Singles (Regular)—Jim Setser, Dayton, Ohio.

Singles (Classic)—Les Zikes, Chicago.

Doubles (Regular)—Bob Metz–Steve Partlow, Dayton, Ohio.

Doubles (Classic)—Bill Bunetta, Fresno, Calif–Marty Piraino, Syracuse, N.Y.

All-Events (Regular)—Bobby Meadows, Dallas, Tex.

All-Events (Classic)—Bill Beach, Sharon, Pa.

Team (Regular)—Roy Black Chrysler, Cleveland.

Team (Classic)—Mussingwear #2, Minneapolis.

Team (Booster)—Leisure Lanes, Kankakee, Ill.

Women's International Bowling Congress

Singles—Barbara Leicht, Albany, N.Y.

Doubles—Jeanette James, Oyster Bay, N.Y.–Dawn Raddatz, East Northport, N.Y.

All-Events—Virginia Park, Whittier, Calif.

Team—Atlanta Bowling Center, Buffalo.

B.P.A.A. Open Champions

Men—Steve Neff, Sarasota, Fla.

Women—Paula Sperber, Miami.

BOXING

World Professional Champions

Heavyweight—Muhammad Ali, Chicago.

Light Heavyweight—Victor Galindez, Argentina, recognized by World Boxing Association; John Conteh, England, recognized by World Boxing Council.

Middleweight—Carlos Monzon, Argentina, WBA; Rodrigo Valdez, Colombia, WBC.

Junior Middleweight—Yu Jae Do, South Korea, WBA; Elisha O'Bed, Bahamas, WBC.

Welterweight—Angel Espada, Puerto Rico, WBA; John Stracey, England, WBC.

Junior Welterweight—Antonio Cervantes, Colombia, WBA; Saensak Muargsurin, Thailand, WBC.

Lightweight—Roberto Duran, Panama, WBA; Guts Ishimatsu, Japan, WBC.

Junior Lightweight—Ben Villaflor, Philippines, WBA; Alfredo Escalera, Puerto Rico, WBC.

Featherweight—Alexis Arguello, Nicaragua, WBA; David Kotey, Ghana, WBC.

Bantamweight—Alfonso Zamora, Mexico, WBA; Rodolfo Martinez, Mexico, WBC.

Flyweight—Erbito Salavarria, Philippines, WBA; Miguel Canto, Mexico, WBC.

Junior Flyweight—Luis Estaba, Venezuela, WBC; class not recognized by WBA.

National AAU Champions

106 Pounds—Claudell Atkins, St. Louis.

112 Pounds—Richard Rozelle, Columbus, Ohio.

119 Pounds—Eiichi Jumaway, Hawaii.

125 Pounds—Dave Armstrong, Tacoma, Wash.

132 Pounds—Jilmer Kenty, Columbus, Ohio.

139 Pounds—Ray Leonard, Palmer Park, Md.

147 Pounds—Clinton Jackson, Evergreen, Ala.

156 Pounds—Charles Walker, Mesa, Ariz.

165 Pounds—Tom Brooks, U.S. Air Force.

178 Pounds—Leon Spinks, U.S. Marines.

Heavyweight—Michael Dokes, Cleveland.

CANOEING

KAYAK

Singles (500 meters)—Steve Kelly, Inwood CC, New York.
Women's Singles (500 Meters)—Linda Murray, Washington.
Singles (1,000 Meters)—Kelly.
Singles (10,000 meters)—Bill Leach, Newport Beach, Calif.
Women's Tandem (500 Meters)—Linda Murray–Ann Turner, St. Charles, Ill.
Tandem (1,000 Meters)—Phil Regosheske–Bruce Barton, Niles Buchanan, Mich.
Tandem (10,000 Meters)—Regosheske–Barton.
Women's Tandem (5,000 Meters)—Loli Flood–Nancy Leahy, Washington.
Fours (10,000 Meters)—New York AC.
Women's Fours (500 and 5,000 Meters)—Julie Jones–Sperry Rademaker–Patience Vanderbush–Ann Turner.

CANOE

Singles (500 Meters)—Roland Muhlen, Cincinnati.
Singles (1,000 Meters)—Muhlen.
Singles (10,000 Meters)—Andy Weigand, Washington.
Tandem (500, 1,000 and 10,000 Meters)—Muhlen–Weigand.
Fours—St. Charles (Ill.) CC.

WHITEWATER

Kayak Singles—Eric Evans, Amherst, Mass.
Women's Kayak Singles—Linda Harrison, Newark, Del.
Canoe Singles—Jamie McEwan, Silver Spring, Md.
Canoe Doubles—John Evans–Carl Toeppner, Mountain, Ranch, Calif.

WILDWATER

Kayak Singles—William Nutt, Etna, N.H.
Women's Kayak Singles—Carol Fisher, Evanston, Ill.

Canoe Singles—A. Button, Minneapolis.
Canoe Doubles—Wally Dyer–Ben Cass, Philadelphia.

CASTING

United States Champions

Grand All-Round—Steve Rajeff, San Francisco.
Women's All-Accuracy—Pauline Cathcart, La Canada, Calif.

COURT TENNIS

U.S. Open—Gene Scott, New York.
U.S. Amateur—Scott.

CROSS-COUNTRY

National AAU—Greg Fredericks, College Station, Pa.
National AAU Team—Colorado Track Club.
National Women's AAU Team—Los Angeles T.C.
NCAA Division I—Craig Virgin, Illinois.
NCAA Division I Team—Texas-El Paso.
NCAA Division II—Ralph Serna, California–Irvine.
NCAA Division II Team—California–Irvine.
NCAA Division III—Vin Fleming, Lowell.
NCAA Division III Team—North Central Illinois.
NAIA—Mike Boit, Eastern New Mexico.
NAIA Team—Edinboro State.
Women's Collegiate (AIAW)—Peg Neppel, Iowa State.
Women's National AAU—Lynn Bjorklund, Albuquerque, N.M.
Women's Collegiate Team—Iowa State.
IC4A—David Merrick, Penn: College Division: Bob Braile, Bucknell.
IC4A Team—Northeastern: College Division: Bucknell.
Heptagonal—Dave Merrick, Penn.
Heptagonal Team—Princeton.

CURLING

World—Switzerland.
U.S.—Seattle Granite Club.
U.S. Women—Wilmette, Ill.

CYCLING

World

Sprint—Daniel Morelon, France.
Women's Sprint—Sue Novarra, Flint, Mich.
Pursuit—Thomas Huschke, East Germany.
Women's Pursuit—Cornelia Van Hoosten-Hage, Netherlands.
Road—Adrianus Gevers, Netherlands.

National Champions

ROAD RACING

Senior (123 miles)—John Howard, Houston, Tex.
Women (35 miles)—Linda Stein, Los Angeles.
Veterans (44 miles)—Nikola Farac-Ban, San Francisco.
Junior (48 miles)—Larry Shields, Goleta, Calif.

TRACK RACING

Sprint—Steve Woznick, Ridgefield Park, N.J.
Women's Sprint—Sue Novarra, Flint, Mich.
Pursuit—Ron Skarin, Van Nuys, Calif.
Women's Pursuit—Mary Jane Reoch, Philadelphia.
Team Pursuit—Southern California.
10 Miles—Leroy Gatto, San Jose, Calif.
Junior—Curtis Miller, San Jose, Calif.

TIME TRIALS

Senior—Wayne Stetina, Indianapolis.
Women—Mary Jane Reoch, Philadelphia.
Junior—Paul Deem, San Pedro, Calif.

DOGS

Major Best-in-Show Winners

Westminster (New York)—Ch. Sir Lancelot of Barvan, Old English sheepdog, owned by Mr. and Mrs. Ronald Vannord, Newmarket, Ontario; 3,035 dogs entered.
Boardwalk (Atlantic City)—Ch. Dersade Bobby's Girl, Sealyham terrier, owned by Mrs. Dorothy Wimer, Churchtown, Pa.; 3,714.
Trenton—Ch. Tarnbreck Cassius, Lakeland terrier, owned by Countess Ercilia LeNy, Milford, N.J.; 3,657.
Westchester (Tarrytown, N.Y.)—Ch. Dersade Bobby's Girl, 2,619.
International (Chicago, fall)—Ch. Dersade Bobby's Girl; 3,857.
Santa Barbara (Calif.)—Ch. Jo-Ni's Red Baron of Crofton, Lakeland terrior, owned by Mrs. Virginia K. Dickson, La Habra, Calif.; 4,442.

National Bird Dog Champions

National Pointer and Setter—Volcanic Express, pointer, owned by Dr. and Mrs. W.L. Humphries, Little Rock, Ark.
National Free-for-All—Attache, pointer, owned by William Jarrett, Indianapolis.
Oklahoma Open—Buckboard, pointer, owned by Dr. D.E. Hawthorne, Tulsa, Okla.
Saskatchewan Open—The Nimrod, pointer, owned by Gary Pinalto, Broken Arrow, Okla.

FENCING

World Champions

Foil—Christian Noel, France.
Foil Team—France.
Epee—Alexander Pusch, West Germany.
Epee Team—Sweden.
Saber—Vladimir Nazlimow, USSR.
Saber Team—USSR.

Women's Foil—Katalin Jencsik-Stahl, Rumania.
Women's Foil Team—USSR.

United States Champions

Foil—Ed Ballinger, Salle Santelli, New York.
Epee—Scott Bozek, Tanner City (Mass.) Fencers.
Saber—Peter Westbrook, Fencers Club, New York.
Women's Foil—Nikki Tomlinson, Liberty Bell, New York.
Foil Team—Fencers Club, New York.
Epee Team—New York AC.
Saber Team—Fencer's Club, New York.
Women's Foil Team—Halberstadt FC, San Francisco.

National Collegiate Champions

Foil—Greg Benko, Wayne State.
Epee—Risto Hurme, New York University.
Saber—Yuri Rabinovich, Wayne State.
Team—Wayne State.
Women's Foil—Vincent Hurley, San Jose, State.
Women's Team—San Jose State.

FOOTBALL

Intercollegiate Champions

Eastern (Lambert Trophy)—Penn State.
Eastern (Lambert Cup)—Lehigh.
Eastern (Lambert Bowl)—Ithaca.
Atlantic Coast—Maryland.
Big Eight—Nebraska and Oklahoma.
Big Sky—Boise State.
Big Ten—Ohio State.
Ivy League—Harvard.
Metropolitan-8—Brooklyn College.
Mid-American—Miami.
Missouri Valley—Tulsa.
Ohio Valley—Tennessee Tech and Western Kentucky.
Pacific-8—California and UCLA.
Pacific Coast AA—San Jose.
Southeastern—Alabama.
Southern—Richmond.

Southwest—Arkansas, Texas and Texas A&M.
Western Athletic—Arizona State.
Yankee—New Hampshire.
NCAA Division II—Northern Michigan.
NCAA Division III—Wittenberg.
NAIA—Texas A&I.
NAIA Division II—Texas Lutheran.

National League

NATIONAL CONFERENCE

Eastern Division—St. Louis Cards.
Central Division—Minnesota Vikings.
Western Division—Los Angeles Rams.
Playoff Wild Card—Dallas Cowboys.
Conference—Dallas Cowboys.

AMERICAN CONFERENCE

Eastern Division—Baltimore Colts.
Central Division—Pittsburgh Steeler.
Western Division—Oakland Raiders.
Playoff Wild Card—Cincinnati Bengals.
Conference—Pittsburgh Steelers.

Super Bowl

Pittsburgh Steelers

Canadian Professional

Grey Cup—Edmonton Eskimos.

GOLF

Men

National Open—Lou Graham, Nashville, Tenn.
National Amateur—Fred Ridley, Winter Haven, Fla.
Masters—Jack Nicklaus, North Palm Beach, Fla.
PGA—Jack Nicklaus.
British Open—Tom Watson, Kansas City, Mo.
British Amateur—Vinny Giles, Richmond.
Canadian Open—Tom Weiskopf, Columbus, Ohio.

Canadian Amateur—Jim Nelford, Vancouver, B.C.

U.S. Public Links—Randy Barenaba, Laie, Hawaii.

USGA Senior—Bill Colm, Pebble Beach, Calif.

USGA Junior—Brett Mullin, Riverside, Calif.

World Cup (pro)—United States.

World Cup Individual—Johnny Miller, Napa, Calif.

Ryder Cup—United States.

U.S. Senior GA—Dale Morey, High Point, N.C.

NCAA Division I—Jay Haas, Wake Forest.

NCAA Division I Team—Wake Forest.

NCAA Division II—Jerry Wisz, California-Irvine.

NCAA Division II Team—California-Irvine.

NCAA Division III—Charles Baskervill, Hampden-Sydney.

NCAA Division III Team—Wooster.

NAIA—Dan Gray, Texas Wesleyan.

NAIA Team—Texas Wesleyan.

World Series of Golf—Tom Watson.

Tournament of Champions—Al Geiberger, Santa Barbara, Calif.

PGA Player of Year—Jack Nicklaus.

Vardon Trophy (Low Average Rounds) —Bruce Crampton, Australia.

PGA Team—Jim Colbert-Dean Refram Wesley Chapel, Fla.

PGA Earnings Leader—Jack Nicklaus.

Women

National Open—Sandra Palmer, Dallas.

National Amateur—Beth Daniel, Charleston, S.C.

LPGA—Kathy Whitworth, Richardson, Tex.

British Amateur—Nancy Syms, Colorado Springs.

Canadian Amateur—Debbie Massey, Bethlehem, Pa.

USGA Senior—Mrs. Albert Bower, Pelham, N.Y.

USGA Girls—Dayne Benson, Anaheim, Calif.

Intercollegiate—Barbara Barrow, San Diego State.

Intercollegiate Team—Arizona State.

North-South—Cindy Hill, Colorado Springs.

Trans-National—Beverly Davis, Jacksonville, Fla.

Eastern—Debbie Massey.

LPGA Earnings Leader—Sandra Palmer.

LPGA Player of the Year—Sandra Palmer.

Vare Trophy—JoAnne Carner.

GYMNASTICS

AAU Champions

MEN

All-Round—Mike Carter, Louisiana State.

Parallel Bars—Shinsuke Shoji, Memphis, Tenn.

Vaulting—Shinsuke Shoji.

Pommel Horse—Russell Hoffman, West Chicago, Ill.

Still Rings—Pete Studenski, Lincoln, Neb.

Horizontal Bar—Tim Shaw, California Gym Club.

Floor Exercise—Ron Gallimore, Tallahassee, Fla.

WOMEN

All-Round—Roxanne Pierce, Philadelphia.

Vaulting—Ann Carr, Philadelphia.

Uneven Parallel Bars—Ann Carr.

Balance Beam—Roxanne Pierce.

Floor Exercise—Ann Carr.

NCAA Champions

All-Round—Wayne Young, Brigham Young.

Floor Exercise—Kent Brown, Arizona State.

Parallel Bars—Yoichi Tomita, Long Beach State.

Still Rings—Keith Heaver, Iowa State.

Pommel Horse—Ted Marcy, Stanford.

Vault—Tom Beach, California.
Horizontal Bar—Rick Larson, Iowa State.
Team—University of California.

Women's Collegiate

All-Round—Cole Dowaliby, Southern Connecticut.
Uneven Parallel Bars—Diane Sepke, Illinois-Chicago Circle.
Balance Beam—Cole Dowaliby.
Floor Exercise—Karen Schuckman, Penn State.
Vault—Tie among Karen Brezack, Clarion State, Laurel Anderson, Seattle Pacific, and Karen Schuckman.

HANDBALL

United States Handball Assn. Champions

FOUR-WALL

Singles—Jay Bilyeu, Fresno, Calif.
Doubles—Marty Decatur–Steve Lott, New York.
Masters Singles—Jack Scrivens, Portland, Ore.
Masters Doubles—Arnold Aguilar-Gabe Enriquez, Los Angeles.
Golden Masters Doubles—Ken Schneider, Chicago–Irv Simon, Los Angeles.
Super Masters Doubles—Bill Keays-Jeff Capell, San Francisco.

National AAU Champions

ONE-WALL

Singles—Ruby Obert, New York.
Doubles—Wally Ulbrich–Joel Wisotsky, New York.
Masters Doubles—Artie Reyer–Joe Danilczyk, New York.

HARNESS RACING

Horse of the Year—Savoir.
Pacer of the Year—Silk Stockings.
2-Year-Old Trotter—Nevele Thunder.
2-Year-Old Pacer—Armbro Ranger.

3-Year-Old Trotter—Bonefish.
3-Year-Old Pacer—Silk Stockings.
4-Year-Old Trotter—Dream of Glory.
4-Year-Old Pacer—Handle With Care.
Aged Trotter—Savoir.
Aged Pacer—Rambling Willie.
Leading Driver (Heats)—Darry Busse.
Leading Driver (Earnings)—Carmine Abbatiello.
Hambletonian—Bonefish.
Yonkers Trot—Surefire Hanover.
Kentucky Futurity—Noble Rogue.
Dexter Cup—Songflori.
Colonial—Meadow Bright.
Little Brown Jug—Seatrain.
Cane Pace—Nero.
Adios—Nero.
Messenger—Bret's Champ.
Roosevelt International—Savoir.
Empire State Trot—Bonefish.
Monticello-OTB Classic—Silk Stockings.

HOCKEY

Stanley Cup—Philadelphia Flyers.
National League—Norris Division: Montreal; Adams: Buffalo; Patrick: Philadelphia; Smythe: Vancouver.
NHL Most Valuable Player—Bobby Clarke, Philadelphia.
NHL Leading Scorer—Bobby Orr, Boston.
World Association—Canadian Division: Quebec; Eastern: New England; Western: Houston.
WHA Most Valuable Player—Bobby Hull, Winnipeg.
WHA Leading Scorer—Andre Lacroix, San Diego.
American League—Springfield.
Central League—Salt Lake City.
North American League—Johnstown.
Southern League—Charlotte.
International League—Toledo.
United States League—Thunder Bay.
World Amateur—Soviet Union; Group B: East Germany.
NCAA—Michigan Tech.
NAIA—St. Scholastica, Duluth.

ECAC Division I:—Boston U.; Division II: Bowdoin; Division III: Bryant.
WCHA—Minnesota.
Allan Cup—Thunder Bay.
Memorial Cup: Toronto Marlboros.

HORSESHOE PITCHING

World Champions

Men—Elmer Hohl, Wellesley, Ontario.
Women—Vickie Winston, LaMonte, Mo.
Senior—Stan Manker, Lynchburg, Ohio.
Junior—Walter R. Williams Jr., Auburn, Calif.

HORSE RACING

Eclipse Awards

Horse of the Year—Forego.
2-Year-Old Colt—Honest Pleasure.
2-Year-Old Filly—Dearly Precious.
3-Year-Old Colt—Wajima.
3-Year-Old Filly—Ruffian.
Older Horse—Forego.
Older Filly or Mare—Susan's Girl.
Sprinter—Gallant Bob.
Grass Horse—Snow Knight.
Steeplechaser—Life's Illusion.

Stakes Winners

Kentucky Derby—Foolish Pleasure.
Preakness—Master Derby.
Belmont Stakes—Avatar.
American Derby—Honey Mark.
Arlington Handicap—Royal Glint.
Coaching Club American Oaks—Ruffian.
Flamingo—Foolish Pleasure.
Gulfstream Handicap—Gold and Myrrh.
Hollywood Gold Cup—Ancient Title.
Jersey Derby—Singh.
Jockey Club Gold Cup—Group Plan.
Santa Anita Derby—Avatar.
National Thoroughbred Championship—Dulcia.
Santa Anita Handicap—Star Dust Mel.

Washington D.C. International—Nobiliary.
Widener—Forego.
Woodward—Forego.
Filly Triple Crown—Ruffian.

Foreign

Ascot Gold Cup—Sagara.
Canadian International—Snow Knight.
Epsom Derby—Grundy.
Epsom Oaks—Juliette Morny.
Grand National Steeplechase—L'Escargot.
King George VI and Queen Elizabeth—Grundy.
Melbourne Cup—Think Big.
Prix de l'arc de Triomphe—Star Appeal.
Queen's Plate—L'Enjoleur.

HORSE SHOWS

American Horse Shows Assn. Champions

Stock Seat—Melinda Robb, Rancho Santa Fe, Calif.
Saddle Seat—Kate Williams, Tulsa.
Hunter Seat—Cynthia Hankins, Furlong, Pa.

National Horse Show Equitation Champions

ASPCA Trophy (Maclay)—Katherine Burdsall, Glastonbury, Conn.
Saddle Seat (Good Hands)—Kate Williams.

ICE SKATING

FIGURE

World Champions

Men—Sergei Yolkov, USSR.
Women—Dianne de Leeuw, Netherlands.
Pairs—Irina Rodnina-Alexander Zaitsev, USSR.
Dance—Irina Moiseeva-Andrei Minenkov, USSR.

United States Champions

Men—Gordon McKellen, Lake Placid, N.Y.

Women—Dorothy Hamill, Riverside, Conn.

Pairs—Melissa Militano, Dix Hills, N.Y.–Johnny Johns, Bloomfield Hills, Mich.

Dance—Colleen O'Connor–Jim Millns, Colorado Springs.

SPEED

World Champions

Men—Harm Kuipers, Netherlands.

Women—Karin Kessow, East Germany.

Sprint—Aleksander Safranov, USSR.

Women's Sprint—Sheila Young, Detroit.

United States Champions

Outdoor—Rich Wurster, Grafton, Wis.

Women's Outdoor—Nancy Swider, Park Ridge, Ill.

Indoor—Bud Campbell, Paramount, Calif.

Women's Indoor—Michele Conroy, St. Paul.

JUDO

National AAU Champions

139 Pounds—Keitch Nakasone, Pacific Assn.

154 Pounds—Paul Maruyama, Armed Forces.

176 Pounds—Steve Cohen, Chicago.

205 Pounds—Tommy Martin, Sacramento, Calif.

Heavyweight—Allen Coage, East Orange, N.J.

Open—D. Davis, Central Assn.

Grand Champion—Tommy Martin.

WOMEN'S SHIA

Under 110 Pounds—Lynn Lewis, New England.

110–120 Pounds—Diane Pierce, Minnesota.

120–130 Pounds—F. Tomlinson, Potomac Valley.

130–142 Pounds—D. Nelson, Pacific.

142–154 Pounds—Bonnie Kortie, Ozark.

Over 166 Pounds—Ebbie Fisher, Pacific.

Open—Maureen Braziel, New York.

Grand Champion—Bonnie Kortie.

JUNIOR COLLEGES

National Junior College Champions

Baseball—Yavapai College.

Basketball—West Texas College.

Bowling—Erie CC, North.

Cross-Country—Joe Ossansky, Southern Michigan; Team: Southern Michigan.

Football—Mesa (Ariz.) Community College.

Golf—Bill Britton, Miami-Dade North.

Golf Team—Miami-Dade North.

Gymnastics—Odessa (Tex.) JC.

Hockey—Canton (N.Y.) ATC.

Judo—Forest Park CC.

Lacrosse—Nassau (N.Y.) CC.

Marathon—John Roscoe, Southwestern Michigan.

Skiing—Champlain College.

Swimming—Indian River (Fla.).

Tennis—Perfecto Alina, Odessa JC.; doubles: Paul Fineman-Virgilio Sison, Odessa.

Tennis Team—Odessa (Tex.) JC.

Track (Indoor)—Essex County (N.J.)

Track (Outdoor)—Mesa (Ariz.) CC.

Wrestling—North Idaho.

Volleyball—Kellogg CC, Battle Creek, Mich.

LACROSSE

NCAA Division I—Maryland.

NCAA Division II—Cortland State.

Club—Mount Washington LC.

North-South Game—North.

LAWN BOWLING

United States Champions

Men—Richard W. Folkins, Sunland, Calif.

Men's Pairs—A. Grimmit–Neil McInnes, Arroyo Seco, Calif.

Women's—Mrs. Dorothy Bacon, Berkeley, Calif.

Women's Doubles—Mrs. Pat Boehm, Tacoma, Wash.–Mrs. Erma Aipist, Berkeley, Calif.

MOTORBOATING

Unlimited Hydroplane Races

President's Cup—Miss Budweiser, Mickey Remund, Palm Desert, Calif., driver.

Gar Wood Trophy—Miss U.S., Tom D'Eath, Fair Haven, Mich., driver.

APBA Gold Cup—Pride of Pay 'N Pak, George Henley, Eatonville, Wash., driver.

Season Champion—Pride of Pay 'N Pak.

Champion Driver—George Henley.

Distance Races

Bacardi Griffith—Bob Nordskag, Van Nuys, Calif.

Bahamas 500—Hal Sahlman, Boca Raton, Fla.

Benihana Grand Prix—Jon Varesa, Fort Lauderdale, Fla.

Marine City Classic—Sandy Saltullo, Fairview Park, Ohio.

U.S. Offshore Champion—Sandy Saltullo.

World Offshore Champion—Wally Franz, Brazil.

MOTORCYCLING

National Champion—Gary Scott, Springfield, Ohio.

Moto-Cross National 250 Champion—Tony Di Stefano, Morrisville, Pa.

Moto-Cross National 500 Champion—Jim Weinert, Laguna Beach, Calif.

PARACHUTING

United States Champions

Overall—Jimmy Davis, Charlotte, N.C.

Women's Overall—Debbie Schmidt, Joliet, Ill.

PLATFORM TENNIS

Doubles—Keith Jennings–Chauncey D. Steele, Boston.

Women's Doubles—Annabel Lang, Plainfield, N.J.-Hilary Hilton, Pacific Palisades, Calif.

POLO

National Champions

Open—Milwaukee.

20 Goals—Dallas.

16 Goals—Tulsa.

Collegiate—University of California, Davis.

RACQUETBALL

Singles—Charlie Brumfield, San Diego.

Women's Singles—Peggy Steding, Odessa, Tex.

Amateur Singles—Jay Jones, Sherman Oaks, Calif.

Women's Amateur Singles—Ruth Knudsen, Salt Lake City.

RACQUETS

World—William Surtees, Chicago.

RODEO

World Champions

All-Round—Leo Camarillo, Oakdale, Calif.
Saddle Bronc Riding—Monty Henson, Mesquite, Tex.
Bareback Bronc—Joe Alexander, Cora, Wyo.
Bull Riding—Don Gay, Mesquite, Tex.
Calf Roping—Jeff Copenhaver, Spokane, Wash.
Steer Wrestling—Frank Shepperson, Midwest, Wyo.
Barrell Racing—Jimmie Gibbs, Valley Mills, Tex.

ROLLER SKATING

World Champions

Singles—Michael Obrecht, West Germany.
Women's Singles—Sigrid Mullenbach, West Germany.
Pairs—Ron Sabo-Darlene Waters, Columbus, Ohio.
Dance—Jane Puracchio-Kerry Cavazzi, East Meadow, L.I.
Freestyle—Leonardo Lienhard, Switzerland.
Women's Freestyle—Sigrid Mullenbach.

United States Champions

Singles—Michael Glatz, San Diego.
Women's Singles—Moana Brigham, San Diego.
Dance—John LaBriola-Debra Coyne, Whittier, Calif.
Mixed Pairs—Ron Sabo-Darlene Waters, Columbus, Ohio.
Figures—Kim Rouse, Akron, Ohio.
Women's Figures—Kathleen O'Brien, Edgewater Park, N.J.
Speed—Tim Small, Fort Lauderdale, Fla.
Women's Speed—Marcia Yager, Cincinnati.

Dance International—Kerry Cavazzi-Jane Puracchio, East Meadow, L.I.

ROWING

World Champions

Singles—Peter-Michael Kolbe, West Germany.
Doubles—Frank and Alf Hansen, Norway.
Eights—East Germany.

WOMEN

Singles—Christine Scheiblich, East Germany.
Eights—East Germany.

United States Champions

Singles—Sean Drea, Ireland.
Singles Dash—Jim Dietz, New York AC.
Doubles—Dietz-Larry Klecatsky, AC.
Pairs with Coxswains—John Mathews–Darryell Vreugenhil-Ken Dreyfuss, coxswain, Vesper.
Quads—New York AC.
Eights—U.S. National Team.
155-Pound Singles—Bill Belden, Undine.
155-Pound Doubles—Klecatsky-Mike Verlin, New York AC.
155-Pound Pairs—Frank Pisoni-Ted Bonanno, New York AC.

Intercollegiate Champions

IRA—Wisconsin; Second Varsity: Wisconsin; Freshman: Penn.
Eastern Sprints—Harvard.
Western Sprints—Washington.
Dad Vail—Coast Guard Academy.

U.S. Women

Singles—Wiki Royden Cambridge, Mass.
Singles Dash—Gail Pierson, Cambridge, Mass.
Doubles—Johane Lepage-Elaine Bourbeau, Quebec.

Pair—Ann and Marie Jonik, Vesper.
Eights—Wisconsin University.

RUGBY

World—South Africa Springboks.
Rugby League, World—England.
Eastern U.S. Club—Providence.

SHOOTING

Grand American Trapshooting Champions

Men—Wayne Hegwood, Jackson, Miss.
Women—Ann Kisner, Muscatine, Iowa.

Skeet Shooting

Men—Robert Paxton, San Antonio, Tex.
Women—Jackie Ramsey, Dallas, Tex.
Junior—Steven Pyles, Temple Hill, Md.
Senior—M.E. Kidd, Monroe, La.

United States Pistol Champions

National—Sgt. Bonnie Harmon, Columbus, Ga.
National Trophy—Hershel Anderson, Tracy City, Tenn.
Women—Sgt. Barbara J. Hile, Columbus, Ga.

United States Rifle Champions

High Power—Gary Anderson, Axtell, Neb.
Women's High Power—Betty Swarthout, Westand, Mich.
Smallbore Position—Lieut. Robert A. Gustin, San Dimas, Calif.
Smallbore, Prone—Maj. Lones Wigger, Carter, Mont.

SHUFFLEBOARD

United States Champions

Winter Open—William Folbert, Cleveland, Ohio.

Women's Winter Open—Mary Eldridge, Lake George, N.Y.
Summer Open—Arthur J. Davis, New Castle, Ind.
Women's Summer Open—Betty Stone, Miami, Fla.

SKIING

World Cup Winners

Men—Gustavo Thoeni, Italy.
Women—Annemarie Proell Moser, Austria.

National Alpine Champions

MEN

Downhill—Andy Mill, Aspen, Colo.
Slalom—Steve Mahre, White Pass, Wash.
Combined—Greg Jones, S. Lake Tahoe, Calif.
Giant Slalom—Phil Mahre, White Pass, Wash.

WOMEN

Downhill—Gail Blackburne, Brunswick, Me.
Slalom—Cindy Nelson, Lutsen, Minn.
Combined—Becky Dorsey, Wenham, Mass.
Giant Slalom—Becky Dorsey.

National Nordic Champions

JUMPING

Class A—Jerry Martin, Minneapolis.
Veteran—Glen Kotlarek, Duluth, Minn.
Junior—Roy Weaver, Iron Mountain, Mich.

CROSS-COUNTRY
MEN

15 Kilometers—Bill Koch, Guilford, Vt.
30 Kilometers—Tim Caldwell, Putney, Vt.
50 Kilometers—Tim Caldwell.

WOMEN

5 Kilometers—Martha Rockwell, West Lebanon, N.H.
10 Kilometers—Martha Rockwell.
20 Kilometers—Martha Rockwell.

Nordic Combined

Overall—Mike Devecka, Bend, Ore.

National Collegiate Championships

Downhill—Mark Ford, Colorado.
Slalom—Peik Christensen, Denver.
Alpine Combined—Mark Ford.
Jumping—Didrick Ellefsen, Colorado.
Nordic Combined—Stig Hallingbye, Wyoming.
Cross-Country—Steiner Hybertsen, Wyoming.
Team—University of Colorado.

SOCCER

United States Champions

North American Soccer League—Tampa Bay Rowdies.
Challenge Cup—Maccabee, Los Angeles.
Amateur Cup—Chicago Kickers.
Junior—Timo's Pizza, St. Louis.

Collegiate Champions

NCAA Division I—San Francisco.
NCCA Division II—Baltimore.
NCCA Division III—Babson College.
NAIA—Quincy College.

Other Champions

English Association Cup—West Ham United.
English League Cup—Aston Villa.
Scottish Association Cup—Glasgow Celtic.
Scottish League Cup—Glasgow Celtic.
European Cup—Bayern Munich.

SOFTBALL

Amateur Softball Assn. Champions

Fast Pitch—Rising Sun Hotel, Reading, Pa.
Women's Fast Pitch—Raybestos Brakettes, Stratford, Conn.
Slow Pitch—Pyramid Cafe, Lakewood, Ohio.
Women's Slow Pitch—Mark's Brothers Dots, North Miami, Fla.
Industrial Slow Pitch—Nassau County Police Dept., Mineola, L. I.
Women's Modified Pitch—Silvestri's, Staten Island.
Little League Girls—Medford, Ore.

SQUASH RACQUETS

Singles—Victor Niederhoffer, New York.
Women's Singles—Virginia Akabane, Rochester.
Doubles—Michael Pierce–Maurice Hecksher 3d, Philadelphia.
Women's Doubles—Carol Thesieres–Jane Stauffer, Philadelphia.
Veterans Singles—Pete Bostwick, Jr., New York.
Veterans Doubles—Don Leggat, Hamilton, Ontario-Charles Wright, Toronto.
Senior Singles—Bob Stuckert, Milwaukee.
Senior Doubles—Eugene O'Conor-Tom Schweitzer, Baltimore.
Collegiate Singles—Juan de Villafranca. U. of Mexico.
Women's Collegiate—Wendy Zaharko, Princeton.
Team—Harvard.

SQUASH TENNIS

Singles—Pedro Baccallao, New York.
Doubles—Baccallao-Joe Homes, New York.

SURFING

National Champions

Men—Aaron Wright, Pedro Point, Calif.
Women—Sally Prange, Honolulu.

SWIMMING

World Championships

MEN

100-Meter Freestyle—Andy Coan, Fort Lauderdale, Fla.
200-Meter Freestyle—Tim Shaw, Long Beach, Calif.
400-Meter Freestyle—Tim Shaw.
1,500-Meter Freestyle—Tim Shaw.
100-Meter Backstroke—Roland Matthes, East Germany.
200-Meter Backstroke—Zoltan Veraszto, Hungary.
100-Meter Breast-Stroke—David Wilkie, Britain.
200-Meter Breast-Stroke—David Wilkie.
100-Meter Butterfly—Greg Jagenburg, West Chester, Pa.
200-Meter Butterfly—Bill Forrester, Jacksonville, Fla.
200-Meter Individual Medley—Andras Hargitay, Hungary.
400-Meter Individual Medley—Andras Hargitay.
400-Meter Freestyle Relay—United States.
400-Meter Medley Relay—United States.
800-Meter Free-Style—West Germany.

WOMEN

100-Meter Freestyle—Kornelia Ender, East Germany.
200-Meter Freestyle—Shirley Babashoff, Fountain Valley, Calif.
400-Meter Freestyle—Shirley Babashoff.
800 Meter Freestyle—Jenny Turrall, Australia.
100-Meter Backstroke—Ulrike Richter, East Germany.
200-Meter Backstroke—Birgit Treiber, East Germany.
100-Meter Breast-Stroke—Hannelore Anke, East Germany.
200-Meter Breast-Stroke—Hannelore Anke.
100-Meter Butterfly—Kornelia Ender.
200-Meter Butterfly—Rosemarie Kother, East Germany.
200-Meter Individual Medley—Kathy Heddy, Summit, N.J.
400-Meter Individual Medley—Ulrike Tauber, East Germany.
400-Meter Freestyle Relay—East Germany.
400-Meter Medley—East Germany.

World Diving

Springboard—Lt. Phil Boggs, U.S. Air Force.
Platform—Klaus DiBiasi, Italy.
Women's Springboard—Irinna Kalina, USSR.
Women's Platform—Janet Ely, Dallas.

National Long-Course Champions

MEN

100-Meter Freestyle—Jim Montgomery, Madison, Wis.
200-Meter Freestyle—Bruce Furniss, Long Beach, Calif.
400-Meter Freestyle—Tim Shaw, Long Beach, Calif.
1,500-Meter Freestyle—Bobby Hackett, Yonkers, N.Y.
100-Meter Backstroke—John Naber, Menlo Park, Calif.
200-Meter Backstroke—John Naber.
100-Meter Breast-Stroke—Rick Colella, Seattle.
200-Meter Breast-Stroke—Rick Colella.
100-Meter Butterfly—Steve Baxter, Santa Clara, Calif.
200-Meter Butterfly—Greg Jagenburg, West Chester, Pa.
200-Meter Individual Medley—Bruce Furniss.
400-Meter Individual Medley—Dave Hannula, Tacoma, Wash.
400-Meter Freestyle Relay—Badger Dolphins, Madison.

400-Meter Medley Relay—Long Beach, (Calif.) S.C.

800-Meter Freestyle—Long Beach S.C.

WOMEN

100-Meter Freestyle—Shirley Babashoff, Fountain Valley, Calif.

200-Meter Freestyle—Shirley Babashoff.

400-Meter Freestyle—Shirley Babashoff.

1,500-Meter Freestyle—Heather Greenwood, Fresno, Calif.

100-Meter Backstroke—Linda Jezek, Santa Clara, Calif.

200-Meter Backstroke—Melissa Belote, Silver Spring, Md.

100-Meter Breast-Stroke—Marcia Morey, Decatur, Ill.

200-Meter Breast-Stroke—Marcia Morey.

100-Meter Butterfly—Camille Wright, New Albany, Ind.

200-Meter Butterfly—Valerie Lee, Mission Viejo, Calif.

200-Meter Individual Medley—Kathy Heddy, Summit, N.J.

400-Meter Individual Medley—Jenni Franks, Wilmington, Del.

400-Meter Freestyle Relay—Mission Viejo, Calif. Nadadores.

400-Meter Medley Relay—Mission Viejo.

800-Meter Freestyle Relay—Mission Viejo.

National Outdoor Diving

MEN

One-Meter—Tom Moore, Westerville, Ohio.

Three-Meter—Lt. Phil Boggs, Air Force Academy.

Platform—Kent Vosler, Eaton, Ohio.

WOMEN

One-Meter—Cynthia McIngvale, Dallas.

Three-Meter—Cynthia McIngvale.

Platform—Janet Ely, Dallas.

National Collegiate Champions

50-Yard Freestyle—Joe Bottom, Southern California.

100-Yard Freestyle—Jonty Skinner, Alabama.

200-Yard Freestyle—George McDonnell, U.C.L.A.

500-Yard Freestyle—John Naber, Southern California.

1,650-Yard Freestyle—Mike Bruner, Stanford.

100-Yard Backstroke—John Naber.

200-Yard Backstroke—John Naber.

100-Yard Breast-Stroke—John Hencken, Stanford.

200-Yard Breast-Stroke—John Hencken.

100-Yard Butterfly—Jeff Roan, Utah.

200-Yard Butterfly—Robin Backhaus, Washington.

200-Yard Individual Medley—Fred Tyler, Indiana.

400-Yard Individual Medley—Lee Engstrand, Tennessee.

400-Yard Freestyle Relay—Indiana.

400-Yard Medley Relay—Southern California.

800-Yard Freestyle Relay—Indiana.

One-Meter Dive—Tim Moore, Ohio State.

Three-Meter Dive—Tim Moore.

Team—University of Southern California.

TABLE TENNIS

World Champions

Singles—Istvan Jonyer, Hungary.

Women's Singles—Yung Sun Kim, North Korea.

Doubles—Jonyer-Gabor Gergely, Hungary.

Women's Doubles—Maria Alexandru, Rumania-Shoko Takahashi, Japan.

Mixed Doubles—Stanislav Gomozkov-Tatjana Ferdman, USSR.

Swaythling Cup (men's team)—China.

Corbillon Cup (women's team)—China.

United States Champions

Singles—Kjell Johansson, Sweden.
Women's Singles—Chung Hyun Sook, South Korea.
Doubles—Dragutin Surbek-Anton Stipancic, Yugoslavia.
Women's Doubles—Ann-Christin Hellman-Eva Stroemvall, Sweden.

TENNIS

International Team Champions

Wightman Cup (Women)—Britain.
Federation Cup (Women)—Czechoslovakia.
Stevens Cup (Seniors)—United States.
World Cup—Australia.

Wimbledon Champions

Singles—Arthur Ashe, Miami.
Women's Singles—Billie Jean King.
Doubles—Vito Gerulaitis, New York-Sandy Mayer, Mendham, N.J.
Women's Doubles—Ann Kiyomura, San Mateo, Calif.-Kazuko Sawamatsu, Japan.
Mixed Doubles—Margaret Court, Australia-Marty Riessen, Amelia Island, Fla.

U.S. Open Champions

Singles—Manuel Orantes, Spain.
Women's Singles—Chris Evert, Fort Lauderdale, Fla.
Doubles—Jimmy Connors, Belleville, Ill.-Ilie Nastase, Rumania.
Women's Doubles—Margaret Court, Australia-Virginia Wade, Britain.
Mixed Doubles—Rosemary Casals, San Francisco-Dick Stockton, Dallas.
Boys Singles—Howard Schoenfield, Beverly Hills, Calif.
Girls' Singles—Natasha Chmyreva, USSR.

Other United States Champions

Team—Pittsburgh Triangles.
Indoor—Jimmy Connors.
Women's Indoor—Martina Navaratilova.
Clay Court—Manuel Orantes.
Women's Clay Court—Chris Evert.
Men's 35—Gene Scott, New York.
Amateur Grass Court—Gonzalo Nunez, Austin, Tex.
Women's Amateur Grass Court—Lele Forood, Fort Lauderdale, Fla.
Amateur Clay Court—Victor Amaya, Holland, Mich.
Women's Amateur Clay Court—JoAnn Russell, Naples, Fla.
Senior Clay Court—Del Sylvia, Knoxville, Tenn.
Women's Clay Court—Nancy Reed, McLean, Va.
Senior Grass Court—Don Gale, Mountain View, Calif.
Junior—Howard Schoenfield.
Junior Women—Beth Norton, Fairfield, Conn.
NCAA—Division I: Billy Martin, UCLA; Division II: Andy Rae, University of San Diego.
NAIA—Dave Petersen, Gustavus-Adolphus.
Women's Collegiate—Stephanie Tolleson, Trinity (Texas).

Other Foreign Opens

Australian Men—John Newcombe.
Australian Women—Evonne Goolagong.
French Men—Bjorn Borg, Sweden.
French Women—Chris Evert.
Canadian Men—Manuel Orantes.
Canadian Women—Chris Evert.

TRACK AND FIELD

Men's National Indoor Champions

60-Yard Dash—Hasely Crawford, Eastern Michigan.
60-Yard High Hurdles—Charles Foster, N. Carolina Central.

600 Yards—Wesley Williams Jr., San Diego.
1,000 Yards—Rick Wohlhuter, U. of Chicago TC.
One-Mile Run—Filbert Bayi, Tanzania.
Three-Mile Run—Miruts Yifter, Ethiopia.
Two-Mile Walk—Ron Daniel, New York AC.
Sprint Medley Relay—Penn State.
One-Mile Relay—Seton Hall.
Two-Mile Relay—U. of Chicago TC.
Long Jump—Arnie Robinson, San Diego.
Shot-put—Al Feuerbach, Long Beach, Calif.
Triple Jump—Tommy Haynes, U.S. Army.
High Jump—Dwight Stones, Long Beach, Calif.
Pole Vault—Roland Carter, Houston, Tex.
35-Pound Weight Throw—George Frenn, Hawaiian Gardens, Calif.

Men's National Outdoor Champions

100 Meter Dash—Don Quarrie, Beverly Hills Striders.
200 Meter Dash—Don Quarrie.
400-Meter Dash—David Jenkins, Britain.
800-Meter Run—Mark Enyeart, Utah State.
1,500-Meter Run—Len Hilton, Long Beach, Calif.
3,000-Meter Steeplechase—Randy Smith, Wichita State.
5,000-Meter Run—Marty Liquori, New York AC.
10,000-Meter Run—Frank Shorter, Gainesville, Fla.
5,000-Meter Walk—Ron Laird, New York AC.
110-Meter Hurdles—Gerald Wilson, Beverly Hills Striders.
400-Meter Hurdles—Ralph Mann, Beverly Hills Striders.
Long Jump—Arnie Robinson, San Diego.
High Jump—Tom Woods, Long Beach Calif. Pacific Coast Club.

Triple Jump—Anthony Terry, San Mateo, Calif.
Hammer Throw—Boris Djerassi, New York AC.
Discus—John Powell, Long Pacific Coast Club.
Javelin—Richard George, Brigham Young.
Shot-put—Al Feuerbach, Pacific Coast Club.

Other Champions

AAU Decathlon—Fred Samara, New York AC.
USTFF Decathlon—Bruce Jenner, San Jose, Calif.
Boston Marathon—William H. Rodgers, Boston.

Women's National Outdoor Champions

100-Meter Dash—Rosalyn Bryant, Chicago.
200-Meter Dash—Debra Armstrong, Washington.
400-Meter Dash—Debra Sapenter, Prairie View, Tex.
800-Meter Run—Madeline Jackson, Cleveland.
1,500-Meter Run—Julie Brown, Los Angeles.
3,000-Meter Run—Lynn Bjorklund, Albuquerque, N.M.
100-Meter Hurdles—Jane Frederick, Los Angeles.
400-Meter Hurdles—Debbie Esser, Woodbine, Iowa.
1,500-Meter Walk—Lisa Metheny, Rialto, Calif.
400-Meter Relay—Tennessee State.
880-Yard Sprint Medley Relay—Sports International, Washington.
One-Mile Relay—Atoms TC., Brooklyn.
Two-Mile Relay—Blue Ribbon TC., Cleveland.
High Jump—Joni Huntley, Oregon TC.
Long Jump—Martha Watson, Lakewood, Calif.
Discus—Jean Roberts, Newark, Del.
Shot-put—Maren Seidler, Chicago.
Javelin—Kathy Schmidt, Los Angeles.

Other Champions

AAU Pentathlon—Jane Frederick, Los Angeles.
AIAW Pentathlon—Mitzi McMillin, Colorado U.
AIAW Team—UCLA.
AAU Marathon—Kim Merritt, Parkside, Wis.
Boston Marathon (First Woman Finisher)—Lisne Winter, Wolfburg, Germany.

National Collegiate Outdoor Champions

100-Yard Dash—Hasely Crawford, Eastern Michigan.
220-Yard Dash—Reggie Jones, Tennessee.
440-Yard Dash—Benny Brown, UCLA.
880-Yard Run—Mark Enyeart, Utah State.
One-Mile Run—Eamon Coghlan, Villanova.
Three-Mile Run—John Ngeno, Washington State.
Six-Mile Run—John Ngeno.
3,000-Meter Steeplechase—James Munyala, Texas-El Paso.
120-Yard Hurdles—Larry Shinn, Louisiana State.
440-Yard Hurdles—Craig Cuadill, Indiana.
440-Yard Relay—Southern California.
One-Mile Relay—Washington.
High Jump—Warren Shanklin, NE Louisiana.
Triple Jump—Ron Livers, San Jose State.
Long Jump—Charlton Ehizuelen, Illinois.
Pole Vault—Earl Bell, Arkansas State.
Discus—Jim McGoldrick, Texas.
Javelin—Keith Goldie, Long Beach State.
Hammer—Boris Djerassi, Northeastern.
Shot-put—Hans Hoglund, Texas-El Paso.
Team—Texas-El Paso.

Other Champions

NCAA Decathlon—Ramo Phil, Brigham Young.
NAIA Team—Southeastern Louisiana.
NAIA Decathlon—James Herron, Cameron State.
NAIA Marathon—Roger Vann, John Brown U.

VOLLEYBALL

U.S. Volleyball Assn. Champions

Open—Charthouse, San Diego.
Women's Open—Adidas VC Anaheim, Calif.
Senior—Captain Jack, Long Beach, Calif.
Collegiate—Pepperdine.

Other National Champions

AAU—Outriggers Canoe Club, Honolulu.
AAU Women—Chimo, Vancouver.
Women's Small College—Texas Lutheran.
NCAA—UCLA.
NAIA—California-Dominguez Hills.
Women's Collegiate—UCLA.
Women's J.C.—Ricks (Idaho)
Professional—Los Angeles Stars.

WATER POLO

World—Soviet Union.
AAU—Concord (Calif.) Aquatics.
Women's AAU—North Miami Beach, Fla.
Collegiate—California-Irvine.
Senior Indoor—New York AC.

WATER SKIING

World Championships

Overall—Carlos Suarez, Venezuela.
Women's Overall—Liz Allan Shetter, Groveland, Fla.

Slalom—Roby Zucchi, Italy.
Women's Slalom—Liz Shetter.
Tricks—Carlos Suarez.
Women's Tricks—Maria Victoria Carrasco, Venezuela.
Jumping—Wayne Grimditch, Hillsboro Beach, Fla.
Women's Jumping—Liz Shetter.
Team—United States.

United States Champions

Overall—Ricky McCormick, Hialeah, Fla.
Women's Overall—Liz Allan Shetter, Groveland, Fla.
Slalom—Kris LaPoint, Castro Valley, Calif.
Women's Slalom—Cindy Todd, Pierson, Fla.
Tricks—Tony Krupa, Jackson, Mich.
Women's Tricks—Liz Shetter.
Jumping—Wayne Grimditch, Hillsboro Beach, Fla.
Women's Jumping—Liz Shetter.
Senior Overall—Ken White, Honolulu.
Senior Women—Barbara Cleveland, Hawthorne, Fla.

WEIGHT LIFTING

National AAU Champions

114 Pounds—Forrest Felton, Savannah, Ga.
123 Pounds—John Yamauchi, Honolulu.
132 Pounds—Dave Hussey, Florissant, Mo.
148 Pounds—Dan Cantore, San Francisco.
165 Pounds—Fred Lowe, Lansing, Mich.
181 Pounds—Peter Rawluk, Los Angeles.
198 Pounds—Michael Karchut, Calumet City, Ill.
242 Pounds—Mark Cameron, Middletown, R.I.
Superheavyweight—Bruce Wilhelm, Phoenix, Ariz.

WRESTLING

National AAU Freestyle Champions

105.5 Pounds—David Range, Cleveland.
114.5 Pounds—John Morley, New York A.C.
125.5 Pounds—Mark Massery, Chicago.
136.5 Pounds—Doug Moses, Waterloo, Iowa.
149.5 Pounds—Gene Davis, Long Beach, Calif.
163 Pounds—Carl Adams, Brentwood, N.Y.
180.5 Pounds—John Peterson, Lancaster, Pa.
198 Pounds—Russell Hellickson, Madison, Wis.
220 Pounds—Greg Wojciechowski, Toledo, Ohio.
Heavyweight—Mike McCready, Dubuque, Iowa.

National Collegiate Championships

118 Pounds—Shawn Garel, Oklahoma.
126 Pounds—John Fritz, Penn State.
134 Pounds—Mike Frick, Lehigh.
142 Pounds—Jim Bennett, Yale.
150 Pounds—Chuck Yagla, Iowa.
158 Pounds—Dan Holm, Iowa.
167 Pounds—Ron Ray, Oklahoma State.
177 Pounds—Mike Lieberman, Lehigh.
190 Pounds—Al Nacin, Iowa State.
Heavyweight—Larry Bielenberg, Oregon State.

YACHTING

U.S. Yacht Racing Union Champions

Men (Mallory Cup)—Chris Pollock, Cedar Point, Conn.
Women (Adams Cup)—Cindy Batchelor, Pettipaug, Conn.
Junior (Sears Cup)—Mike Alexander, Coconut Grove, Fla.
O'Day (Single-handed)—Sam Altrueter, Fair Haven, N.J.
Smythe (Junior Single-handed)—Shawn Kempton, Ocean Gate, N.J.

Prince of Wales Trophy (Club)—California Y.C., Los Angeles.

Women's Double-handed—Nell Taylor-Sally Lindsay, Branford, Conn.

Junior Double-handed—Dan Hathaway-Scott Young, Dallas.

National Sea Exploring—South Central Region.

Collegiate Champions

Single-handed (Foster Trophy)—Sam Altrueter, Tufts.

Outstanding Sailor—Sam Altrueter.

Overall Team—Tufts.

Women's Team—Princeton.

Distance and Ocean Races

Annapolis-Newport—Salty Goose, Robert Derecktor, Mamaroneck, N.Y.

Block Island—Charisma, Jesse Philips, Dayton, Ohio.

Los Angeles-Honolulu—Chutzpah, Stuart Cowan, Honolulu.

Marblehead-Halifax—La Forza del Destino, Norman Raben, Bedford Village, N.Y.

Newport-England—Robin, Ted Hood, Marblehead, Mass., Lee Van Gemert, skipper.

Other Cups and Championships

Canada Cup—Golden Dazy, U.S.; Don Driner

Admirals Cup—Britain.

Southern Ocean Racing Conference—Stinger, Dennis Conner, San Diego.

Congressional Cup—Dennis Conner.

WHO'S WHO IN
BEST SPORTS STORIES—1976

WRITERS IN BEST SPORTS STORIES—1976

THE PRIZE WINNERS

ROBERT M. LIPSYTE (Pride of the Tiger), winner of this year's magazine award, is a free-lance writer who was formerly sports columnist for *The New York Times*. A three-time previous winner in the *Best Sports Stories* annuals, he has published a novel, *Liberty Two,* and a nonfiction work, *Sports World/An American Dreamland.* Last year he taught a course in sports journalism in New York University's graduate school of journalism. He won this anthology's feature award in 1967 and 1969, both times with stories on rookies. He won the news-coverage award in 1965 for his story on the Clay (Muhammed Ali)-Liston fight.

MAURY ALLEN ("An Event for the Ages"), winner of the news-coverage award, has been a sports reporter for the *New York Post* since 1962. He began his newspaper career with the *Seymour* (Ind.) *Times* after army service, went to the *Levittown* (Pa.) *Times,* and then worked for *Sports Illustrated.* He then went to the sports desk of the *New York Post.* He has authored many sports books and his latest, *Where Have You Gone, Joe DiMaggio?,* was warmly received by the critics. Because of his perceptive and interesting sports analysis he is much in demand by many of the nation's better periodicals.

WELLS TWOMBLY (There Was Only One Casey), winner of the news-feature award, can no longer be described as the house's peripatetic author. For a decade he wandered around, starting in New England at Willimantic (Conn.), going far West to Hollywood, down South to Houston, and up North to Detroit, each time with a different paper's sports desk. In 1970, when he won this book's news-coverage prize with the story of the upset of the New York Jets over the Baltimore Colts, he gathered his family once more and discovered gold with the *San Francisco Examiner.* He now writes a sports column and in addition has written a number of sports books. He also free-lances for many major magazines and travels very little now.

OTHER CONTRIBUTORS (In Alphabetical Order)

BOB ADDIE (The Quiet Golfer from Nashville) is one of the fine veteran writers in this country and won the feature award of *Best Sports Stories* in 1963 with his sensitive account of blind children at a baseball game. He was graduated from the University of Alabama and began his newspaper career with the old New York *Journal American*. Later he was taken on by *The Washington Post* and is now a sports columnist there. In 1967 he was president of the Baseball Writers Association of America. In addition to his feature award in 1963, his articles have merited many appearances in *Best Sports Stories*.

PETE AXTHELM (Ruffian's Last Race) has been sports editor of *Newsweek* since 1970. He joined that magazine in 1968 and his star rose fast to the point where he is generally recognized as one of the major sports-writing talents in this country. Previously, he wrote for *Sports Illustrated* and before that was a writer and racing columnist for the now-defunct New York *Herald Tribune*. Besides contributing stories to numerous magazines, he is the author of four books, all of which received warm critical acclaim. One book in particular, *The City Game* (Harper's Magazine Press), is regarded as the definitive work on Harlem basketball.

CATHERINE BELL (Virginia Wade: Whatever Became of Her "Brilliant Future"?) covers women's tennis. She was born in England, grew up in Tasmania, Australia, and is a graduate in psychology of the University of Tasmania. She now lives in London, where she is an associate editor of *Lawn Tennis* magazine and a free-lance writer. She has been writing a series of biographical sketches while in America for *Tennis* magazine on the many fine, emerging women tennis players, and is also co-authoring a book on that sport with Rosie Casals. This makes her second appearance in *Best Sports Stories*.

FURMAN BISHER (A Landslide It Wasn't) is the sports editor of *The Atlanta Journal*. He has been honored by *Time* magazine as one of the outstanding sports columnists in this country and has merited many inclusions in *Best Sports Stories*. Besides his newspaper work, he is in great demand by many of the major magazines and *The Sporting News*. He has also written a number of sports books, his latest being *Arnold Palmer—The Golden Year*.

THOMAS BOSWELL (All New England Feels Feverish) has been a sports reporter with *The Washington Post* since 1971. His major beats are major-league baseball (World Series and playoffs), tennis (Forest Hills), and general assignment coverage of the Washington Redskins, Washington Bullets, college football, and basketball. He is a graduate of Amherst College, class of 1969. This is his first appearance in *Best Sports Stories.*

ROYAL BROUGHAM (Shelby's Moment of Glory), called the dean of American sports writers in active service—64 years on one newspaper, *The Seattle Post-Intelligencer*—has covered most of the world's important stories, dating from the miracle decade of the 1930s, when so many great athletes made the headlines. He is eighty-one and still counting.

SI BURICK (The Old Cat-and-Mouse Game) has been sports editor of the *Dayton Daily News* for 46 years. He has been honored as Ohio Sportswriter of the Year for each of the past 13 years and has been a frequent contributor to *Best Sports Stories.* He has covered baseball's spring training camps for 38 years and has sat in on virtually every major sports event, missing only two Kentucky Derbies since 1929 and two World Series since 1930. He was the 1972 president of the Football Writers Association of America and the 1971 president of the National Sportscasters and Sportswriters Association. He is the author of *Alston and the Dodgers,* a biography of Los Angeles Dodgers manager Walter Alston.

BUD COLLINS (Ashe's Lucky Saturday) has been a sports and general columnist for *The Boston Globe* for 12 years, and a tennis telecaster on national networks for the same period. A native of Ohio, he graduated from Baldwin-Wallace College, started his newspaper career with the *Boston Herald,* and built character for such as the eminent Yippie, Abbie Hoffman, during five years as tennis coach at Brandeis. This is his fourth appearance in *Best Sports Stories.*

BILL CONLIN (Rose Sticks It to the Red Sox) has been with the *Philadelphia Daily News* for 12 years after four years with the *Evening Bulletin* of the same city. He first appeared in *Best Sports Stories* in 1963 with a basketball piece and shared the news-coverage prize with Bob Lipsyte in 1965 for his story on the Penn State upset of Ohio State. He covers the Phillies, Penn State football, and all major football. In addition to conducting a Philadelphia radio sports show, he also does basketball announcing.

GLENN DICKEY (A Throwback to Football's Stone Age) graduated from the University of California at Berkeley in 1958 and hit the newspaper circuit immediately, becoming the sports editor of the Watsonville *Register-Pajoronian* in 1963. He then went to the sports desk of the *San Francisco Chronicle* and in 1971 he became a sports columnist with that paper and has remained there. He is the author of two books, *The Jock Empire* and *The Great No-Hitters.* His third book, *The Influence Peddlers in Sports,* is due in 1976. He is also a prolific major magazine sports contributor. This marks his fifth appearance in *Best Sports Stories.*

FRANK DOLSON (Swarthmore Finally Has Champagne) has merited many appearances in this sports anthology. He was graduated from the University of Pennsylvania in 1954, spent six months with *Sports Illustrated,* and in 1955 joined the *Philadelphia Inquirer.* He wrote an occasional column at first, but his fine talents merited his being given a regular column assignment in 1966.

LARRY ELDRIDGE (Muhammad Ali Takes on Harvard). After five years with the *Philadelphia Inquirer* and 11 with The Associated Press, he joined *The Christian Science Monitor* staff as a columnist in 1971, becoming sports editor last June. He has covered such events as the 1972 Olympics (both Sapporo and Munich), the Fischer-Spassky chess match in Iceland, the Super Bowl, the World Series, and Forest Hills. This is his first appearance in *Best Sports Stories.*

GERALD ESKENAZI (Namath's Mother Also Scores) has been a reporter for *The New York Times* since 1963. He covered major-league hockey for six years and has written eight books on the sport. He currently covers the New York Jets and is working on a book about the football Giants of the 1950s. He lives in Roslyn, Long Island, with his wife and three children. He has appeared in *Best Sports Stories* on many occasions.

STANLEY FRANK (Name the U.S. Congressman Who Holds the NFL Record for the Most Fumbles Recovered, Lifetime) is a veteran sports writer who has spent most of his life in the environs of New York City and has probed deeply into his assignments on the local and national scene. Most of his newspaper work was done with the *New York Post,* both as a reporter in the sports department and as a columnist. He has been a free-lance writer now for many years and has appeared many times in *Best Sports Stories.*

JOE GERGEN (A Grand Finale) has been with *Newsday* for eight years, this last year as sports columnist. A 1963 graduate of Boston College, he spent five years with United Press International in New York before joining *Newsday* in 1968. He has covered all major sports for *Newsday* with emphasis on baseball and professional football. In 1971 he received the National Headliner Award as the outstanding sports writer in the country. This marks his fourth inclusion in *Best Sports Stories.*

WILL GRIMSLEY (China Through Different Eyes) has covered the globe in pursuit of stories for The Associated Press. He has reported on five Olympic Games, made 12 trips to Australia for Davis Cup tournaments, and has had numerous reportorial chores in every major world capital. He also has had time enough to write three books—*Golf: Its History, People and Events; Tennis: Its History, People and Events;* and *Football: Greatest Moments of the Southwest Conference.* He also was supervising editor of *Century of Sports,* a popular book that sold close to 100,000 copies in 1971. This marks his sixth appearance in *Best Sports Stories.*

PAUL HENDRICKSON (He's Not as Simple as ABC) has been a feature writer for *The National Observer* since December 1974. He is a 1967 graduate of St. Louis University, earned a master's degree at Penn State, and has worked for *Holiday* magazine and the *Detroit Free Press*. He has free-lanced extensively. This is his second appearance in *Best Sports Stories*.

PHIL HERSH (They Do It to Hear Bubbles) is twenty-nine and may be better known for a midsummer night's disagreement with Ralph Houk, but most of his time is placidly spent as a sports writer for the *Baltimore Evening Sun*. During his three years in Baltimore, Hersh has covered everything from eighty-seven-year-old whitewater canoeists to pro football.

DAVE HIRSHEY (Million-Dollar Question: Bucks or Books?) is a 1971 graduate of Dickinson College with a major in English. He went to work for the *New York Daily News* at age twenty-one, becoming the youngest sports reporter in New York. He began by covering soccer, roller derby, and racing. He now covers all sports, specializing in college football, college basketball, and tennis as well as general features. This marks his third appearance in *Best Sports Stories*.

STAN HOCHMAN (Bernie Parent Misses the Boat) has had his stories enhance this sports anthology for many years and his fine work has regaled Philadelphia and its environs, too. After 12 years as a baseball writer and columnist for the *Philadelphia Daily News*, he was named sports editor in 1971. He is a former schoolteacher who left his classroom for the sports desk. His articles are not confined to the event itself, but there is also always a consistent concern with the human angle of the athletes and their efforts.

MARK JACOBSON (Trying Out for the Jets) is twenty-eight and was born in Manhattan. He attended the University of Wisconsin, New York University, the University of California at Berkeley, and the San Francisco Art Institute. Jacobson produced psychedelic light shows at the Whiskey a Go-Go on Sunset Strip and drove a cab in New York City from 1972 to 1974. He has made two underground feature-length films—*The Birds Coit Tower* and *The Fool Killer*—and has written two plays—*Arnie Con Carne* and *Shaving Cream Fight in Madison*. A free-lance writer since 1974, he has published articles in *New York* magazine, *The Village Voice*, *High Times*, *Monster Times*, and *Crawdaddy*. This is his first appearance in *Best Sports Stories*.

ROGER KAHN (Can Sports Survive Money?) has won three magazine awards in this sports anthology: the first in 1960, the second in 1969, and the last in 1970 with his fine analysis of Willie Mays as both player and person entitled, "Willie Mays, Yesterday and Today." He began his newspaper career as a copy boy, then became a sports reporter with the late New York *Herald Tribune*, went to *Newsweek* as sports editor, and then to *The Saturday Evening Post* before settling down as a regular sports columnist with *Esquire*. He is a graduate of NYU, free-lances a great deal, and has authored many books, one of which, *The Boys of Summer,* became a best seller and was warmly received by critics and readers.

DAVID KINDRED (A Rookie League) is thirty-four and has worked for the Louisville newspapers since 1966. He became sports editor of the *Louisville Times* in 1969, spent a year in the paper's Washington bureau in 1972, and has been sports editor of *The Courier-Journal* since. Three times Kentucky Sports Writer of the Year, he won a National Headliner Award for general interest columns in 1971. He's the author of a book, *Basketball: The Dream Game in Kentucky.* His stories have appeared in *Best Sports Stories* three times.

HARVEY KIRKPATRICK (Wayne Estes's Final Game) is a native of Englewood, Colo., and a graduate of the University of Denver. He embarked upon his professional career in 1961 as sports information director at his alma mater and from 1964 through 1969 served in the same capacity at Utah State University. He since has been associated with pro hockey and basketball franchises in Salt Lake City. At present he is president of his own public relations firm, Win, Inc., and is a licensed real-estate salesman. This is his first appearance in *Best Sports Stories.*

TONY KORNHEISER (Little Looie) has worked at *Newsday* for the past five years as a sports reporter, a rock music critic, and the lifestyle specialist for the daily magazine section. His stories have appeared in *Rolling Stone, New York,* and *Sport* magazine. For the past three years he has been a regular contributor to the *Street & Smith Basketball Annual,* where this story appeared. He and his wife, Karril, live in Long Beach, N.Y. This is his fourth appearance in *Best Sports Stories.*

HAL LEBOVITZ (The Lady in Red) is a graduate of Western Reserve University who started his career as a high school chemistry teacher, but because of his avid interest in athletics became a sports writer. He started work for the *Cleveland News* and then went to the *Cleveland Plain Dealer,* where he is now the sports editor. His column "Hal Thinks" is supplemented by his "Ask Hal" and both have earned him numerous writing honors as well as a devoted reading public. He is a past president of the Baseball Writers Association of America and has merited many inclusions in *Best Sports Stories.*

ALLEN LEWIS (It Was Tiant's Show) has been covering sports for the *Philadelphia Inquirer* for more than 30 years, concentrating on baseball for the last two decades. Upon graduation from Haverford College, where he was sports editor of the school paper, he worked briefly for a Connecticut weekly and the now-defunct *Philadelphia Ledger* before serving over four years in uniform. For more than 10 years he was chairman of Baseball's Scoring Rules Committee. This is his fifth appearance in *Best Sports Stories.*

JOAN LIBMAN (Women's Golf: The Rewards Are Elusive) was hired as a reporter for *The Wall Street Journal*'s San Francisco news bureau in 1974.

Formerly she had been employed as a television news reporter in Oakland, Calif. She has a bachelor's and master's degree in history from Cal State, and is thirty-one and single. This is her first appearance in *Best Sports Stories.*

BARRY LORGE (Orantes's Triumph: Portrait of Ecstasy), a native of Worcester, Mass., is a 1970 graduate of Harvard College, where he majored in government. He started writing sports for the *Worcester Telegram & Gazette* while he was in school, happened on to the tennis beat, and since 1971 has been a free-lancer specializing in tennis. He has covered the sport in more than a dozen countries for a number of publications. In 1975 he achieved the grand slam, covering the Australian, French, Wimbledon, and U.S. opens. He is a contributing editor for *Tennis* magazine, and his stories appear frequently in *The Washington Post.*

RON MARTZ (Football Trophies: Their Stories) has been in the newspaper business only five years following an honorable discharge from the Marine Corps and two years at the University of Houston. He worked at *The Fort Pierce* (Fla.) *News Tribune* as general assignments reporter and wire editor for two years; at *Cocoa* (Fla.) *Today* as sports writer and later assistant sports editor for two years before joining *The St. Petersburg Times* as a sports writer in 1974. This is his second appearance in *Best Sports Stories.*

REGIS MCAULEY (Cure for the Blues) will be installed as national president of the Football Writers Association of America at its annual meeting August 1976. He has been a sports writer for 32 years, past sports editor of the *Cleveland News* and *Cleveland Press,* and after serving 25 years with those newspapers came to Tucson in 1969 and was named sports editor of the *Tucson Daily Citizen* in 1974. He has won three American Newspaper Guild Awards for his stories. This is his first appearance in *Best Sports Stories.*

NEIL MILBERT (The Great Dictator of the Thoroughbred World) covers racing, professional and college football as well as boxing for the *Chicago Tribune.* A graduate of Marquette University, he served in the Marine Corps and worked for WEMP Radio (Milwaukee), the *Ottumwa* (Iowa) *Courier,* and the *Jersey City* (N.J.) *Journal* before joining the *Chicago Tribune.* He has made three appearances in *Best Sports Stories.*

HUBERT MIZELL (Play-by-Play Before Its Heyday) is thirty-six and sports editor of *The St. Petersburg* (Fla.) *Times* and a former feature sports writer for The Associated Press in Miami and New York. He has covered almost all of the world's great sports events, including the Olympic Games, and was included in *Best Sports Stories—1974.* Mizell, who is also a contributing editor to *Golf Digest* magazine, began his career on the *Florida Times-Union* in Jacksonville at age seventeen.

JIM MURRAY (A Hard Man to Find) writes a daily syndicated column that is distributed by the *Los Angeles Times.* His perceptive and humorous thrusts have caused him to be named America's Sportswriter of the Year for eight consecutive years by the National Sportscasters and Sportswriters Association. He was born in Hartford, Conn., graduated from Trinity College, and started his writing career with the *New Haven* (Conn.) *Register.* In 1944 he went to work for the *Los Angeles Examiner* and in 1953 was one of the founders of *Sports Illustrated.* In 1961 he returned to the *Los Angeles Times* as its premier sports columnist. He has won the National Headliners Award in 1965. He is also the author of two books, both anthologies of his own writing. This marks his second appearance in *Best Sports Stories.*

MURRAY OLDERMAN (The Ultimate Pol) is a sports editor of Newspaper Enterprise Association (NEA) and also sports cartoonist for that syndicate. This talented writer and graphic artist is also the former president of the Football Writers Association of America. His work appears in some 500 newspapers throughout the country. Prior to joining NEA, he worked for the McClatchy Newspapers of California and the *Minneapolis Star-Tribune.* He is a native of New York State and received his education at Missouri, Stanford, and Northwestern. His work has merited several appearances in *Best Sports Stories.*

WALLY PROVOST (How Ivan Does It), sports columnist, is a 25-year veteran of the *Omaha World-Herald,* where his assignments have ranged from courthouse reporter to sports editor. He attended the University of Nebraska and Milwaukee State Teachers College, served in the China-Burma-India theater during World War II, and is a four-time winner of the Nebraska Sports Writer of the Year award. This is his first appearance in *Best Sports Stories.*

JOHN S. RADOSTA (The Indy "Float") was graduated from New York University in 1935 and was a reporter for the New York *Herald Tribune* from 1935 to 1941. In World War II he was a correspondent-editor of *The Stars and Stripes.* Since joining *The New York Times* in 1945, he has done every kind of writing and editing. He has been a sports writer since 1967, specializing in motor sports, golf, and ice hockey. He is the author of *The New York Times Guide to Auto Racing,* published in 1971, and won the magazine award this sports anthology offers in 1975.

NORD RILEY (Fishing with My Father—and Other Outlandish Partners) is appearing in *Best Sports Stories* for the first time. A graduate of the University of Chicago, "I worked once, in 1937, but got over it and have free-lanced ever since," he says. He has contributed to most national magazines with short stories and articles. He also did TV writing for a few years and has written two novels and a play. He has been traveling in Europe since 1969.

DICK SCHAAP (That Thrilla in Manila), currently editor of *Sport* magazine, has had wide experience with all forms of communications. A graduate of Cornell University, he was sports editor of *Newsweek* before becoming a columnist and then city editor for the defunct New York *Herald Tribune*. He is a newscaster for NBC-TV and was a visiting columnist for the *Washington Star* for 10 weeks in 1975. He is the author of 19 books, the best known being *Instant Replay* and the most recent being *Sport*, a collection of his newspaper, magazine, and book work spanning 20 years.

JOHN SCHULIAN (The Mystery Man of the Blazers) is a thirty-year-old rookie sports writer for *The Washington Post*, specializing in professional football and basketball and offbeat characters. Before moving to the *Post* in September 1975, he spent five years as a rewrite man, feature writer, and rock-and-roll columnist for the *Baltimore Evening Sun*. Schulian, who has a B.A. from Utah and an M.S. from Northwestern, has free-lanced for many magazines, including *Sports Illustrated*. This is his second appearance in *Best Sports Stories*.

NICK SEITZ ("The Only-Ness") is one of the few writers who has hit the ten-time mark in this sports anthology. He is now the editor of *Golf Digest*. His alma mater was the University of Oklahoma, where he majored in philosophy. Then, at the age of twenty-two, he became editor of the *Norman* (Okla.) *Transcript*. His majoring in philosophy was excellent background for his golf articles, which not only concern themselves with the techniques of the game but also with the frustrations and tribulations of ordinary mortals who are constrained to watch the epic golf events on the tube and then attempt to emulate them. He has won numerous prizes in golf and basketball writing contests.

BLACKIE SHERROD (Defense, the Old Equalizer). It is a rare year when *Best Sports Stories* does not contain an article by this fine veteran writer of the Southwest. Although most of his work is done through his columns, where his wit and perception are highly appreciated, this year the editors have chosen a news coverage piece to regale readers. He is the executive sports editor of the *Dallas Times Herald* and has garnered just about every important sports-writing prize in this country. His reputation as a master of ceremonies, banquet speaker, radio and TV commentator is a major facet of Sherrod's talents.

JOHN SIMMONDS (The Cardiac Kids End an Incredible Season) has been in the sports department of *The Oakland Tribune* for the last 15 of the 20 years that he has worked with that paper. His coverage of basketball began in 1961 with the old American Basketball League, in which the San Francisco Saints were formed; he stayed on with the Warriors to become his paper's top writer of pro basketball activities. This past year he was named as *The Oakland Tribune*'s assistant sports editor. This is his first appearance in *Best Sports Stories*.

JOE SOUCHERAY (Mama Clears the Smoke) is twenty-six years old, a sports feature writer and general news columnist on *The Minneapolis Tribune*. He was graduated from the College of St. Thomas in St. Paul, Minn., and joined the *Tribune* in 1973. Soucheray has covered a variety of sporting events—from the Winnipeg 500 Snowmobile Race to the Connors-Newcombe tennis match in Las Vegas. His column appears weekly in the "Thursday" section of *The Minneapolis Tribune*. This is his second appearance in *Best Sports Stories*.

ART SPANDER (Play That Again, Sam), a 1960 UCLA graduate with a B.S. in political science, has been on the *San Francisco Chronicle* for 11 years after periods with the *Santa Monica Evening Outlook* and Los Angeles bureau of UPI. He has specialized in golf and pro basketball, but also covered every other sport from ballooning to volleyball. Spander has won numerous writing awards, including one for best coverage story in the 1971 edition of *Best Sports Stories*. He has appeared in this anthology five times. He also won the San Francisco Press Club first prize for best sports story and twice took first place in the Golf Writers Association of America writing contest.

PHOTOGRAPHERS IN BEST
SPORTS STORIES—1976

THE PHOTO WINNERS

GEORGE D. WALDMAN (Head in Groin, Shoe in Belly, Cleats in Face & Other Items) is the winner of the action-photo award in *Best Sports Stories —1976*. He is a native of Colorado, thirty-two years old, and chief photographer for the *Colorado Springs Sun,* a 30,000-circulation daily. He has a degree in journalism and brief experience as a reporter as well as four years as a photographer. His background includes four years as a weather observer in the U. S. Air Force, three of them in Athens, Greece. He has been a camera salesman, ditch digger, milk man, busboy and has held endless jobs as a laborer.

CLETUS M. (PETE) HOHN ("Now the Way to Prevent a Slice. . . .") the feature photo winner, has been a photographer for the *Minneapolis Tribune* for 20 years. A University of Minnesota graduate in 1953 in photo-journalism, Hohn first worked for the *Rochester* (Minn.) *Post-Bulletin.* This is his second appearance in *Best Sports Stories.*

OTHER PHOTOGRAPHERS (In Alphabetical Order)

MICHAEL A. ANDERSON (The Mighty Luis at Bat) has been a general assignment photographer for the *Boston Herald American* and *Sunday Herald Advertiser* for the past seven years. He is a past national treasurer of the National Press Photographers Association and last year received the NPPA Joseph Costa Award. He has been New England Press Photographer of the Year twice and has appeared in *Best Sports Stories* five times.

JOHN E. BIEVER (Aaron Doesn't Break Only Home-Run Records) graduated with a B.A. from the University of Wisconsin, Milwaukee, and has been a staff photographer with *The Milwaukee Journal* for three years. He has had photos in *Best Sports Stories* four times previously, including the best action photo in 1973.

RON BURDA (Saving Face) has been a photo-journalist for seven years, five years at the *San Jose Mercury-News.* He has a B.S. from Brigham Young University and an M.S. in mass communications from San Jose State University.

RICHARD DARCEY (Golden State Played 12 Feet Tall) is a two-time winner in the photo section of *Best Sports Stories,* once in 1967 and later in 1972. Both shots were action photos. He is director of photography at *The Washington Post,* where he has been since 1948. In 1956 he began to cover major-league sports and his past honors have included *Look*'s top sports picture of the year award and prizes in the National Press Photographers' competition.

KAREN ENGSTROM (Two to Tangle) has been a news photographer at *The Portland Oregonian* for one year. She was previously vacation replacement photographer at *The Seattle Times.* She worked a year as a medical photographer at the University of Washington Medical School. Prior to that she was a commercial artist and lithographer. She is the first female photographer to appear in *Best Sports Stories.*

JOHN P. FOSTER (A Family Affair) is a stringer for *The Seattle Times* who has been teaching photo-journalism at Central Washington State College, Ellensburg, Wash., for the past 10 years. He has business-journalism and master's degrees from Indiana University and was editor of the weekly *Hancock Journal* in Greenfield, Ind. He was chief photographer for the *Roswell* (N.M.) *Daily Record* and later a photographer for the *Indianapolis News.* This is his second appearance in *Best Sports Stories.*

MARVIN M. GREENE (Almost Measured by a Foot), who holds a B.F.A. from the Cleveland Institute of Art, has been a staff photographer and picture and graphics editor for the *Cleveland Plain Dealer.* He was a naval photographer during World War II. This is his first appearance in *Best Sports Stories.*

HARRISON A. HOWARD (A Mother's Kiss) tried almost two years to get a shot of a dam and foal. He has been a journalist 25 years and covered everything from high school to college sports, auto racing and harness racing, even owning a stable of his own. He attended the University of Alabama, Butler University, and Ohio Christian, earning a bachelor's degree in journalism, and has been employed at *The Indianapolis Star* 13 years.

RON JETT (The Feminine Touch) is a staff photographer for the *Sarasota* (Fla.) *Journal.* He began as a part-time circulation helper, then copy boy, and then photographer with the *Tampa Times.* He got a chance to go to Hawaii to work for the *Honolulu Advertiser,* where he received all formal training in photography and returned to the *Tampa Tribune* and then to the *Sarasota Journal.*

ROBERT JOHNSON ("What Team You Playin' With?") is a staff photographer for *The Nashville Tennessean.* He attended the University of Tennessee and broke into photography by taking pictures to accompany sports articles written by his father. This is his third appearance in *Best Sports Stories.*

CHARLES KIRMAN ("Hang On, I'm Coming") received a B.S. with honors in the field of professional photography from Rochester Institute of Technology in 1972. Since then he has been employed as a staff photographer for the *Chicago Sun Times.* He has received over 35 photo-journalism awards since joining the *Sun Times,* and in 1975 he won the Illinois Press Photographer of the Year award. He appeared in *Best Sports Stories* in 1974 and 1975.

RICHARD MACKSON ("First and Ten, Let's Do It Again"), is twenty-one and has been a staff photographer for the *Santa Monica Evening Outlook* since he was sixteen years old. He is an occasional photographer for *Sports Illustrated* and the league photographer for the Inter-National Volleyball Association. This is his second appearance in *Best Sports Stories.*

FRED MATTHES (A Nightmare Start) has been a staff photographer at the *San Jose Mercury-News* for 15 years. He started as a student in photography at City College of San Francisco, then went to International News Photos. Upon the merger with United Press, he spent a couple of years in industrial photography until his present job.

RICH MCCARTHY (A Bitter End in End Zone) was a navy staff photographer covering action in Vietnam during the Tet Offensive of 1968 before joining the staff of the *San Diego Evening Tribune* in 1970. McCarthy has a degree in journalism from San Diego State University and is president of the California Press Photographers Association.

TOM MERRYMAN (Polarity) worked in a news agency and portrait studio until he went into service with a Photo Recon Squadron in World War II. He has been with the *Cedar Rapids Gazette* for 21 years and is the chief photographer for that paper. His sport shots have merited several inclusions in *Best Sports Stories.*

WILLIAM MEYER (No Last Hurrah) is a twenty-six-year-old staff photographer for the Journal Company, publishers of *The Milwaukee Journal* and *The Milwaukee Sentinel.* He started with the paper after graduation from the University of Wisconsin, Milwaukee, in 1971. His pictures have been published in the last three *Best Sports Stories.*

JOHN PINEDA (A Winning Story by Sports Editor) is a Chicagoan who joined the *Miami Herald* photo staff in 1955. He is a past president of the Miami Press Photographers Association and was a director of the National Press Photographers Association in 1971–72.

JAMES ROARK ("Gotcha!") won the *Best Sports Stories—1975* feature photo award on his first try. He is a Chicagoan who completed the Famous Photographers School course and then joined the *Los Angeles Herald-Examiner* as a copy boy. He then became a staff photographer there and for the past three years has been the staff sports photographer.

ELWOOD P. SMITH (The Moose Shuffle) has been a photographer for the *Philadelphia Daily News* since 1939. He went to the *Philadelphia Bulletin* for a few years after serving in the U.S. Marine Corps as a photographer and then returned to the *Daily News*. Smith won the black-and-white action photo prize in the 1974 Football Hall of Fame photo contest.

W. F. (BILL) THOMPSON (Ref Makes Like the Statue of Liberty) is a Texas-born photographer who did his first camera work with the Marine Corps. From 1951 to 1965 he was with United Press International in Austin and at present he is a staff photographer with *The Houston Post*.

DAVE WEINTRAUB (Bored Blazers in a Laugher) twenty-six years old, was born in New York City. He moved to Portland after graduation from Columbia in 1970 with a B.A. in English. Photography has always been his hobby, and in 1974 he went to *The Oregon Journal* looking for work. He was hired as a copy boy in October and made a part-time staff photographer in January 1975.

JOHN H. WHITE (Man Left at Starting Gate) was a winner in this anthology's photo section in 1972 with his shot of a young girls' foot race. He attended Piedmont Community College in North Carolina, then joined the Marine Corps, being discharged with the rank of sergeant. After a short stint in a photo studio in Charlotte, N.C., he joined the *Chicago Daily News* in 1969, and he has been with them ever since. This shot marks his third appearance in *Best Sports Stories*.

THE YEAR'S
BEST SPORTS PHOTOS

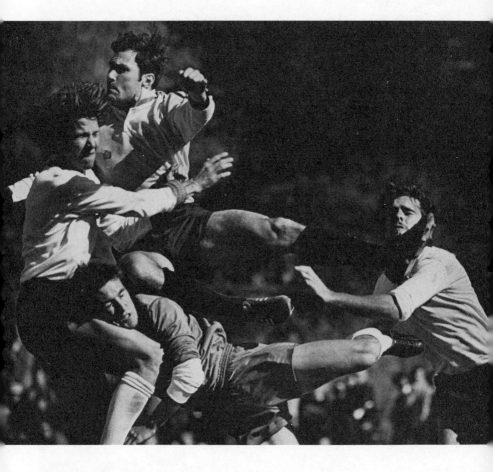

HEAD IN GROIN, SHOE IN BELLY, CLEATS IN FACE & OTHER ITEMS

by George D. Waldman, *Colorado Springs Sun*. This is the winner in the action photo division. The photographer has caught the violent action of four players in a midair collision in a soccer game between the Air Force Academy and Colorado College. The Air Force goalie at top flies over teammate Dwight Landman to punch out goal shot by opposition. Putting the squeeze on goalie Greg Schulze and his teammates are Colorado's Brad Turner (left) and Kornel Simons (right). The flurry of action, the grimacing and total effort of all involved convinced the judges that this shot was the most meritorious. Incidentally Colorado won, 1–0. Copyright ©, 1975, *Colorado Springs Sun*.

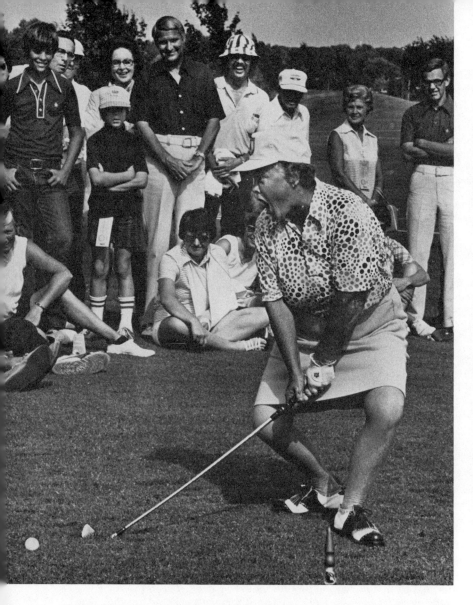

"NOW THE WAY TO PREVENT A SLICE. . . ."

by Cletus M. (Pete) Hohn, *Minneapolis Tribune*. Patty Berg, veteran pro golfer from Minnesota, is giving a golf lesson. Her clinics in this area are most instructive and amusing. Copyright ©, 1975, *Minneapolis Tribune*.

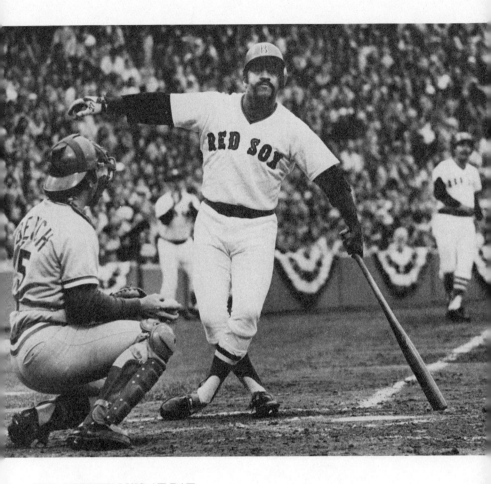

THE MIGHTY LUIS AT BAT

by Mike Anderson, *Boston Herald American.* This photo depicts Red Sox pitcher Luis Tiant, certainly one of the heroes of the last World Series and famed for his corkscrew windup on the mound, repeating that same gesture while batting for the first time in two years (because of the American League's designated hitter rule). Johnny Bench watches in silent awe. Copyright ©, 1975, The Hearst Corporation—Boston Herald American/Advertiser Division.

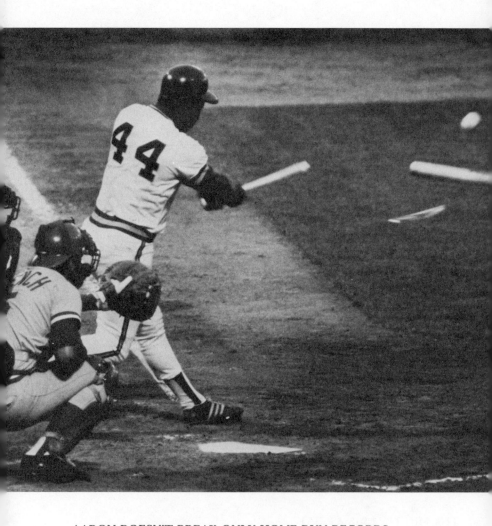

AARON DOESN'T BREAK ONLY HOME-RUN RECORDS

by John E. Biever, *The Milwaukee Journal.* The great home-run king, while swinging at a pitch in the All-Star game of 1975, had his bat disintegrate into three pieces. Aaron was pinch hitting in the third inning and it marked his twenty-fourth All-Star game appearance, tying him with Willie Mays and Mickey Mantle for most All-Star games played. Copyright ©, 1975, *The Milwaukee Journal.*

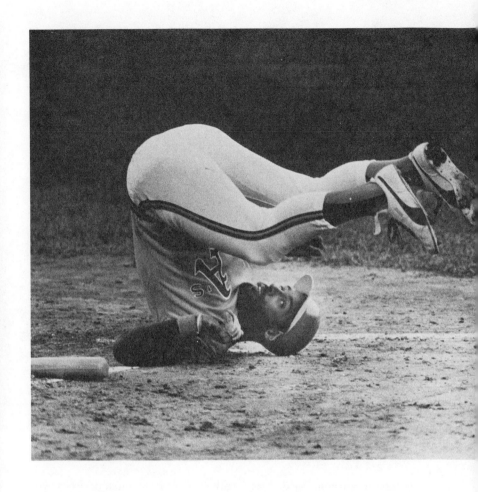

SAVING FACE

by Ron Burda, *San Jose Mercury-News*. Bill North, center fielder for the
Oakland A's, tumbles backward to avoid a pitch thrown to the region of his
face. The action occurred in the decisive game of the American League
playoff and Boston went on to win and play the Cincinnati Reds in the
World Series. Copyright ©, 1975, *San Jose Mercury-News*.

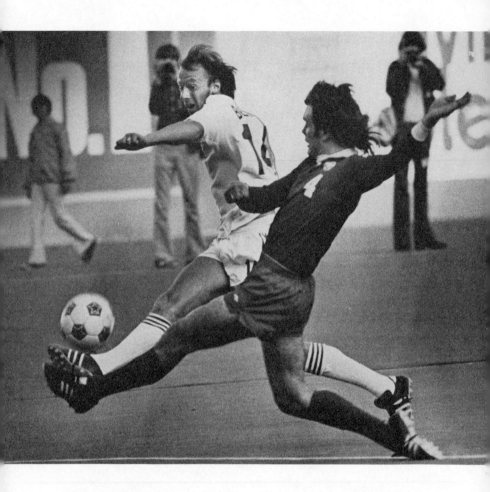

TWO TO TANGLE

by Karen Engstrom, *The Portland Oregonian*. The photographer catches two soccer players with a picturesque dip and sway attempting to control an elusive ball. The action occurred in the North American Soccer League at Portland. Vancouver's Bobby Lenarduzzi and Portland's forward Tony Betts appear right in step, toward either the goal or Fred Astaire's dancing school. Reprinted by permission.

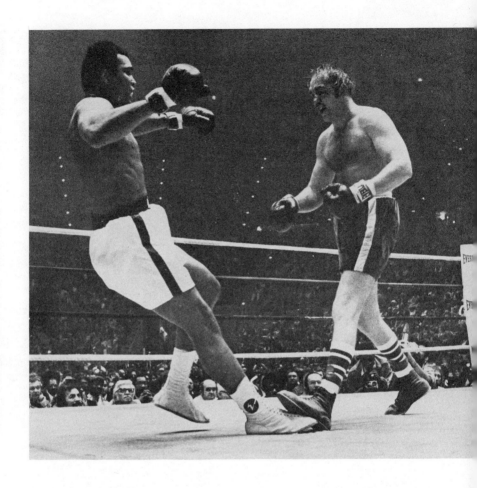

ALMOST MEASURED BY A FOOT

by Marvin M. Greene, *Cleveland Plain Dealer*. It was toe to toe in the ninth round on March 24, 1975, when Chuck Wepner almost took Ali's measure by stepping on his foot, causing him to go down. Referee Tony Perez ruled that Wepner had floored Muhammad. However, Ali claimed he tripped and fell because Wepner was standing on his corns . . . as this picture clearly shows. Copyright ©, 1975, Plain Dealer Publishing Co.

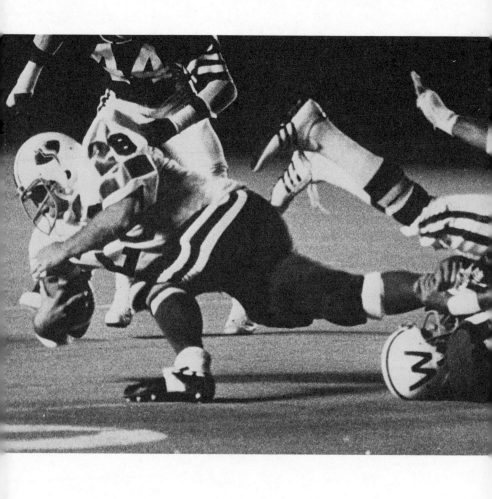

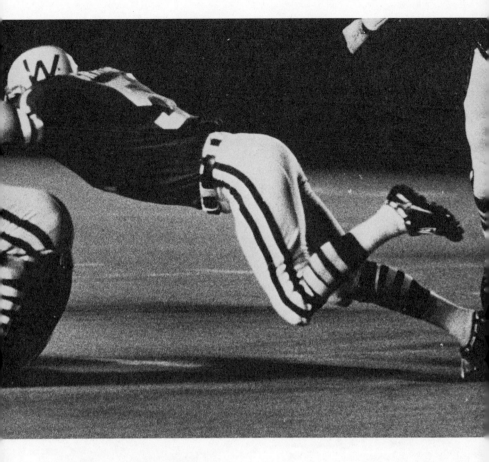

"HANG ON, I'M COMING"

by Charles Kirman, *Chicago Sun Times*. Harry Howard desperately clutches at leg of Portland ball-carrier Jim Evanson while Chicago's Dean Baird (51) flies at play from behind. Copyright ©, 1975, *Chicago Sun Times*—Charles Kirman.

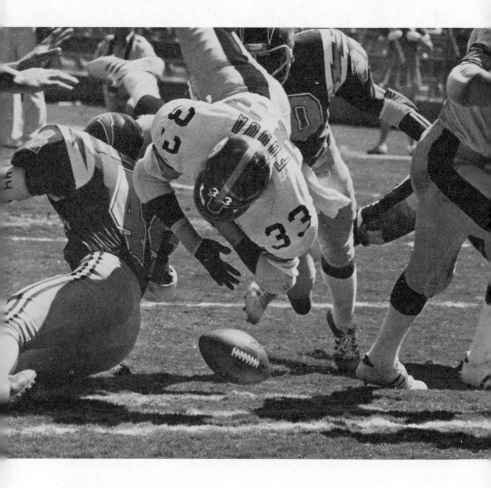

BITTER END IN END ZONE

by Rich McCarthy, *San Diego Evening Tribune.* Frenchy Fuqua, No. 33 of the Pittsburgh Steelers, fumbles the ball in the end zone after taking it in from five yards out. However, teammate Gerry Mullins recovered for the Steelers and got credit for the TD. The opponents were the San Diego Chargers, who lost the game. Copyright ©, 1975, *San Diego Evening Tribune.*

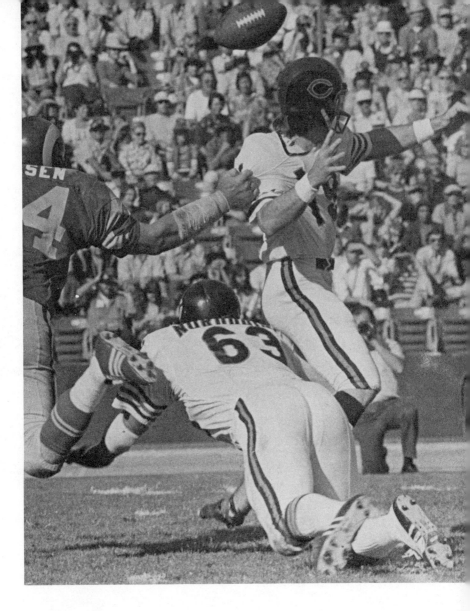

"GOTCHA!"

by James Roark, *Los Angeles Herald-Examiner*. One can just hear that triumphant cry—one that Merlin Olsen of the Los Angeles Rams must have uttered many times—"Gotcha!" as he grabs the passing arm of hapless Chicago Bear quarterback Gary Hoff and forces a turnover. Copyright ©, 1975, *Los Angeles Herald-Examiner*.

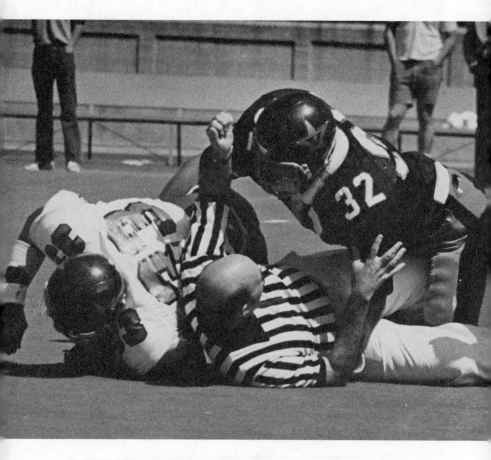

"WHAT TEAM YOU PLAYIN' WITH?"

by Robert Johnson, *The Nashville Tennessean*. Official Jack Cochrane got caught in a pass play with two Vanderbilt players who were trying to break it up. The play was broken and so nearly was the official. Copyright ©, 1975, *The Nashville Tennessean*.

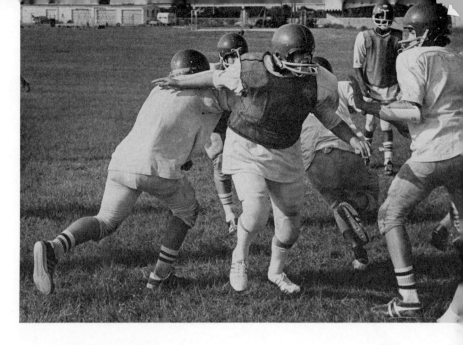

THE FEMININE TOUCH

by Ron Jett, *Sarasota Journal.* With a tender touch, Brenda Hand of a Sarasota, Fla., school team knocks an opposing linesman to the ground and is ready to take on the blocker who is protecting the runner. He decided to go around the other end. Copyright ©, 1975, *Sarasota Journal.*

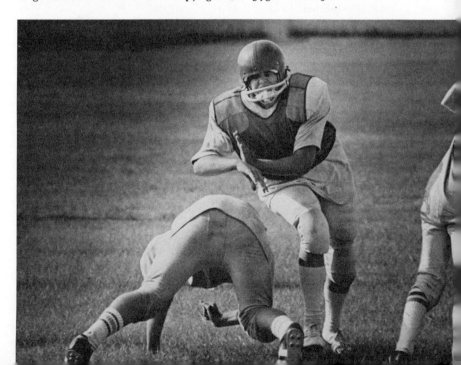

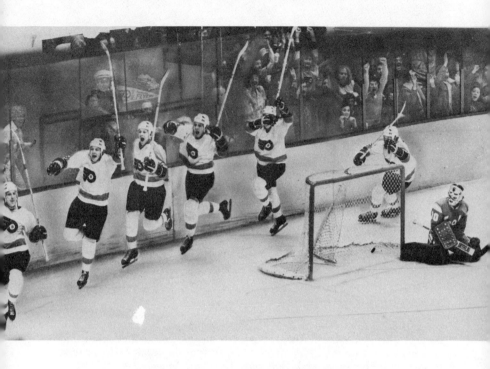

THE MOOSE SHUFFLE

by Elwood P. Smith, *Philadelphia Daily News*. The sequence camera catches the stages of Audie "Moose" Dupont's ritualistic victory "shuffle" around the rink after scoring a winning goal for the championship Philadelphia Flyers. Gary Simmons of the losing team, the Seattle Seals, doesn't look too appreciative of the festivities. Copyright ©, 1975, *Philadelphia Daily News*.

A WINNING STORY BY SPORTS EDITOR

by John Pineda, *Miami Herald*. Earlie Fires, the spectacled jockey, looks on in amazement as his rival, Sports Editor, passes him to win the race. Fires was sure Sports Editor was left for dead when he was forced wide at the turn. But complacency disappeared when Earlie saw first-place money fading. Copyright ©, 1975, The Miami Herald Publishing Co.

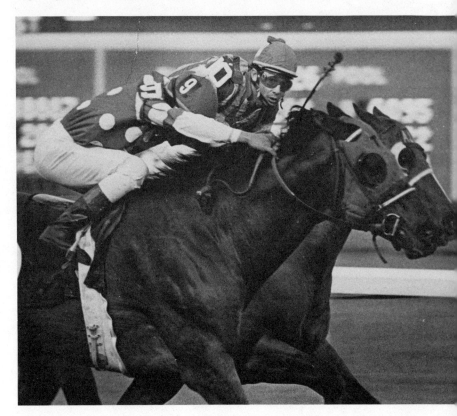

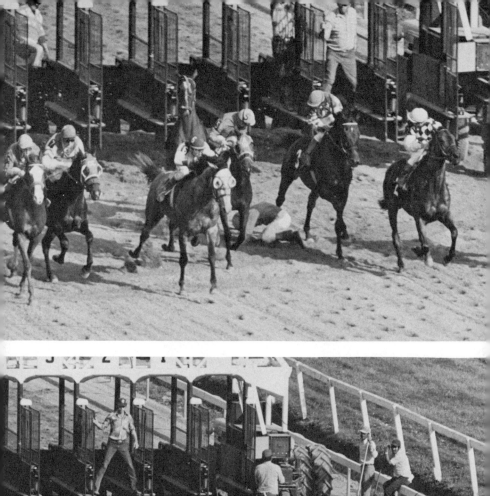
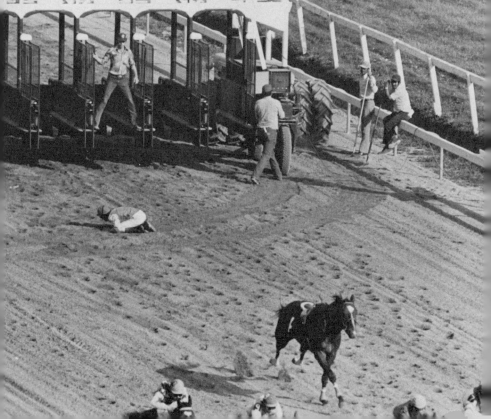

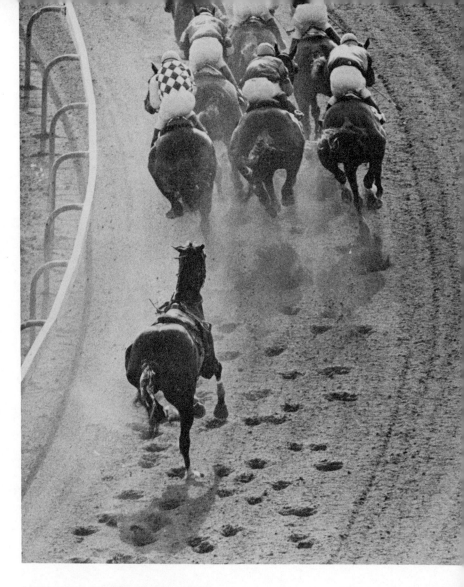

MAN LEFT AT STARTING GATE

by John H. White, *Chicago Daily News.* The horses were off and running during the fifth race at Hawthorne racetrack, but a switch occurred and jockey Geary Louviere was left at the starting gate—minus his horse. The other riders turned their mounts away from the fallen Louviere and he was left alone, unhurt but somewhat chagrined. Meanwhile, his horse, Royal Defender, decided to finish the race without him. Copyright ©, 1975, *Chicago Daily News*—John White.

A MOTHER'S KISS

by Harrison A. Howard, *The Indianapolis Star.* Only two hours old, little Spring Glory gets careful attention from her standard-bred pacing dam, Windale Donna, shortly after she was foaled. Since horses just don't stand around in one spot long enough after foaling, the photographer was lucky indeed to catch this scene. Copyright ©, 1975, Harrison A. Howard.

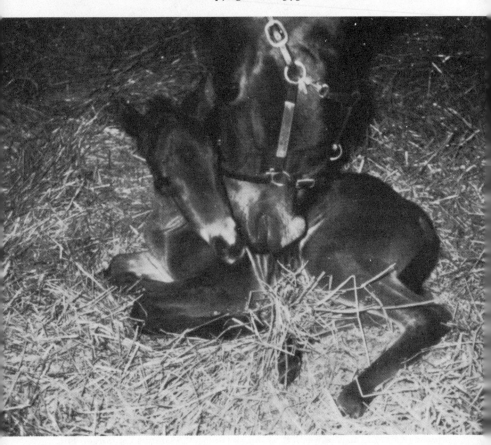

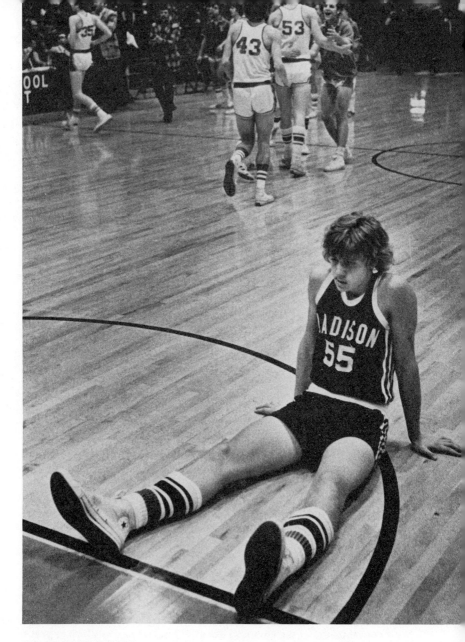

NO LAST HURRAH

by William Meyer, *The Milwaukee Journal.* A desolate basketball player sits unhappily while the opposing team celebrates its victory in the Wisconsin high school basketball tournament. Dan McCoy of Milwaukee Madison is the unhappy player and at the other end of the court the victors from Milwaukee Marshall are effusively congratulating each other. Copyright ©, 1975, *The Milwaukee Journal.*

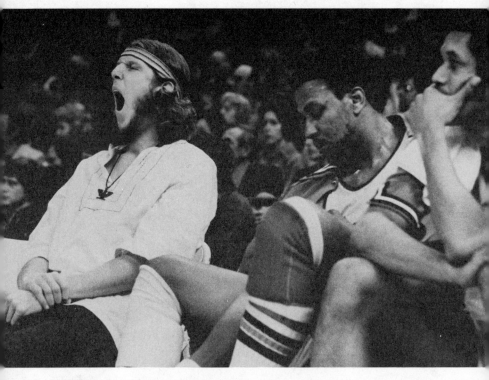

BORED BLAZERS IN A LAUGHER

by Dave Weintraub, *The Oregon Journal.* A "laugher" occurs when a team gets so far ahead that everybody can relax and substitutes earn their keep for a change. However, "laugher" can hardly describe the Blazers' bench as Portland poured it on the Los Angeles Lakers, 126–97. The mighty yawn is by Bill Walton and the somnolent players are Lloyd Neal (nodding) and John Johnson (daydreaming). Copyright ©, 1975, *The Oregon Journal,* Portland, Ore.

REF MAKES LIKE THE STATUE OF LIBERTY

by W. F. (Bill) Thompson, *The Houston Post.* Perhaps the photographer was not thinking of the immortal words of Emma Lazarus which appear on the Statue of Liberty "Give me your tired, your poor," but at the base or foot of the referee is a hapless victim of circumstance and all that is lacking is a lighted torch. The incident took place at a Southwest Basketball Conference game between Rice and Texas Christian. Copyright ©, 1975, *The Houston Post.*

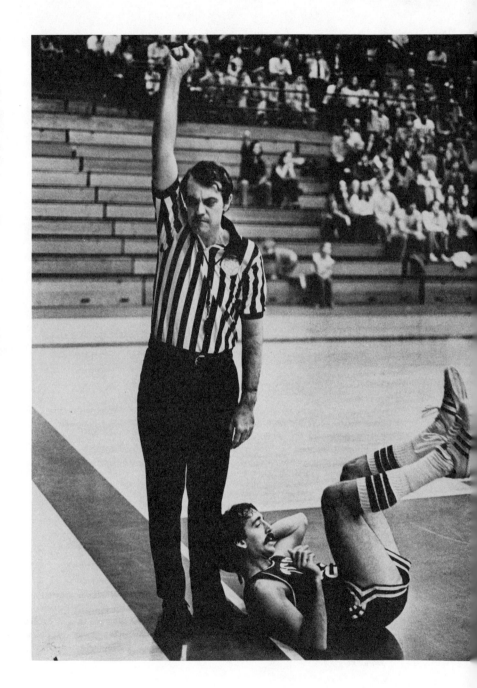

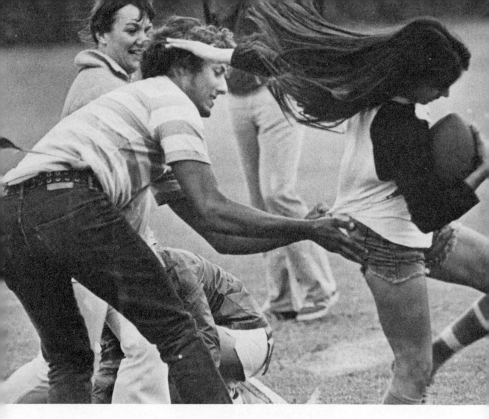

"FIRST AND TEN, LET'S DO IT AGAIN"

by Richard Mackson, *Santa Monica* (Cal.) *Outlook.* This shot ranks high in the feature division. It gracefully illustrates the joys of co-ed sports. The time, score, and names of the participants are irrelevant. The joy and spirit of the picture aren't. The girl in the picture was the leading ground gainer of the day. The leading pass receiver was also female. Copyright ©, 1975, Richard Mackson, Santa Monica, California.

GOLDEN STATE PLAYED 12 FEET TALL

by Richard Darcey, *The Washington Post.* Warriors rookie guard Phil Smith, 6-foot-4, leaps to block the rim as Bullets' guard Kevin Porter can't get off a lay-up. Action occurred in game four of the NBA championship series at Capital Centre. Copyright ©, 1975, *The Washington Post.*

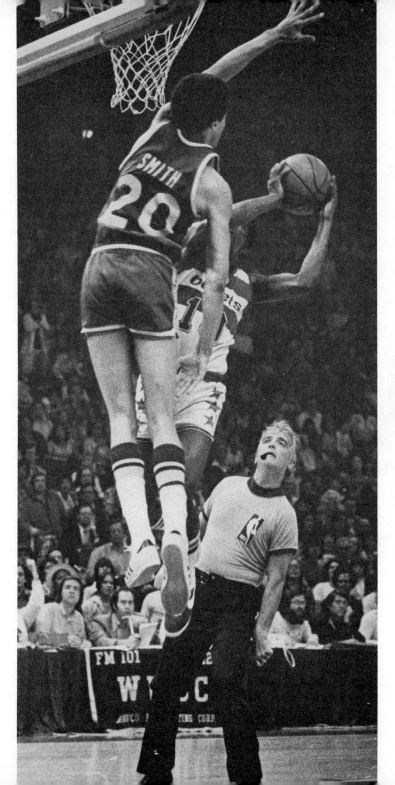

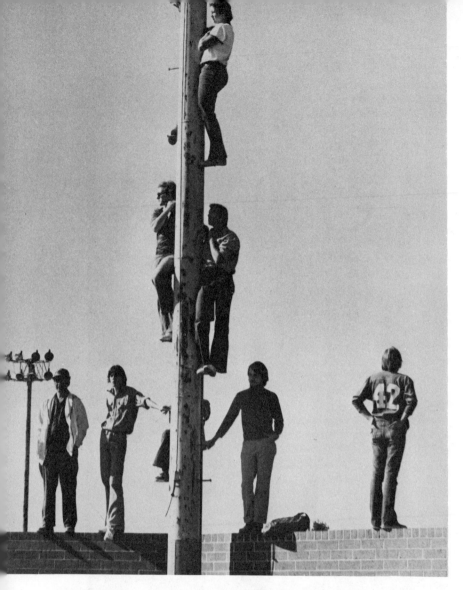

POLARITY

by Tom Merryman, *Cedar Rapids Gazette*. Seven young men have climbed
poles and a roof to watch a bona fide football game played by authentic
gridders. Off to the side stands a recluse, No. 42, contemplating a group
of girls engaging in the same exercise, but to him a bit more fascinating.
Action occurred during one of the Iowa University games and the spectators were those who didn't get into the game but watched anyway. Copyright ©, 1975, *Cedar Rapids Gazette*.